WEINER'S HERBAL

WEINER'S HERBAL

THE GUIDE TO HERB MEDICINE

Michael A. Weiner, M.S., M.A., Ph.D.

with

Janet Weiner

And with chemical
and pharmacological findings
by

Norman R. Farnsworth, Ph.D.

Illustrations for expanded section courtesy of Nature's Herbs

Quantum Books
6 Knoll Lane
Mill Valley, Ca 94941

WEINER'S HERBAL: THE GUIDE TO HERB MEDICINE
BY: MICHAEL A. WEINER, Ph.D. & JANET WEINER

2ND Edition, 1990

Publication Date: October, 1990
First Printing: October, 1990
Second Printing: March, 1991
Third Printing: January, 1992

Copyright © 1990 by Michael A. Weiner
All rights reserved
Printed in the United States of America
Quantum Books
6 Knoll Lane, Suite D
Mill Valley, CA 94941
Telephone (415) 388-1006
FAX (415) 388-2257

1st Edition 1980
Originally published by
Stein and Day Publishers
Scarborough House
BriarCliff Manor, NY 10510

Library of Congress Cataloging in Publication Data

Weiner, Michael A.
    Weiner's Herbal. The Guide to Herb Medicine
    1990 Edition

    Includes Index.
    1. Herbs—Therapeutic use. 2. Therapeutics
    3. Botany, Medical.

ISBN #
0-912-845-03-1

For
Russell
and
Rebecca

Contents

WEINER'S HERBAL

INTRODUCTION
RATIONAL HERBALISM

Between thinking that we know and thinking that we don't know, we exist; functioning harmoniously if we intuitively comply with the laws of nature, falling ill if we do not comply or if we are subjected to accident or pestilence. Between laboratory science and the marketplaces of superstition, the nonmedical population seeks the calm and cure.

Where do those of us interested in rational herbalism turn when so many scientists offer us little intelligible information, and healers often offer "miracles" only at a stiff fee? Is there a way to heal ourselves using the best advice from folkloric medicine, reinterpreted through the findings of twentieth-century analytical procedures?

Simple complaints should often be self-treated, but of course, "simple" complaints which persist may require more than a simple guidebook to medicinal herbs. Nevertheless, herbs sustained our ancestors into this century and still provide the chief form of medicine for most of the world's people. Hundreds of millions of poor in underdeveloped countries and millions more of relatively well-off people in the Soviet Union, France, Britain and other Western European nations still rely upon the earth's cures.

Although folklore rarely carries completely useless information through the ages, we've probably inherited *some* superstitious medical ideas and treatments. Added to this load of superstition are the new claims for cure thrown up wherever a "healer" happens to practice.

There is no way to analyze every claim for the reputed healing properties of various herbs. Each environment produces its own medicine bag, offering herbs useful in that niche for people who seldom travel far from home. We must also accept that healers can sometimes effect "cures" through their own charismatic powers. These facts, however, do not necessarily make for useful contributions to *world* medicine; that is, plant drugs useful for broad populations in various ecological niches.

Certainly Indian Snakeroot, Coca, curare, Ipecac, Cinchona, Foxglove, vincristine, and vinblastine have proven themselves in many countries and climes. No doubt other such broadly useful drugs remain to be uncovered from the vast mine of medicinal herbs growing all over the world—some known to local groups and some yet unrecognized. But we must restrain our optimism before rushing too hastily into the bush. Although modern medicine has its faults, many of our technological treatments have their place in the overall scheme of health care. It should be our aim to bring the more useful herbs into the mainstream of contemporary medicine.

How many of our once useful plant medications

1

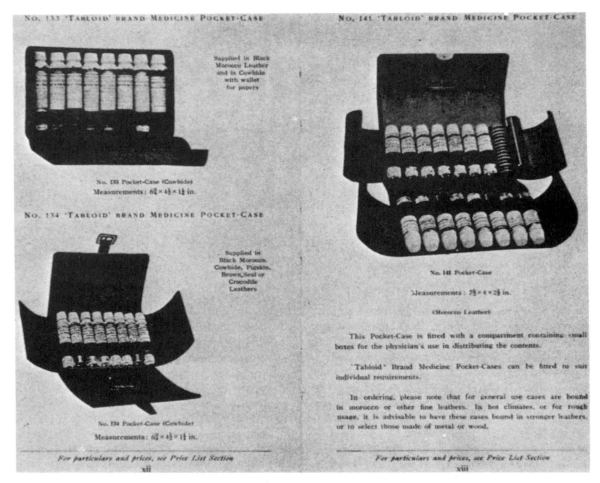

are now precluded from general practice? How many "proven" remedies are in disrepute? Looking through the 1908 edition of the Burroughs Wellcome *Excerpta Therapeutica*, we find that a tablet composed of the "active principles of kola nut and coca leaves" (caffeine and cocaine) was prescribed regularly. "Formerly known as *'Tabloid Forced March,'* it was said to allay thirst and hunger and sustain strength under mental or physical strain." The physician is instructed that "coca is a stimulant, tonic and restorative, which decreases the sensation of fatigue in prolonged muscular exertion or mental effort."

"Direction—One, dissolved in the mouth every hour, when undergoing continued mental strain or physical exertion."

Are we to believe that our grandparents were addicted to this "dangerous" drug, or to other equally potent and effective medications presently forbidden in general medical practice? This is doubtful. Yet, this drug was dropped from medical practice for its stimulant effects. Other useful botanicals were eliminated over the years, drugs which might profitably serve us again. In the following pages we present some useful botanical alternatives or adjuncts to synthetic drugs.

Herbs serve us not only as medicine, but also as nutritious foods. Many are rich in vitamins and minerals as well as in the "major" nutrients (protein, carbohydrate—especially fiber—and fat, and ash). The following table summarizes the findings of Dr. James Duke and K. Wain, which is the first analysis of herbs for nutrients ever conducted on this scale.

2

Nutritional Components of Herbs per 100 Grams of Plant Part

Common Name	Latin Binomial	Part*	Calories	Water (%)	Protein (g)	Fat (g)	Carbo-hydrate (g)	Fiber (g)	Ash (g)	Calcium (mg)	Phos-phorous (mg)	Iron (mg)	Sodium (mg)	Potas-sium (mg)	Carotene (IU)	Thia-mine (mg)	Ribo-flavin (mg)	Niacin (mg)	Ascorbic Acid (mg)
Anise	*Pimpinella anisum*	S	415	11.0	19.0	24.7	45.3	—	—	698	—	34.8	—	—	—	—	—	—	0
Arrowroot	*Maranta arundinacea*	R	157	57.2	2.4	0.1	39.0	1.9	1.3	20	24	3.2	—	—	0	0.08	0.03	0.07	9
Burdock	*Arctium lappa*	R	89	76.5	2.5	0.1	20.1	1.7	0.8	50	58	1.2	30	18.0	0	0.25	0.08	0.30	2
Butternut Chestnut, Spanish	*Juglans cinerea*	S	629	3.8	23.7	61.2	8.4	—	2.9	—	—	6.8	—	—	—	—	—	—	—
	Castanea satival	S	194	52.5	2.9	1.5	42.1	1.1	1.0	27	88	1.7	6	45.4	—	0.22	0.22	0.60	—
Dandelion	*Taraxacum officinale*	L	45	85.6	2.7	0.7	9.2	1.6	1.8	187	66	3.1	76	39.7	8400	0.19	0.25	—	35
Elder	*Sambucus canadensis*	F	72	79.8	2.6	0.5	16.4	7.0	0.7	38	28	1.6	—	30.0	360	0.07	0.06	0.50	36
		L	—	47.8	10.2	2.1	37.9	15.7	2.0	—	—	—	—	—	—	—	—	—	—
Fennel	*Foeniculum vulgare*	L	31	89.2	2.9	0.5	5.6	0.5	1.8	114	54	2.9	—	33.8	2610	0.12	0.15	0.70	34
Flax	*Linum usitatissimum*	S	498	6.3	18.0	34.0	37.2	8.8	4.5	271	462	43.8	—	—	0	0.17	0.16	1.40	—
Ginger	*Zingiber officinale*	B	22	93.0	0.,8	0.6	4.2	1.2	1.4	42	55	0.7	—	47.5	—	—	—	—	—
		R	46	87.4	1.6	0.8	9.2	1.3	1.0	19	32	1.3	7	31.6	55	0.01	0.03	1.70	4
Gotu Kola	*Centella asiatica*	L	34	89.3	1.6	0.6	6.9	2.0	1.6	170	30	3.1	—	41.4	6580	0.15	0.14	1.20	4
Indian Corn	*Zea mays* subsp. *mays*	G	134	62.5	4.2	1.7	30.7	1.1	0.9	5	126	0.9	3	25.9	160	0.20	0.11	1.50	8
		S	349	13.6	9.1	4.2	71.7	2.3	1.4	14	245	2.8	5	—	270	0.29	0.11	2.10	0
		X	319	20.6	7.4	2.8	68.3	2.9	0.9	—	210	2.9	—	—	0	0.00	0.16	3.00	—
Marijuana	*Cannabis sativa*	S	421	13.6	27.1	25.6	27.6	20.3	6.1	120	970	12.0	—	—	51	0.32	0.17	2.10	0
Mugwort	*Artemisia vulgaris*	L	35	87.3	5.2	0.8	4.5	3.4	2.2	82	40	1.5	—	—	2140	0.15	0.16	3.00	72
Mulberry, Black	*Morus nigra*	F	42	87.9	1.4	0.3	9.8	0.7	0.6	24	26	3.0	30	12.3	15	0.04	0.08	0.70	39
Mustard, White	*Sinapis alba*	S	469	5.0	26.4	36.3	28.2	5.2	4.1	410	613	29.0	—	—	630	0.40	0.31	7.30	0
Nightshade, Black	*Solanum nigrum*	L	44	85.0	4.6	0.4	8.4	1.1	1.6	216	88	4.2	—	—	1650	0.12	0.24	1.30	30
Onion	*Allium cepa*	L	26	92.2	1.8	0.6	4.7	1.1	0.7	42	43	3.4	—	—	308	0.05	0.11	0.70	39
		Q	39	89.6	1.5	0.2	8.3	1.0	0.4	34	42	1.4	—	—	0	0.04	0.04	0.40	13
		R	38	88.6	1.6	0.2	9.0	0.7	0.6	30	44	1.10	9	16.6	—	0.06	0.04	0.20	9
Opium	*Papaver somniferum*	S	—	4.3	24.4	49.1	20.1	5.8	6.0	1450	880	11.1	—	—	0	1.18	1.20	1.28	—
Papaya	*Carica papaya*	F	45	87.1	0.5	0.1	11.8	0.5	0.5	24	22	0.7	4	22.1	710	0.03	0.05	0.40	73
		G	26	92.1	1.0	0.1	6.2	0.9	0.6	38	20	0.3	7	21.5	15	0.02	0.03	0.30	40
		L	74	77.5	7.0	2.0	11.3	1.8	2.2	344	142	0.8	16	65.2	11565	0.09	0.48	2.10	140
Passion-flower	*Passiflora incarnata*	F	111	72.5	2.3	3.3	21.0	7.3	0.9	14	43	1.6	—	—	—	—	—	—	—
Peperomia	*Peperomia Pereskiifolia*	L	25	92.2	0.5	0.3	5.9	1.0	1.1	124	34	3.2	8	27.7	2500	0.03	0.07	0.60	10
Plantain	*Plantago major*	L	61	81.4	2.5	0.3	14.6	—	1.2	184	52	1.2	16	27.7	2520	—	0.28	0.80	8
Pome-granate	*Punica granatum*	F	72	80.0	1.0	0.6	17.7	1.1	0.7	13	23	0.7	7	37.9	—	0.07	0.01	0.30	7
		S	—	35.0	9.4	6.9	35.0	22.4	1.5	—	—	—	—	—	—	—	—	—	—
Prunus SP.	*Prunus sp.*	F	49	86.1	0.6	0.2	12.5	1.1	0.6	10	12	0.6	—	—	770	—	—	—	—
Red Pepper	*Capsicum abyssinicum*	F	106	72.8	3.0	2.4	20.2	9.2	1.6	19	110	5.6	—	—	1410	—	0.30	1.60	147
Rhubarb	*Rheum officinale*	Z	16	94.9	0.5	0.1	3.8	0.7	0.7	51	25	0.5	—	—	20	0.01	0.02	0.10	10
Safflower	*Carthamus tinctorius*	S	482	4.8	12.6	27.8	50.5	25.1	4.3	126	310	9.7	—	—	0	0.59	0.14	0.50	0
Shepherd's Purse	*Capsella bursa-pastoris*	L	33	88.2	4.2	0.5	5.2	1.2	1.9	208	86	4.8	—	39.4	2590	0.25	0.17	0.40	36
Tamarind	*Tamarindus indica*	F	214	38.7	2.3	0.2	56.7	1.9	2.1	81	86	1.3	3	57.0	10	0.22	0.08	1.10	3
		G	71	79.5	2.4	0.1	17.2	0.8	0.8	58	29	0.7	3	31.6	10	0.15	0.05	0.40	12
		I	75	80.0	2.5	1.8	15.0	1.2	0.7	53	44	1.4	5	25.4	205	0.08	0.12	1.20	12
		L	78	77.2	5.1	1.0	16.1	1.3	0.6	24	52	2.0	8	27.3	2510	0.10	0.11	1.50	6
Walnut, Black	*Juglans nigra*	S	628	3.1	20.5	59.3	14.8	1.7	2.3	—	570	6.0	3	46.0	180	0.22	0.11	0.70	—
Yellow Dock	*Rumex crispus*	L	21	92.6	1.5	0.3	4.1	0.9	1.5	74	56	5.6	—	—	2770	0.06	0.08	0.40	30

Source: Dr. James Duke and K. Wain

* *Part Code:*

A Aril	G Green fruit; green pulp	K Dry fruit	O Oil	S Seed, mature seed	X Seedling
B Bud, shoot	H Heart	L Leaf	P Pulp of fruit; mature pulp	U Cooked seed	Z Leaf stalk
E Epidermis; bark	I Inflorescence	M Cooked leaf	Q Green root	V Dry seed	
F Fruit; mature fruit	J Juice	N Dry leaf	R Root	W Green seed	

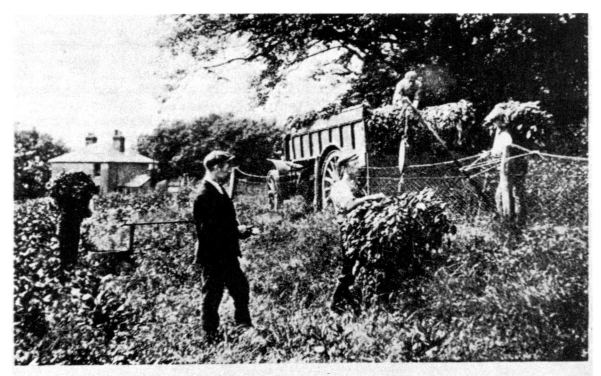

LOADING BELLADONNA

The yield ranges from 1-1 2 to 5 tons per acre. The freshly-cut herb is weighed in bundles and carried straight to the laboratories in a motor trolley. A portion of the leaves is dried in a few hours in specially-ventilated chambers. The roots, which are collected in the autumn, are sliced in order to accelerate the drying, and so prevent any undesirable change taking place.

Some may ask whether any of our plant drugs are as "strong" as our industrially produced medicines, as quick in action, and as compatible with our contemporary way of life.

Obviously, Valium, Thorazine, and other synthetic calming agents act more quickly than Valerian, Passionflower, or Vervain. But, which medicine you choose in times of extreme need depends upon how well you understand human physiology. "What goes up must come down." Similarly, what brings you down too rapidly must also bring you back to the level of anxiety you were attempting to escape.

Subtlety of action is the key to most herbal medicine. Effects are often *not* dramatic, especially when self-treating minor complaints, but neither are most side effects usually overly powerful.

Whether you prefer popping a pill, taking an herbal extract or capsule, or slowly preparing an infusion is a matter of choice. Reason suggests, though, that the gradual cure will be the more effective. Real, major ills require slow treatment, while imagined or hypothetical ills will often respond to "instant" cures, only to return as soon as the initial dose wears off.

Many of us have a tendency toward being that "self-centered little clod of ailments and grievances" described by George Bernard Shaw. For medical complaints of this nature the only cure is prayer and fasting (from negative activities). For the vast spectrum of other ills herbal remedies very definitely have a place in modern medicine.

One sometimes hears that plant remedies by themselves, withdrawn from the traditional social and religious context, are ineffective fragments of a total healing picture. This criticism, while *valid* for people *within* ethnic groups, such as American Indian tribes which are still intact, is *invalid* for people *outside* any group from which these remedies may have originated. For example, the chemical *d*-tubocurarine, found in curare, a potent South American arrow poison, will paralyze you whether you are a Brazilian Indian, a Mescalero Apache, or one of the technological masses. It doesn't have to be utilized as part of a larger ethnological picture; you don't need any rituals. If you take curare you're going to be affected by it. The drug will have its effects whether taken in the complex native form or as a chemical isolated from the plant.

Similarly, the chemical constituent of willow bark—salicin, a relative of salicylic acid, which is a constituent of aspirin—lowers fevers of the Indian who receives it as part of a complex socio-religious healing ritual, as it lowers the fever for the alienated concrete dweller. In most cases medicinal constituents are impartial to the context in which the needy patient takes them.

Conversely, crude drugs which are known to be efficacious are sometimes ineffective in their component parts. Ginseng has been shown to have definite antistress properties in many experiments, yet such activity has never been confirmed when isolated chemical parts of the whole root have been subjected to pharmacological trials.

Cybernetic Angels and Recreational Eating

Nature does not deceive us. By attempting to feed and heal ourselves as though we were cyber-

netic angels when we are physiologically closer to the wolf than to the bird, we deceive ourselves. Our absurd desire to transcend the zoological order is reflected in our diets. Seemingly endless quantities of meat, refined sugar, white flour, salt, and chemical additives continue to take their toll, while some of us pretend not to know. A vast array of synthetic foods attests to man's capacity for self-deception—a capacity, in fact, which is unknown elsewhere in the living world. We see the origin of what we might call "recreational eating" at the zoo. There candied popcorn must be mighty appealing to the orangutan who's trapped within the confines of a cage. Although he ought to be fed according to jungle laws, the boredom of captivity exacts its toll, and junk food begins to look good to him. Yet the price for this nutritional transgression is paid by the deceived creature within a few hours. We have made a habit of deceiving ourselves and have so reinforced our distorted dietary ideas as to have conveniently forgotten the causes of our illnesses in many cases, many of which are the result of our foods and sheer gluttony. The orangutan can't fool himself like that. He hasn't been practicing long enough.

Human systems abused for many years will not usually respond easily to herbal remedies. Our synthetic medicines are in fact similar to the compounds which cause many of our ills in that their effects are extreme and they act dramatically. Too many of us demand constant stimulation for our overworked, jaded nervous systems. Enter herbal medicines, and we find a blasé reaction in many people. For herbs to be effec-

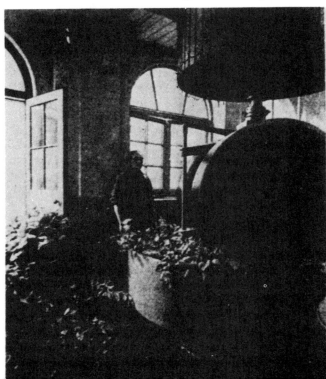

FRESH
BELLADONNA
LEAVES

About to be expressed for juice and for making the green extract. It is extremely important that this be done promptly to avoid fermentation and consequent deterioration of the product. The fresh herb is gathered as soon as the sun is up, and expressed and treated before sunset.

'WELLCOME'
CHEMICAL
WORKS

5

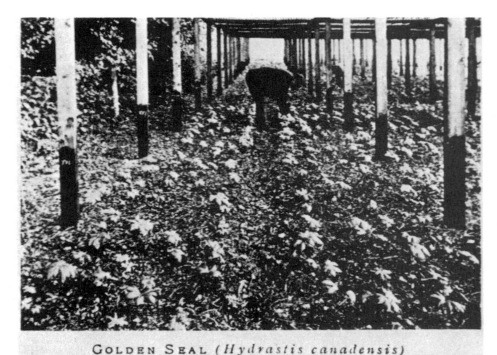

GOLDEN SEAL *(Hydrastis canadensis)*
The same plant under a specially-designed lattice structure, which ensures the
requisite amount of shade.

tive, where cosmopolitan lifestyles are the norm, we must at the same time wean ourselves from the overly processed, highly imbalanced foods.

By approaching herbal medicine from this vantage point, truly effective alternative healing can be realized. In simpler terms, the solution is not merely to unleash herbal medicine on the general public and proclaim it the solution to our ills. Our systems are not the natural systems that herbal medicines evolved with, so a slow weaning process is often in order.

A Failure of the Scientific Method

There was a rabbi in Jerusalem who was talking about Jewish mysticism. He was a mystic himself; he wasn't just a student of the subject. The rabbi was asked what he thought about the people who were scientific scholars of the subject of Jewish mysticism, and he said, "Well, they are accountants. . . .Well, that is like accountants, they know where the wealth is, its location and its value, but it doesn't belong to them. They cannot use it." That analogy applies to some of the

scientific approaches to herbs by scientists who are much like these accountants. They know that there's something in those plants, they may know where the wealth is, they may be able to locate it, but they can't use it.

There are, for example, approximately 1,400 scientific papers in the literature on Ginseng. The root displays documented antistress properties, yet no one has been able to break the code—decipher its active principle or principles. Here is one problem of the scientific method in a field (herbs) that doesn't easily lend itself to piecemeal analysis. Western science looks at a plant that works and reasons, "Let's break it apart and find out what part of it works, let's remove that, let's make a drug out of it." As an example, we have cocaine. The Coca plant has numerous alkaloids. When they work together an effect different from that of the individual alkaloid, cocaine, is produced. So a person who chews Coca leaf is not simply chewing cocaine. Trying to break plants down into a single "active" medicinal element is often a fruitless approach.

The Mother of All Medicines: Placebo

Let's evaluate the achievements of that great drug, perhaps the mother of all medicines—the placebo. How do we explain cures based upon imaginary medicine? If we are too gross, too jaded, to respond to subtle medicines such as herbs, how do we account for our frequent responses to mere suggestions of a medicine? Are the Christian Scientists correct when they tell us to remember that we cannot be ill since we are pure in spirit? Well, this may work to some extent, but remember that the graveyards are filled with many a person who denied his ills to his stoic end. Deny though we may, diseases work according to their own rhythms. Even trout develop liver cancer at times. This despite the fact that they are not divorced from their own kind—that is, they are not alienated creatures, nor are they leading too hectic an existence so far as we know. The point is, microbes *do* exist, despite our best attempts at psychosomatic therapeutics. And, of course, so do higher laws.

We must never be too sure of ourselves, nor of our medical systems. Everything appears to be subject to higher laws which are merely felt down here, and it is in this area of feeling that we must seek our confirmation, for intuitively we are beginning to reawaken to these higher laws in which natural medicines such as plants play a role.

Cynics may believe that herbs are pure placebos without any medical value whatever. Yet, even in a synthetic age such as ours, the constituents of approximately 25 percent of all prescriptions written derive from the higher species of plants. That's fairly significant in an age when plants have been kicked out of the picture by pharmaceutical advertisers. Moreover, plant medicines are the only drugs available for the majority of the world's people, without the chemist's genius. In China, where thousands of years of practice have elevated herbalism to a science, a disorder treated only by surgery in the West is effectively cured by an herbal remedy: Acute appendicitis is medicated with traditional drugs (which must sound like "Ripley's Believe It or Not" to most Westerners). According to a National Academy of Sciences Trip Report on China, since the Revolution as many as twenty thousand cases

of appendicitis treated with herbs have reflected an overall cure rate of 90 percent! Simple nonperforative appendicitis is generally cured within an average of three and a half days, according to this report. If peritonitis arises, antibiotics such as penicillin and surgery are then employed. Here we see a perfect blending of herbal and technological medicine.

Of the various herbal remedies used to treat appendicitis in China, Rhubarb (*Rheum tanguticum*) is the common ingredient in all prescriptions. It contains anthraquinones, which explain the laxative effect. Tannins, which are also present in rhubarb, then serve to arrest the cathartic action started by the other chemical. Other plants in the remedies may offer antibacterial effects and circulatory stimulation. Interestingly, the Chinese medical doctors take an approach opposite from that of our physicians, who strictly contraindicate cathartics in acute appendicitis. In the West, when you have appendicitis physicians tell you never to take a laxative. Chinese medical doctors use the opposite approach. But the patient doesn't just take a laxative; it would kill him. As explained above, the herbs also have tannins in them which stop the effect of the laxative, just at the right time. The herbal remedy also contains antibacterial properties, which eventually act on the infection.

This is only one example of a philosophical difference which enables one school of practice to effectively employ herbs for a condition which the other generally considers to be strictly in the surgeon's realm.

The Ideal Herbalist

Returning to our accountant analogy, we see that there are people who know where the wealth is, its location and value, but are unable to use it. It's time, then, to define different degrees of possible involvement with herbs.

Among them are the herbalist, the herbal pharmacist, the herbal physician, the herb scientist, the herb journalist, and the herb tradesperson. These are nonhierarchical categories, encompassing different ways of looking at the world of herbs.

We may define an herbalist as a person who

knows where the treasure is and can utilize and tap into it, perhaps more so than the herb pharmacologist (who approaches herbs from the scientific viewpoint). Anyone who attempts to alleviate or cure an ailment through the use of plant remedies might be considered an herbalist. This implies that if you read a book on herbs and prescribe a plant remedy to somebody and it works, you may consider yourself an herbalist. But think about this. Any number of practicing herbalists, anywhere in the world, can give you their point of view about many plant remedies. Yet how wide can the experience of one practitioner be? Can this experience equal the collective wisdom of centuries compiled through an exhaustive scientific search of current findings worldwide? That's where the herb scientist comes in—a person who collates these reports and who finds patterns in usage.

Following is a list of things the ideal herbalist should know. An examination for the ideal herbalist might test whether he can:

1. Identify the root samples of six species of plants.
2. Identify six similar leaf samples.
3. Accurately describe the known medicinally active constituents of five common herbs.
4. Describe the effects of the known medicinally active constituents of twenty-five herbs within the body. (For example, what effect does the salicin in the Willow bark have in the human body?)
5. State which foods are to be avoided with each of ten common herbs.
6. Describe the symptons of diseases which cannot be treated by herbs.
7. Demonstrate the preparation of a compound infusion, a compound decoction, and a compound tincture.
8. Correctly describe each organ system of the human body, and trace the pathway of any two herbs through the body.
9. State which of the hundred most popular herbs in the world are to be avoided during pregnancy, and the reasons why.
10. Finally, the ideal herbalist can describe the principal schools of herbal thought as prac-

ticed in China, England, France, Germany, the Soviet Union, and the United States.

THE ALTERNATIVE HEALTH MOVEMENT

I recently received an inquiry from the publisher of a widely circulated alternative health newsletter. A very famous American herbalist was about to make a number of claims for the use of medicinal plants for women's problems. The publisher asked for confirmation or denial from the scientific literature of the efficacy of these folk remedies.

Subsequent research rendered an answer the enterprising publisher didn't want to hear. He was unwilling to jeopardize his profits by disagreeing with a viewpoint he knew his readers would embrace.

What should we say of a plant for which thousands of people claim a beneficial effect when the scientific literature maintains that laboratory findings do not support such use? Even though we'd all like to see that people get whatever help there is to be had, this does not mean we should enter such plants into the world armamentarium, thereby elevating every folkloric remedy to the stature of a universal medicine. The object of this book is to promote the use of herbal remedies, and to restore to medical practice those truly useful herbs that have been abandoned without sufficient cause over the years. This herbal does, however, include negative evaluations of the efficacy of certain plants where warranted. Each plant entry in this work contains the most historically consistent traditional uses and, when available, a scientific update which summarizes the most recent available experimental findings. This book, then, is the first comprehensive modern and scientific contribution to herbal literature. The volume is no mere rehash of uses that have appeared in generations of herbals, borrowed one from another, and with no basis for experimental or clinical experience to back up the claims.

The great interest in and practice of alternative medicine is no doubt due to the widespread notion that the medical establishment is mercenary, but how can we be certain that alternative health practitioners are themselves not guilty of this motive? Certainly the fee schedules are not much lower than those levied by licensed, educated health professionals. Too many "alternative healers" have undertaken little if any serious study. In fact, many self-styled herbalists in America have simply read one or two popular books and then gone on to prescribe, treating people for every kind of infirmity from halitosis to cancer! Are we to believe that these people are divinely inspired, that precisely because they are uneducated they have a secret design for methods of healing unknown to licensed, educated professionals?

Still, how do we explain the reputed herbal and other cures of so many serious ailments, including cancer? As long ago as 1835 Dr. Bigelow, quoted in Stephenson and Churchill's *Medical Botany* had at least a partial answer:

> Those persons who know how seldom genuine cancers occur in comparison with reported ones, will be more ready to allow it the character of curing ulcerous, than really cancerous afflictions. There are undoubtedly many ulcers, and those frequently of a malignant kind, which are benefited by antiseptic stimulants; and to such the Pyrola [Spotted Wintergreen, *Chimaphila umbellata*] may be useful. But of its efficacy in real cancer we require more evidence than is at present possessed, before we ascribe to it the power of controlling so formidable a malady.

This plant contains ericolin, arbutin, chimaphilin, urson, tannin, and gallic acid, and we believe that the tannins are largely responsible for any beneficial effects the herb may have in treating ulcerous conditions. As we see, the cure of "cancer" by herbalists may often be the treatment of a simple skin condition or ulcer.

Why the perceivable drift toward disavowing modern medicine in favor of prescientific systems? We see increasing death rates from degenerative diseases, despite our scientific medicine and nearly unlimited research funds. Why do some of us look to the past for our future in medicine? Perhaps it is the same existentialist posture which

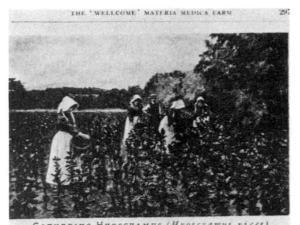

THE 'WELLCOME' MATERIA MEDICA FARM

GATHERING HYOSCYAMUS (*Hyoscyamus niger*)

Hyoscyamus niger, one of the most difficult plants with which the herb farmer has to deal, is grown from seed sown about March or April. The young plants show above ground at the end of May or beginning of June. In the autumn they are separated if too close together. In the following May an aerial stem is developed, which rapidly grows until it reaches the height of three or four feet. The flowering takes place in June or July, when the crop is harvested.

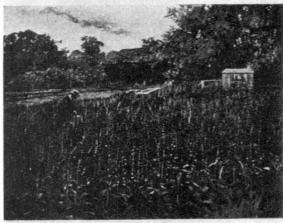

DIGITALIS (*Digitalis purpurea*) IN FLOWER

Digitalis purpurea is obtained from carefully-selected wild seed, and any variations from the wild type are struck out. Great care is taken in collecting and drying the leaves, otherwise the medicinal activity would be adversely affected. Blighted, faded or defective leaves are rejected, and only the finest preserved for use.

has us fleeing from so much else of what passes for "modern" in our technological societies.

Weiner's Herbal gives you information on plants with beneficial properties worth noting, while also commenting on plants of previously reputed value which we feel are no longer appropriate in folk medicine, due to their toxicity or ineffectiveness. Many of our experimental evaluations are inconclusive. We don't mean to discourage sincere folk practitioners, however, who through careful clinical trials have found these plants efficacious. Where the scientific method fails and the cure works, most people conclude that the cure is right. Healing is not the same as science. As previously explained, science is often unable to explain why plant remedies work. The methods of science themselves very often inhibit a true understanding of the action of herbs. That's because the entire plant is rarely if ever tested, but only a component of the plant—and in its dried state at that—and usually against simple animal systems rather than on humans suffering from the illness. In this sense, herbalism is, at its best, a practice between science and religion—and at its worst, between mysticism and astrology. Man often imagines he has broken free of the zoological order, yet every day he is reminded of his foundation in the physical plane. Minor or major aches and pains, desires and agonies, all serve to bring him back to earth.

To keep ourselves physically healthy, it is obviously wise to avoid whatever is injurious to the body and to cultivate habits conducive to major health and vigor. Herbal medicine by itself, in fact any medicine by itself, will not assure well-being. Cultivate a total health picture: principally, reasonable dietary habits, exercise, and adequate rest. If you fall ill and the diet and rest are not the cure, you may turn to herbal medicine. If herbs fail to turn the tide, seek the advice of a sensitive, Western-trained allopathic physician who is disposed to as little drug therapy as possible. You may instead prefer a homeopath. Failing with these methods, we still have radical medicine at our disposal, including surgery, radiation, and other technological innovations. This is a proper view then, of a scheme for medical care in which herbs have an integral place.

LABORATORY SCIENCE AND HERBS
by Dr. N. R. Farnsworth

To correlate results from animal experiments with effects in humans is often difficult, but there does seem to be an observable relationship in most cases. If there is no method for testing a substance in animals, it follows that one cannot project an herb's utility or lack of it for humans. There is no way, for example, to use animals to test the aphrodisiac qualities of a substance. Herbalists have claimed that at least 1,074 plant species are useful as emmenagogues—agents that will induce menstruation. However, there are no agents currently used by the medical profession for which this claim is allowed by the Food and Drug Administration. Does this mean that such agents do not exist? Of course not. It simply means that there isn't yet sufficient proof that an agent will exert this effect in humans and still be safe enough for general use.

Large numbers of plants are claimed to be useful as "carminatives" for "stomach disorders." It is again difficult to establish whether or not these plants have real effects since the malady is not identified specifically enough. One example will suffice. People all over the world commonly drink cinnamon tea as a refreshing beverage, or for "stomach disorders." Japanese scientists recently studied this practice and, using a number of elegant pharmacological tests on animals, they examined each of the known major chemical constituents of cinnamon for their effects on the stomach and intestinal tract. One of these chemical compounds, cinnamaldehyde or cinnamic acid aldehyde, when given orally to several species of animals, markedly relaxed the smooth muscle of the intestinal tract and reinforced the normal rhythm of other muscles.

The proportionately larger doses of cinnamaldehyde required to work the same effect in humans, however, would require the consumption of an extraordinary amount of cinnamon tea. The fact that humans do experience the effect is most logically explained by the conclusion that cinnamaldehyde may have a cumulative effect. That is, several doses may have to be taken until enough of the cinnamaldehyde accumulates in the body to give the effect. Many modern prescription drugs must be taken for a few days before their effect is felt by an individual.

A second possibility is that humans may not require as much cinnamaldehyde as animals, in order to obtain the same effect. There are many examples of common drugs that act similarly. Common tea contains not only cinnamaldehyde,

How To Use This Book

First reread the caveat at the end of the preceding introduction.

The text is composed of articles on plants, arranged in alphabetical order by common name, with other common names sublisted (the first name is cross-referenced in the Plant Index). The Latin binomial and plant part used—in some cases, several of each—are also keyed above each article, which opens with a detailed "Botanical Description."

Botanical descriptions are primarily drawn from the following: the *United States Dispensatory*, 20th ed. (U.S.D); Bentley's *Medicinal Plants* (Bentley); Neal's *In Gardens of Hawaii* (Neal). These sources, as well as other floras, are given in full in the Bibliography.

As R. Sharrock observed three hundred years ago in "The History of the Propagation and Improvement of Vegetables by the Concurrence of Art and Nature," "Few scientists produce work 'overgarnished with Rhetorical Tropes, which like flowers stuck in a window . . . create a darkness in the place'" (quoted in Agnes Arber, *The Mind and the Eye*, p. 52): These highly detailed botanical descriptions may seem superfluous to those interested in the medicinal aspects of herbs. Nevertheless, these plant descriptions will be useful to those interested in identifying herbs brought in from the field, where many plants of similar appearance are too often mistakenly identified and thus wrongly employed in medicine.

In the following Therapeutic Index, traditional uses and maladies are keyed to the plants that have been employed in conjunction with them.

In the text of each article (next section), "Medicinal Uses" incorporates beneath one heading traditional and experimental findings where available; while the "dose" information repeats reported traditional doses; *do not consider them instructions or prescriptions*. Most entries are as described in the United States Dispensatory (20th ed.); others are adapted from Meyer's *The Herbalist*. Some of the terms used in this context are explicitly defined below:

Fluidextracts contain alcohol as a solvent, where each milliliter represents 1 gram of the drug.

Tinctures are *diluted* alcoholic solutions of herbs, the standard strength being 10 percent for powerful drugs and 20 percent for less powerful ones.

Decoctions are made by *boiling* the herb in a covered container, 1 teaspoonful of the ground herb in approximately 1½ pints of water, for about 30 minutes, at a slow boil. The liquid is then allowed to cool slowly in the *closed* container. Decoctions are for tougher plant parts, such as

13

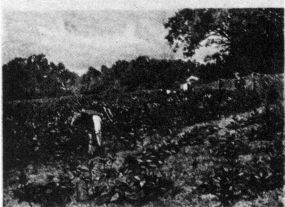

A FIELD OF DATURA METEL

This handsome plant is interesting, as recent investigation has shown that it contains Hyoscine, Hyoscyamine and Atropine in proportions differing from those occurring in other solanaceous plants.

A FIELD OF BELLADONNA (Atropa belladonna)

Atropa belladonna is grown from genuine wild seed. The best crops of leaves are obtained in the second, third or fourth year of the plant's growth, and it is at this period that the alkaloidal content is greatest.

seeds, stem, stembark, and juice from tubers.

Infusions are prepared from softer plant parts such as leaves, flowers, twigs, and the juice from fleshy leaves. Approximately ½ ounce of plant material is *steeped* for 5 to 20 minutes in approximately 1 pint of boiled water.

Juices from tubers and fleshy leaves are mixed with water, fruit juices, other mild herb "teas," aromatics, or carminatives, and sipped directly.

As a final note it is important to remember that in the golden age of botanical medicine, the late nineteenth century, few people actually prepared herbal remedies themselves. The skills of the trained physician/herbalist were called upon, and

most herbal remedies were administered in the form of tinctures. Since few highly trained herbalists are in practice today, many people are learning to prepare herbs themselves. This guidebook will aid the reader who is searching for a rational approach to earth's medicines.

GLOSSARY OF MEDICAL TERMS

Reprinted with permission from *Taber's Cyclopedic Medical Dictionary*, 10th edition, F. A. Davis Co., Philadelphia, 1969.

ABORTIFACIENT: A drug which causes abortion.

ALTERATIVE: Agent which tends gradually to alter a condition.

AMENORRHEA: Absence of or suppression of menstruation.

ANODYNE: Any medicine which allays pain.

ANTHELMINTICS (VERMIFUGES): Medicines capable of destroying or expelling worms which inhabit the intestinal canal.

ANTISCORBUTIC: A remedy for or counteractant to scurvy.

APERIENT: An extremely mild, weak laxative.

AROMATIC: Used chiefly to expel gas from stomach and intestines. Also employed to make other medicines, less agreeable in taste and smell, more palatable, due to the fragrant smells and tastes of the aromatics.

ASTRINGENT: Tightens and contracts skin and/or mucous membranes. Externally as lotions and gargles; internally to check diarrhea.

CALMATIVE: Simply a calming agent, not necessarily sedative.

CARMINATIVE: Substance which removes gases from the gastrointestinal tract.

CATHARTIC: (1) Laxative and Aperient—*Mild* promotion of evacuation of the bowels by action on alimentary canal. (2) Purgative—Induces copious evacuation of the bowels, generally used to treat stubborn constipation in adults.

CHOLAGOGUE: Agents that increase the flow of bile into the intestines.

CORDIAL: A refreshing medicine which is held to revive the "spirits," being cheering, invigorating, and exhilarating.

DEMULCENT: Those medicines, used *internally*, that possess soothing, mucilaginous properties, shielding surfaces and/or mucous membranes from irritating substances.

DEPURATIVE: Agents that purify or cleanse, generally: "depurate a wound" or "depurate a fluid."

DIAPHORETIC: Agent which increases perspiration. Commonly used as an aid for relief of common cold, administered hot, before bedtime.

DIURETIC: Medicine which increases urination, often combined with demulcents.

"DOCTRINE OF SIGNATURES": An ancient medical theory that "like cures like."

DYSMENORRHEA: Painful or difficult menstruation.

EMETIC: A medicine that provokes vomiting.

EMMENAGOGUE: A substance with medicinal properties designed to assist and promote the menstrual discharges.

EMOLLIENT: Generally of oily or mucilaginous nature, used *externally* for its softening, supple, or soothing qualities.

EXPECTORANT: Medicine that promotes the discharge of matter from the lungs, whether it be mucus, pus, or any other morbid accumulation.

FEBRIFUGE: Any medicine that mitigates or dispels fever.

LAXATIVE: Increases the peristaltic motion of the bowels, without purging or producing a fluid discharge. Never to be used when pregnant.

NERVINE: Having a soothing influence and quieting the nerves without numbing them.

PECTORAL: A medicine adapted to cure or relieve complaints of the breast and lungs.

PURGATIVE: Agent which induces copious evacuation of the bowels. Generally used only for stubborn cases, such as chronic constipation among adults. Never to be used when pregnant.

REFRIGERANTS: Cooling beverages.

RELAXANTS: Relaxing muscle fiber and alleviating spasm; allaying nervous irritation due to excitement, strain, or fatigue.

RUBEFACIENT: External application which produces redness of the skin, by virtue of drawing the blood and fluids toward the skin's surface; helpful in treatment of boils and blisters.

SEDATIVE: Allays irritability or nerve action.

STIMULANT: Any agent temporarily increasing activity of cardiac, bronchial, gastric, cerebral, intestinal, nervous, motor, vasomotor, respiratory, or secretory organs.

SUDORIFIC: Causes copious perspiration.

VERMIFUGE: See ANTHELMINTICS.

VULNERARY: Application for external wounds.

15

WEINER'S HERBAL THERAPEUTIC INDEX

please refer to indices to locate plants
SECTION I INDEX, pages 211-214
SECTION II INDEX, pages 273-275

ABDOMINAL PAINS
  Anemone
  Hops (external application)
ABORTIFACIENTS (ABORTION INDUCERS)
  Goldenseal
  Cotton Root
  Mistletoe
  Rue
  Savin
ADAPTOGENS
  Bupleurum
  Ginseng, Korean
  Ginseng, Siberian
AGUE
  Cayenne
  Feverfew
AIDS/ARC
  Astragalus
  Chinese Cucumber
  Seaweeds
ALLERGIES
  Garlic
  Quercetin
ANAPHRODISIACS (TO LESSEN SEXUAL DESIRE)
  Water Lily, White
  Willows
ANODYNES (PAIN RELIEVERS)
  Anemone
  Barberry
  Belladonna (external application)
  Bloodroot (external application)
  Coca
  Cohosh, Black
  Cowslip
  Flax (external application)
  Ginger
  Guaraná
  Hops (external application)
  Kava-Kava
  Lettuce

  Marijuana
  Marshmallow
  Mullein
  Mustard (external application)
  Poplar Buds (external application)
  Scullcap
  Thyme (external application)
  Willow
  Wintergreen
  Witch Hazel (external application)
  Wormwood (external application)
ANTI-INFLAMMATORIES
  Astragalus
  Bupleurum
  Cayenne
  Garlic
  Ginger
  Schisandra
  Turmeric
  Willow, White
ANTISCORBUTICS (SCURVY REMEDIES)
  Adder's Tongue
  Rose
  Yellow Dock
ANTISPASMODICS
  Chamomile, German & Roman
  Club Moss
  Cohosh, Black
  Feverfew
  Foxglove
  Goldenseal
  Grindelia
  Marijuana
  Mistletoe
  Motherwort
  Mugwort
  Mullein
  Passionflower
  Peppermint
  Pleurisy Root
  Safflower
  Scullcap
  Skunk Cabbage
  Yam
APHRODISIACS
  Damiana
  Ginseng
  Kava-Kava
  Kino

Bloodwood (see KINO article)
Magnolia
Orchids
APPETITE STIMULANTS
   Yellow Gentian
   Holy Thistle
   Ipecac
   Marijuana
   Mustard
   Quassia
   Sweet Fern
AROMATICS AND CARMINATIVES (*SEE* FLATULENCE)
   Angelica
   Anise
ARTHRITIS
   German Chamomile
   Fennel
   Ginger
   Juniper Berries
   Lavender
   Magnolia
   Manna
   Motherwort
   Pennyroyal
   Peppermint
   Sassafras
   Spearmint
   Star Anise
   Turpentines
   Willow, White
   Wintergreen
   Wood Betony
   Yarrow
ASTHMA
   Balsam of Peru
   Ephedra
   Eucalyptus
   Ginkgo
   Grindelia
   Horehound
   Yellow Jasmine
   Licorice
   Maidenhair Fern
   Marijuana
   Mistletoe
   Nettle
   Pennyroyal
   Sarsaparilla

Senega Snakeroot
Skunk Cabbage
Sumac
Thyme
Wall Germander
Yerba Santa
ASTRINGENTS
   Angelica
   Barberry
   Butternut
   Cherry Laurel
   Chestnut, Spanish
   Cinchona
   Dogwood
   Ginseng, Red American
   Goldenseal
   Henna
   Kino
   Madder
   Oak, White
   Plantain
   Pomegranate
   Red Raspberry
   Rhubarb
   Rose
   Sassafras
   Squaw Vine
   Strawberry Leaf
   Sumac
   Tormentil
   Wall Germander
   Wintergreen
   Witch Hazel
   Wood Betony
   Yarrow
   Yellow Dock
BACK, SORE (LUMBAGO)
   Belladonna (external application)
   Hops (external application)
   Mustard (external application)
   Papaya
   Star Anise
BACTERIAL AND/OR FUNGAL INFECTIONS
   Barberry
   Burdoc
   Couch Grass
   Eucalyptus
   Garlic
   Goldenseal

THERAPEUTIC INDEX

Henna
Juniper Berries
Kava-Kava
Marigold
Mathake
Mulberry, Black
Oak, White
Onion
Pau d'arco
Sassafras
Shepherd's Purse
Star Anise
Thyme
Tormentil
Wall Germander
Yarrow
BOILS
Arrowroot
Devil's Claw
Elecampane
Ivy
Lobelia
Mullein
Onion Pansy
Papaya
Plantain
Slippery Elm
Water Lilies
Yarrow
BREAKBONE FEVER
Boneset
BREASTS, MILK SECRETION
Fennel
Wintergreen
BREASTS, SORE
Bittersweet
BRONCHITIS
Acacia
Balsam of Peru
Ephedra
Eucalyptus
Grindelia
Horehound
Licorice
Marigold
Onion
Pleurisy Root
Senega Snakeroot
Thyme

Turpentines
Wall Germander
Wild Cherry
Yerba Santa
BRUISES
Arnica
Bittersweet
Burdock
Comfrey (external application)
Madder
Marigold
St. John's Wort
Wormwood
Yarrow
BURNS
Acacia
Aloes
Burdock
Goldenseal
Grindelia
Marigold
Mullein
Nettle
Nightshade, Black
Onion
Turpentines
Yarrow
CANCER
Angelica
Astragalus
Chamomile
Garlic
Henna
Horehound
Juniper Berries
Mezereon
Mushrooms
Onion
Pau d'arco
Periwinkle, Tropical
Seaweeds
Solomon's Seal
Turmeric
CATHARTICS (*SEE* CONSTIPATION,
LAXATIVES)
Broom
Buckbean
Buckthorn
Cascara

18

Castor Oil
Elder
Orris
Pansy
Pleurisy Root
Rhubarb
Senna
Tamarind
Toad Flax
Wormwood
CHEST COMPLAINTS
Coltsfoot
Licorice
Mullein
Myrrh
Ohio Buckeye (see HORSECHESTNUT article)
Pansy
Poplar Buds
Sweet Fern
CHILDBIRTH
Cohosh, Blue
Feverfew
Groundsel
Madder
Mistletoe
Mugwort
Red Raspberry
Squaw Vine
CHRONIC FATIGUE SYNDROME
Echinacea
Ginkgo
Ginseng, Korean
Mushrooms
Schisandra
Seaweeds
COLDS
Anemones
Betel Nut Palm
Boneset
Citrus
Echinacea
Ginger
Ginkgo
Ginseng
Maidenhair Fern
Mullein
Onion
Pennyroyal
Yerba Santa

COLIC
Angelica
Anise
Catnip
Chamomile, Roman
Fennel
Ginger
Marijuana
Mullein
Pleurisy Root
Rhubarb
Star Anise
Thyme
Turpentines
Yams
CONSTIPATION (STRONGER LAXATIVES LISTED HERE)
Acacia
Agar-Agar
Aloe
Boneset
Butternut
Cascara
Castor Oil
Dandelion
Quassia
Rhubarb
Senna
Turpentines
CONTRACEPTIVES
Mistletoe
COUGH
Acacia
Catnip
Chestnut, Spanish
Coltsfoot
Couch Grass
Ephedra
Flax
Grindelia
Horehound
Licorice
Maidenhair Fern
Mullein
Nettle
Pleurisy Root
Skunk Cabbage
Slippery Elm
Sweet Fern

THERAPEUTIC INDEX

Club Moss
Cohosh, Blue
Couch Grass
Dandelion
Fennel
Feverfew
Foxglove
Gotu Kola
Groundsel
Holly
Holy Thistle
Juniper Berries
Kava-Kava
Madder
Mistletoe
Mullein
Nettle
Onion
Oregon Grape
Orris
Pipsissewa
Sassafras
Shave Grass
Skunk Cabbage
Squaw Vine
Star Anise
Toad Flax
Turpentines
Wall Germander
Wintergreen
Yam
DROPSY
Buckbean
Burdock
Elder
Elecampane
Foxglove
Indian Corn
Licorice
Madder
Meadow Saffron
Orris
Shave Grass
Skunk Cabbage
Toad Flax
Wall Germander
EARACHE
Fennel

EMETICS (TO PRODUCE VOMITING)
Adder's Tongue
Blood Root
Boneset
Broom
Buckbean
Chamomile, Roman
Elder
Foxglove
Holly
Holy Thistle
Ipecac
Mistletoe
Mustard
Orris
Pansy
Pleurisy Root
Quassia
Skunk Cabbage
Solomon's Seal
Wintergreen
Wood Betony
EMOLLIENTS (EXTERNALLY SOOTHING AGENTS)
Acacia
Agar-Agar
Aloes
Anemones
Arnica
Balsam of Peru
Coltsfoot
Flax
Fleawort (see PLANTAIN article)
Indian Corn
Marigold
Marshmallow
Mistletoe
Mullein
Pansy
Plantain
EMPHYSEMA (CATARRH: DRY COUGHING)
Boneset
Buckbean
Flax
Grindelia
Payaya
Rose Buds
Sassafras

Juniper Berries
Meadow Saffron
Mullein
Nettle
Pennyroyal
Savin
Wall Germander
Wood Betony
GUMS, BLEEDING
Grounsel
HAYFEVER
Ephedra
Grindelia
HEADACHE
Balm
Cowslip
Chamomile, Roman
Feverfew (migraine only)
Ginger
Guaraná
Lavender
Willow, White
Wood Betony
HEART AND RELATED CARDIO-VASCULAR
DISORDERS
Anemones
Asarabacca
Bilberry
Broom
Coca
Ephedra
Foxglove
Garlic
Ginger
Marigold (for high blood pressure)
Mistletoe (for high blood pressure)
Motherwort
Onion
Pennyroyal
Sassafras
Solomon's Seal
Wild Cherry
Wonder Violet (see PANSY article)
HEMMORHAGE
Acacia
Coca
Goldenseal
Groundsel
Ipecac

Kino
Mistletoe
Nettle
Savin
Tormentil
Turpentines
Witch Hazel
Yarrow
HEMORRHOIDS
Butcher's Broom
Buttercups
Horsechestnut
Mullein
Nightshade, Black
Oak, White
Toad Flax
Witch Hazel
Yarrow
HICCOUGH
Mustard
HYPERACTIVITY
Chamomile
Hibiscus
Passionflower
HYPOGLYCEMIA
Licorice
INDIGESTION
Angelica
Boneset
Catnip
Cayenne
Chamomile, German & Roman
Dandelion
Elecampane
Yellow Gentian
Ginger
Goldenseal
Holy Thistle
Ipecac
Juniper Berries
Lettuce
Mustard
Papaya
Peppermint
Quassia
Spearmint
Star Anise
Sweet Fern
Toad Flax

THERAPEUTIC INDEX

LIVER DISORDERS
- Anemones
- Butternut
- Dandelion
- Foxglove
- Horehound
- Marigold
- Milk Thistle
- Oregon Grape
- Pansy

LUNG AILMENTS
- Acacia
- Club Moss
- Coltsfoot
- Elecampane
- Ephedra
- Flax
- Horehound
- Mullein
- Myrrh
- Nettle
- Pennyroyal
- Pleurisy Root
- Rose
- Senega Snakeroot
- Wall Germander
- Wonder Violet (see PANSY article)

MALARIA
- Boneset
- Cinchona
- Dogwood
- Eucalyptus
- Fennel
- Feverfew
- Yellow Gentian
- Holly
- Horehound
- Magnolia
- Mugwort
- Oregon Grape
- Wall Germander
- Willows
- Wormwood

MENSTRUAL TROUBLES
- Aloe
- Angelica
- Burdock
- Catnip
- Chamomile
- Cohosh, Black
- Cohosh, Blue
- Elecampane
- Ergot
- Feverfew
- Ginger
- Goldenseal
- Groundsel
- Henna
- Madder
- Motherwort
- Mugwort
- Passionflower
- Pennywort
- Rue
- Safflower
- Savin
- Squaw Vine
- Turpentines
- Willows
- Wintergreen
- Yarrow

MENTAL DISTURBANCES
- Anemone
- Hops
- Marijuana
- Passionflower
- Sweet Fern

MOUTH INFECTION
- Anemones
- Groundsel
- Marshmallow
- Mulberry, Black
- Myrrh
- Sumac
- Tormentil
- Yellow Dock

MOUTH WASHES, GARGLES
- Anemone
- Barberry
- Groundsel
- Oak, White
- Orris
- Pomegranate
- Sumac
- Tormentil

MUSCLE PAINS
- Marijuana
- Mustard

THERAPEUTIC INDEX

NAUSEA
   Cayenne
   Ginger
   Goldenseal
   Ipecac
   Red Raspberry
   Spearmint
NERVES
   Agave
   Anemone
   Hops
   Lavender
   Marijuana
   Mistletoe
   Motherwort
   Nettle
   Orchids
   Passionflower
   Rue
   Scullcap
   Valerian
   Wild Cherry
   Wood Betony
NOSEBLEED
   Comfrey
   Marijuana
   Pennyroyal
PARALYSIS
   Cowslip
   Guarana
PIMPLES
   Elecampane
   Solomon's Seal
PLEURISY
   Holly
   Pleurisy Root
POISON IVY, POISON OAK (*SEE* ALSO RASHES)
   Grindelia
   Sassafras
POISON ANTIDOTES
   Arrowroot
   Ipecac
   Nettle
PURGATIVES (*SEE ALSO* CATHARTICS)
   Aloes
   Barberry
   Bloodroot
   Boneset
   Buckbean

   Buckthorn
   Elder
   Foxglove
   Holly
   Mistletoe
   Morning Glory
   Pomegranate
   Senega Snakeroot
   Sweet Fern
   Wood Betony
RASHES
   Club Moss
   Grindelia
   Marshmallow
   Safflower
   Skunk Cabbage
   Tormentil
RHEUMATISM
   Bittersweet
   Burdock
   Club Moss
   Cohosh, Black
   Devil's Claw
   Elder
   Horsechestnut
   Magnolia
   Meadow Saffron
   Pipsissewa
   Poplar Buds
   Prickly Ash
   Sarsaparilla & Mexican Sarsaparilla
   Sassafras
   Savin
   Skunk Cabbage
   Soapwort
   Star Anise
   Turpentines (external application)
   Witch Hazel (external application)
   Wormwood (external application)
   Yam
RUBEFACIENTS (TO REDDEN THE SKIN)
   Anemone
   Buttercups
   Cayenne
   Ginger
   Mustard
   Myrrh
   Nettle
   Rue

Savin
Thyme
SCABIES
  Buckbean
  Foxglove
SCARLET FEVER
  Cayenne
SEASICKNESS
  Cayenne
  Ginger
SEDATIVES
  Anemones
  Betel Nut Palm
  Chamomile, German
  Cohosh, Black
  Cowslip
  Gotu Kola
  Hops
  Kava-Kava
  Lettuce
  Horsechestnut
  Marigold
  Marijuana
  Mistletoe
  Motherwort
  Mugwort
  Passionflower
  Scullcap
  Valerian
  Witch Hazel
  Yarrow
SKIN DISEASES
  Anemone
  Balsam of Peru
  Bittersweet
  Bloodroot
  Burdock
  Club Moss
  Comfrey
  Elder
  Elecampane
  Eucalyptus
  Flax
  Foxglove
  Goldenseal
  Grindelia
  Henna
  Ivy
  Kino

Madder
Marshmallow
Nettle
Nightshade, Black
Onion
Oregon Grape
Pansy
(Mexican) Sarsaparilla
Sassafras
Savin
Skunk Cabbage
Soapwort
Solomon's Seal
Toad Flax
Turpentines
Water Lilies
Wormwood
Yarrow
Yellow Dock
SLEEPLESSNESS
  Catnip
  Cowslip
  German Chamomile
  Hops
  Marijuana
  Passionflower
  Valerian
SMALL POX
  Holly
  Tormentil
SNAKE BITE
  Nettle
  Senega Snakeroot
  Virginia Snakeroot
SNUFFS
  Asarabacca
  Comfrey
  Horse Chestnut
SORE NIPPLES (NURSING MOTHERS)
  Acacia
SORES, EXTERNAL
  Balsam of Peru
  Bloodroot
  Devil's Claw
  Foxglove
  Ginseng, Red American
  Ivy
  Marigold
  Pipsissewa

THERAPEUTIC INDEX

Plantain
Wall Germander
STIMULANTS
Angelica
Bloodroot
Cacao
Cayenne
Chamomile, Roman
Coca
Coffee
Cola
Damiana
Dogwood
Elecampane
Eucalyptus
Fennel
Ginger
Ginkgo
Ginseng, Korean
Guaraná
Ivy (external application)
Juniper Berries
Kava-Kava
Khat
Magnolia
Myrrh
Onion
Pennyroyal
Peppermint
Prickly Ash
Schisandra
Spearmint
Star Anise
Tea
Wall Germander
Wintergreen
STOMACH TROUBLES
Angelica
Chamomile, Roman
Cherry Laurel
Dandelion
Elecampane
Feverfew
Flax
Holy Thistle
Ipecac
Juniper Berries
Lettuce
Marshmallow

Mustard
Myrrh
Papaya
Pennyroyal
Peppermint
Quassia
Rurbarb
Spearmint
Sweet Fern
Thyme
Tormentil
Wild Cherry
SUNBURN
Aloes
Balsam of Peru
Horsechestnut
Marigold
Solomon's Seal
SWELLINGS
Burdock
Fennel
Foxglove
Hops
Pansy
THROAT, SORE
Acacia
Barberry
Ginseng, Red American
Holly
Horehound
Kino
Licorice
Marshmallow
Mulberry, Black
Mullein
Pomegranate
Slippery Elm
Sumac
TONICS
Bearberry
Boneset
Buckbean
Cinchona
Damiana
Dandelion
Devil's Claw
Dogwood
Elecampane
Feverfew

THERAPEUTIC INDEX

Medicinal Plants of the World

ACACIA
Acacia vera, A. arabica, A. senegal

PARTS USED: Bark exudate
OTHER COMMON NAMES: Gum Arabic, Egyptian Thorn

Botanical Description: *Acacia vera*. This is a tree of middling size, with numerous scattered branches, of which the younger are much bent and covered with a reddish-brown bark. The leaves are alternate and bipinnate, with 2 pairs of pinnae, of which the lower are usually furnished with 10 pairs of leaflets, the upper with 8. The leaflets are very small, oblong-linear, smooth, and supported upon very short footstalks. On the common petiole is a gland between each pair of pinnae. Both the common and partial petioles are smooth. Two sharp spines, or rather prickles, from ¼ to ½ inch long, of the color of the smaller branches, and joined together at their base, are found at the insertion of each leaf. The flowers are yellow, inodorous, small, and collected in 2 to 5 globular heads. The fruit is a smooth, flat, 2-valved legume, divided by contractions occurring at regular intervals into several roundish portions, each containing a single seed. This species flourishes in Upper Egypt and Senegal, and is scattered over the intervening portion of the African continent.

A. arabica. This species, though often little more than a shrub, attains in favorable situations the magnitude of a considerable tree, being sometimes 40 feet high, with a trunk a foot or more in diameter. The leaves are alternate and doubly pinnate, having from 4 to 6 pairs of pinnae, each of which is furnished with from 10 to 20 pairs of minute, smooth, oblong-linear leaflets.

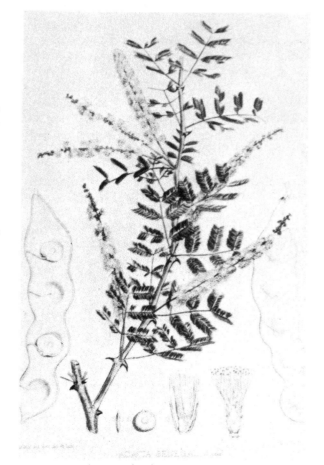

ACACIA: There is full justification for the use of gum acacia as a demulcent, since the gum swells on contact with water, develops a tenacious character, and coats and soothes mucous membranes.

31

The common petiole has a gland between the lowest pair of pinnae, and often also between the uppermost pair. Both the common and partial petiole as well as the young branches are downy. The prickles are straight and disposed as in *A. vera*. The flowers are also thus arranged, and the fruits of both are of a similar shape. *A. arabica* is perhaps the most widely diffused of the gum-bearing species. It grows in Upper and Lower Egypt, Senegal, and other parts of Africa, flourishes also in Arabia, and is abundant in India, where its gum is used for food by the natives.

Besides the two species above described, a third also affords considerable quantities of gum: *A. senegal*, a small tree, inhabiting the hottest regions of Africa, and said to form vast forests in Senegal.

The gum-bearing Acacias are all thorny or prickly trees or shrubs, calculated by nature for a dry and sandy soil, and flourishing in deserts where few other trees will grow. (U.S.D.)

Medicinal Uses: The gummy Acacia exudate, soluble in water, is used for its demulcent properties (soothing to mucous membrane surfaces). For shielding sore throat due to cough, a dried piece of Acacia gum is allowed to dissolve slowly in the mouth, maintaining a constant supply to the irritated area. Bronchial passages are similarly relieved by sucking on such a natural lozenge.

Externally, an application of powdered gum has been employed to check hemorrhage from leech bites. Applied in its mucilaginous state, it has been used to soothe burns and scrapes, as well as the sore nipples of nursing mothers.

Probably the principal medicinal use of the gum has been as a vehicle for other medicines, as in the suspension of insoluble powders, in lozenges, and other uses.

There is full justification for the use of acacia (gum arabic) as a demulcent, since when the gum comes into contact with water it swells, develops a tenacious character, and coats and soothes mucous membranes. The gum consists of a mixture of high-molecular-weight carbohydrate substances. When taken internally they are broken down to simple sugars (e.g., glucose) which are well known to have nutrient value. Further, since gum arabic also swells to some extent when taken orally, it has been used as a mild laxative, although not extensively in recent years.

Dose: The gum is given either in powder or dissolved in almond milk or similar flavored beverages: ½ ounce of the gum to a pint of liquid.

ADDER'S TONGUE
Erythronium americanum

PARTS USED: All parts active; leaves preferred.
OTHER COMMON NAMES: Dog-Tooth Violet, Serpent's Tongue, Yellow Snowdrop, Rattlesnake Violet, Yellow Snakeleaf

Botanical Description: This is an indigenous perennial bulbous plant, sometimes called, after the European species, Dog-Tooth Violet. The bulb, which is brown externally, white and solid within, sends up a single naked slender flower-stem with an obtuse callous point, and 2 smooth, lanceolate, nearly equal leaves, sheathing at their base, and of a brownish-green color diversified by numerous irregular spots. The flower is solitary, nodding, yellow, with oblong lanceolate petals obtuse at the point, a club-shaped undivided style, and a 3-lobed stigma.

E. americanum grows in woods and other shady places throughout the northern and middle United States. It flowers in the latter part of April or early in May. All parts of it are active. (U.S.D.)

Medicinal Uses: The bulbs of this plant have been recorded as emetic (producing vomiting) and as a substitute for Colchicum in the treatment of gout. It has also been reported to be a remedy, in the fresh state, for scurvy.

The plant derives its name from the coloring and shape of the leaf, which resembles an adder's tongue. It is possible that the traditional use of the plant as an external application for the treatment of wounds derived from its appearance, which would suggest that it be used in snakebites and, by extension, in other wounds and ulcers. At any rate, various oil infusions and ointments made from the leaf and spike have been used to treat wounds, and poultices of the fresh leaves have been applied to soothe and heal bruises.

Experimentally, Adder's Tongue has been found to contain alkaloids, and since the plant is closely related to other plants that produce colchicine, it may be presumed that colchicine is present in Adder's Tongue. Colchicine is a specific agent used for the diagnosis and treatment of gout. However, it is extremely toxic, and caution must be exercised concerning the ingestion of even the smallest amount of any plant containing colchicine.

Dose: 1.3 to 2.0 grams of the bulb will produce rapid vomiting. Since the leaves are stronger in action, very cautious doses are recommended by practitioners, starting with 0.25 gram one time per day, and observing the results. If tolerated, the dose is often increased to 0.50 gram per day, but not to exceed 0.75 gram. The fresher the plant material, the greater is the danger of toxicity due to higher alkaloid content.

AGAR-AGAR
Gelidium, Gracilaria, and *Pterocladia* spp.

PARTS USED: Whole plant

Botanical Description: Quite a number of the algae belonging to the Rhodophyceae, growing on the coast of southern and eastern Asia and elsewhere, contain large quantities of mucilage which is extracted and sold under the name of agar-agar (or simply agar). The algae are collected, spread out upon the beach until they are bleached, and then dried. They are then boiled with water and the mucilaginous solution strained through a cloth. The filtrate is allowed to dry thoroughly and harden in the sun. The algae are usually collected during the summer and fall, bleached, and dried, but the process of the manufacture of agar-agar does not take place until cold weather and usually extends from November to February. (U.S.D.)

The following species are sources of agar-agar, with their collection areas indicated:

Gelidium cartilaginium: off coast of South Africa, Mexico, and United States;
G. corneum: off coast of South Africa, Portugal, Spain, and Morocco;
G. amansii, G. liatulum, G. lingulatum, G. pacificum: off coast of Japan;

G. pristoides: off coast of South Africa;
G. sesquipedale: off coast of Portugal and Morocco;
Gracilaria confervoides: Southern Hemisphere;
Pterocladia capillacea: Egypt, Japan, New Zealand, Australia;
Pterocladia lucida: New Zealand.

Medicinal Uses: Agar, widely used in the treatment of chronic constipation, is "the dried mucilaginous substance extracted from marine algae growing along the Eastern coast of Asia." The collection process described above has doubtless been improved with modern technology, but the essential steps remain the same.

Agar is a type of seaweed that has been used for its emollient, demulcent, and mildly laxative effect. This sea plant has a very high concentration of polysaccharide mucilage, which swells and is very slimy when moistened. This mucilage is responsible for the laxative effect of agar, exerting a type of lubricant effect.

When used as a laxative, agar should be taken with large amounts of water, and never dry. It usually will not produce a laxative effect with a single dose, but must be used regularly.

Dose: Agar may be eaten daily as a cereal in the amount of 7 to 15 grams. Milk and honey are usually added to improve taste. Its function is very similar to that of vegetable cellulose foods and of bran, which figure so prominently in today's marketing of high-fiber-content cereals and breads. As a good bulk laxative, it may also be added to cereals, soups, cakes, or any other food without altering its effect. Results should be obtained in 3 to 7 days. If the constipation is stubborn, Cascara bark (see article) is added to precipitate action. This addition was often started at ½ gram and slowly increased to no more than 2 grams daily.

AGAVE
Agave americana

PARTS USED: Sap
OTHER COMMON NAMES: Century Plant

Botanical Description: The name Century Plant was

given to this denizen of hot deserts because under cultivation in the North Temperate Zone the flowers were so seldom seen that at one time they were supposed to appear only once in a hundred years. Actually, the plant may flower after about 10 years and then die. Its home, as of all Agaves, is some warm part of America. It is a large rosette, consisting of 30 to 60 huge, thick, narrow, perennial leaves (3 to 6 feet long, 6 to 9 inches at their widest, above the middle), which are straight or curved back at the tip and extend stiffly and obliquely from a stem that is short or almost lacking. Leaf margins are indented between sharp teeth. Flowers develop on a polelike stem rising 24 to 36 feet high, are borne in clusters near the ends of horizontal branches, and are yellow, 3 inches long, the stamens twice as long as the 6 funnel-shaped flower segments. Seeds may develop but not bulbils. In some forms, the leaves are striped or edged with yellow or white. (Neal)

Medicinal Uses: The fermented and distilled sap of the Agave is called *pulqué*, a favorite intoxicant of Mexican Indians (originally used to treat nervous conditions!). *Pulqué* continues to figure prominently, along with tequila, as a comercially produced alcoholic beverage in Mexico.

The Aztecs utilized egg whites and Agave sap in mixing wound remedies in ancient Mexico. They also used a remedy consisting of crushed Agave leaves, extracts from the Bladderwort, and fresh-ground Maize, all dissolved in warm water and given as an enema to cure dysentery and diarrhea.

Enema syringes were made from the bladders of animals and small birds, which were used as the pouch for the medicine; protruding from the small opening would be a hollow reed or hollow bird's leg through which the healing potion would enter the anus.

Agave leaf juice has soothing and demulcent properties and would thus form a protective coating over inflamed tissues of the stomach and intestinal tract. This would then result in a quieting effect on the stomach, and reduce irritation in the intestine that might be caused by diarrhea or dysentery.

Dose: Approximately 60 milliliters of the sap, swallowed when fresh.

ALOE
Aloe spp.

PARTS USED: Fleshy leaves

Botanical Description: The several Aloes are succulents cultivated for ornamental purposes. Their stems range from long to short to none at all. Their thick, pointed leaves, from triangular to sword-shaped, are crowded along the top of their stems. Most have spiny edges. There are about 180 species, of different sizes and forms. With their stiffness and radial symmetry, they fit well into rock gardens, and since their home is the African desert, they grow well in direct sunlight. Red-, yellow-, or paler-striped flowers rise from the heart of the leaves, hanging from a rather tall stem, branched or unbranched, as a cluster of narrow tubes, which spread slightly at the throat.

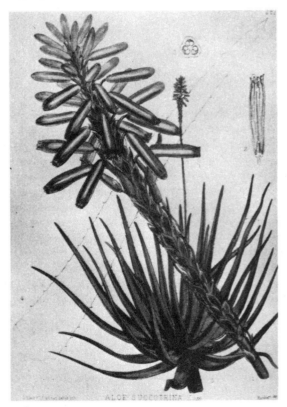

ALOE: Used for treating burns since the time of Cleopatra, this remarkable plant was found to be effective in treating radiation burns in the early 1950s.

The true Aloe (*Aloe barbadensis;* synonym, *A. vera*) yields "Barbados aloes." The leaves are pale green, 1 to 2 feet long and 2 to 3 inches wide at the base, tapering gradually to the pointed tip, edges spiny, and they form a close rosette on a very short stem. The flowers, borne on the upper part of a slender stem about 3 feet high, are yellow, 1 inch long, accompanied by scattered small bracts, the stamens protruding. Various forms of the species vary in size of leaves and color of flowers, in one form the outer lobes being red and the 3 inner lobes yellow. A South African Aloe (*A. succotrina*) yields "bitter aloes." The plant differs from the true Aloe in having a distinct stem up to 4 feet long, alternately branched, the flowers red, the stamens not protruding, and the flower bracts large, ovate, and numerous, concealing the upper part of the flower stem. (Neal)

Medicinal Uses: There are many varieties of the Aloe. Their first known use as medicinals came in 333 B.C., when Alexander the Great heard of this plant and sent a commission to the island of Socotra to investigate and return with samples.

During the 1800s and early 1900s, much of the aloes exported to Europe came from plants cultivated in the Dutch West Indies on the islands of Aruba and Barbados. These are variously identified as Curaçao Aloe, *A. vera,* and Barbados Aloe. African Aloe varieties are Cape Aloe, Uganda Aloe, and Natal Aloe, collectively referred to in commerce as Zanzibar Aloe.

For the treatment of *chronic* constipation *only,* aloes were felt to be particularly effective, as their action is largely limited to the colon. However, they were not recommended as a general laxative. As the action produced by aloes often caused griping (painful muscle spasms of the bowels), it was common to include a carminative such as Fennel to soothe the side effects of this purgative action.

Aloes were also often utilized to treat various forms of amenorrhea (absent or suppressed menses).

Externally we use the Aloe's mucilage raw from the fresh plant as an analgesic for burns, scrapes, sunburn, and insect bites, as well as to promote healing of such injuries. A fleshy stalk is broken off, the skin of the plant is split to expose the interior, and the edges are spread apart for effective wrapping of the afflicted area. One stalk can be used piece by piece till gone, as it forms its own natural container as the plant skin's surface dries and forms a seal which preserves the remainder of the stalk.

Very significantly, a university research team has found the mucilaginous Aloe to be the most effective treatment for minor radiation burns.

The leaf juice of *A. ferox* and *A. vera,* when incorporated into a water-soluble ointment base or used as the fresh juice, has well-established emollient effects on the skin. Such preparations are widely used to treat minor sunburn cases, and also to treat burns from X-ray treatment of cancer and related diseases. The active principle has not been identified, but is probably a polysaccharide that forms a protective and soothing coating when applied to the skin. If the juice is dried and then applied to burns, it is not effective.

If the leaves of various *Aloe* species are extracted in a special way, and the resulting product is concentrated, a mixture of anthraquinones results. This mixture is known in the United States of America and Canada as "aloes" or "aloin," and it is well established to be an effective laxative in humans. The laxative effect is much stronger than that produced by Senna or Cascara products.

Dose: As a purgative, aloes were administered in the form of a tincture or extract, the dose being 100 to 300 milligrams.

CAUTION: Do not use during the menstrual period, nor while pregnant. Do not use for hemorrhoids.

ANEMONE
Anemone, spp.

PARTS USED: Root and flower
OTHER COMMON NAMES: Windflower, Pulsatilla, Lily-of-the-Field, Pasque Flower

Botanical Description: The plants are common throughout Europe and should be employed in the fresh condition. The drug is collected at the time of flowering of the plants, from March to May.

The genus *Anemone* is composed of small herbal

plants growing in almost all the temperate countries of the world.

The leaves and flowering scapes are matted, silky-villous; basal leaves with petioles up to 30 centimeters in length, the latter hollow, often purplish in color, the blades twice or thrice deeply 3- or 4-parted or pinnately cleft, the lobes linear and acute, the base of the petiole more hairy than above and frequently attached to the short rootstock; flowering scapes up to 30 centimeters in length, solid in the lower portion and hollow in the upper part, with sessile, involucral dissected leaves near the flower, occasionally with remains of the dull purple hairy sepals and the dense-woolly, plumrose-tailed akenes. Nearly odorless; taste very acrid.

A. ludoviciana, an American species growing in Minnesota and other parts beyond the Mississippi, was employed in that area.

It is probable that the American *A. quinquefolia*, at first described as a variety of *A. nemorosa*, has similar properties. The American Pasque Flower (*A. patens* var. *wolfgangiam*), formerly known as *A. patens* var. *nuttaliana*, was recognized as a source of the drug Pulsatilla. This plant is also designated as *Pulsatilla hirsutissima*. (U.S.D.)

Medicinal Uses: In ancient texts of Greek and Chinese healers we find continual reference to the healing virtues of the lovely Anemones. Dioscorides revered *A. nemorosa*, *A. stellata*, and *A. coronaria* in the form of external plasters or baths for skin ulcers and inflamed eyes. Pliny advocated their use for toothache and swollen gums. The Chinese employed *A. pulsatilla* for ailments ranging from dysentary to madness.

Today, Pulsatilla continues to be very widely relied on as a homeopathic remedy for various mental symptoms and psychosomatic illnesses; it is also a frequently employed homeopathic remedy for the common cold.

Liverleaf (*A. hepatica*) is so named because its leaves resemble the shape of the liver; according to the "doctrine of signatures" ("like curing like"), this particular Anemone, as a tonic, will consequently aid liver disorders.

There are several other Anemones: *A. ludoviciana* (American Pulsatilla), *A. pratensis* (European Pulsatilla), *A. ranunculoides* (Yellow Wood Anemone), and *A. appennina* (Blue Anem-

one). These are also employed in folk medicines in various capacities. Some have been as alternatives, depressants, demulcents, and vulneraries, and others were once employed as a primary treatment in early cases of tuberculosis.

Many *Anemone* species have been studied in the laboratory, both for their chemical content and for the effects of their extracts in animals and in the test tube. They are all remarkably similar in their chemical and pharmacological properties, a majority of the effects being explained by the presence of a simple chemical compound known as protoanemonin, which is converted to the active substance anemonin.

Anemonin is highly active against a large number of different disease-producing microorganisms, has sedative properties, lowers blood pressure, stimulates the gallbladder, relaxes smooth muscle of the gut, allays pain, and in pure form will produce a vesicant (blistering) effect on the skin or mucous membranes. This latter effect has not been observed when sufficiently dilute water extracts of the *Anemone* species are used, because the anemonin itself is diluted. There is enough of this substance present, however, to slightly irritate the mucous membranes, giving rise to an expectorant, and perhaps a diuretic, effect as well.

Dose: Of the dried powder, the dose is 0.13–0.2 gram, although larger amounts may possibly have been taken safely; of the fluidextract, made from the fresh herb, 4.6–7.8 milliliters, divided over 24 hours.

ANGELICA
Angelica archangelica, A. atropurpurea
(MASTERWORT)

PARTS USED: Root, Herb, and Seed
OTHER COMMON NAMES: Garden Angelica, Archangel, Masterwort, Purple Angelica.

Botanical Description: *Anglica archangelica*. The Garden Angelica has a long, thick, fleshy, biennial root, furnished with many fibers, and sending up annually a hollow, jointed, round, channelled, smooth, purplish

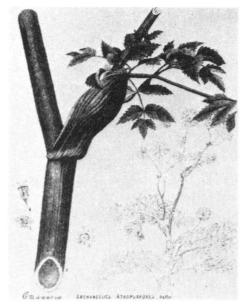

ANGELICA (MASTERWORT): Like Anise, this species has been found a useful remedy suitable for relieving infant flatulence and colic. Angelica oil is characteristic in Benedictine, Chartreuse, and other liquors.

stem, which rises 5 feet or more in height, and divides into numerous branches. The leaves, which stand upon round fistulous footstalks, are very large, doubly pinnate, with oval lanceolate, pointed, acutely serrate leaflets, of which the terminal one is 3-lobed. The flowers are small, greenish-white, and disposed in very large, many-rayed, terminal umbels, composed of numerous dense, hemispherical umbellets.

This plant is a native of the north of Europe, but is also found in the high, mountainous regions in the southern section of that continent, such as Switzerland and among the Pyrenees. It has become an object of culture in various parts of Europe, and may occasionally be met with in the gardens of this country as well. It flowers during the summer. The whole plant diffuses a fragrant odor, and possesses aromatic properties; but only the root and seeds are official.

Angelica atropurpurea. This indigenous species of Angelica, sometimes called Masterwort, has a perennial purplish root, and a smooth herbaceous stem, the dark color of which has given rise to the trivial name of the plant. The leaves are ternate, and supported by very large inflated petioles. The partitions of the leaf are nearly quinate, with ovate, acute, deeply serrate, some-

what lobed leaflets, of which the 3 terminal are confluent. The flowers are greenish-white.

The Purple Angelica extends throughout the United States from Canada to Carolina, growing in meadows and marshy woods, and flowering in June and July. It is smaller than *A. archangelica,* with a less succulent stem. The whole plant is official. It has a strong odor, and a warm aromatic taste. The juice of the recent root is acrid, and is said to be poisonous; but the acrimony is dissipated by drying. (U.S.D.)

Medicinal Uses: Like Anise, this mild remedy is used in relieving infant flatulence and colic. Adults find Angelica helpful in the abatement of heartburn. It is also employed for its aromatic, stimulant, carminative, diaphoretic, and diuretic effects. In the *British Flora Medica* we find the following report: "The Laplanders considered this plant as one of the most important productions of their soil. During that part of the year which they pass in the woods, they are subject to a severe kind of colic, against which the root of Angelica is one of their chief remedies. They also frequently mix the unexpanded umbels with the leaves of the Sorrel and boiling them down in water to the consistence of a syrup, mix it with reindeer's milk, and thus form a stomachic and astringent medicine."

European Angelica is considered superior to the American strain.

Economically, Angelica is cultivated principally for the essential oils from its fruit and roots, which are used in the perfumery, cosmetic, and distillery industries. The oil is characteristic in Benedictine, Chartreuse, and some gins.

Dose: The recommended medicinal dosage was 1 teaspoon of *seeds* per 1 cup boiling water, to be drunk at room temperature, 1 to 2 cups per day.

Root: 1 teaspoon of root, boiled in a covered container with 1 pint water for about ½ hour, at a slow boil. Liquid allowed to cool slowly in the *closed* container. Drunk cold, 1 swallow or 1 tablespoon at a time, 1 to 2 cups per day.

Herb: Approximately ½ ounce of herb to 1 pint of water. Water boiled separately and poured over the plant material and steeped for 5 to 20 minutes, depending on the desired effect. Drunk hot or warm, 1 to 2 cups per day.

ANISE
Pimpinella anisum

PARTS USED: Seeds

Botanical Description: This is an annual plant, about 1 foot in height, with an erect, slightly scabrous, striated, and branching stem. The leaves are petiolate, the lower roundish-cordate, entire or irregularly 3-lobed, the upper 3-parted or ternate. The flowers are white, and in terminal compound umbels, destitute of involucres.

Anise is a native of Egypt and the Levant, but has been introduced into the south of Europe: it is cultivated in various parts of that continent. It is also cultivated occasionally in the gardens of this country. The seeds are abundantly produced in Malta and Spain. The Spanish seeds are smaller than the German or French, and are usually preferred.

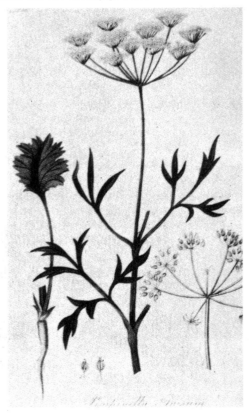

ANISE: One of the earliest aromatics, this elegant plant was utilized by the ancient Egyptians, is spoken of by Theophrastus, and was cultivated in the imperial farms of Charlemagne.

Anise seeds are small, oval, striated, somewhat downy, attached to their footstalks, and of a greenish-brown color, with a shade of yellow. Their odor is fragrant and increased by friction; their taste warm, sweet, and aromatic. These properties, which depend on a peculiar volatile oil, are imparted sparingly to boiling water, freely to alcohol. The volatile oil exists in the envelope of the seeds, and is separated by distillation. Their internal substance contains a bland fixed oil. By expression, a greenish oil is obtained, which is a mixture of the two. The seeds are sometimes adulterated with small fragments of argillaceous earth; and their aromatic qualities are occasionally impaired, in consequence of a slight fermentation which they are apt to undergo in the mass, when collected before maturity. (U.S.D.)

Medicinal Uses: Anise is used to remedy infant colic and flatulence. (Also increases milk secretion for nursing mothers.) Due to its pleasant aroma, it was often added to other preparations to make them more palatable, mainly masking disagreeable odors. (These properties are known as carminative and aromatic.)

According to the 1918 *U.S. Dispensatory,* "It is one of the oldest aromatics, having been used by the ancient Egyptians; is spoken of by Theophrastus; and was cultivated in the imperial German farms of Charlemagne."

The seeds are the source of oil of Anise, utilized extensively in flavoring, especially liquors. Containing 80- to 90-percent anethol, and methyl clavicol, Anise seeds have also been shown to have insecticidal activity.

Dose: Steep 1 teaspoon of crushed seeds per cup boiling water, 3–5 minutes. Drink cold, 1 to 2 cups per day, 1 tablespoon at a time.

ARNICA
Arnica montana

PARTS USED: Leaves and flowers
OTHER COMMON NAMES: Leopard's Bane, Mountain Tobacco

Botanical Description: This is a perennial, herbaceous plant, having a woody, brownish, horizontal root, end-ing abruptly, and sending forth numerous slender fibers of the same color. The stem is about a foot high, cylindrical, striated, hairy, and terminating in 1, 2, or 3 peduncles, each bearing a flower. The radical leaves are ovate, entire, ciliated, and obtuse; those of the stem, which usually consist of two opposite pairs, are lance-shaped. Both are of a bright green color, and somewhat pubescent on their upper surface. The flowers are very large, and of a fine orange-yellow color. The calyx is greenish, imbricated, with lanceolate scales. The ray consists of about 14 ligulate florets, twice as long as the calyx, striated, 3-toothed, and hairy at the base; the disc, of tubular florets, with a 5-lobed margin.

This plant is a native of the mountainous districts of Europe and Siberia, and is found in the northern regions of the United States, west of the Mississippi. (U.S.D.)

Medicinal Uses: While Arnica is a very valuable remedy for *external* complaints, for instance, as a healing application for wounds and bruises or as a salve for irritated nasal passages and chapped lips, it is only to be used internally by a trained homeopath, in minute dosage. Used properly, it is one of the leading homeopathic remedies, especially for injuries and shock. Administration of Arnica in overdose can result in swift and agonizing death. Nevertheless, Arnica has been used internally in the past in a wide variety of diseases characterized by debility and torpor, in which presumably the stimulant and irritant properties of the plant were of value.

Arnica flowers have also been used in herbal medicine externally as emollients and vulneraries and to reduce inflammation in the nasal passages. Internally, herbal preparations have been used for high blood pressure, various heart disorders, and stomach ailments. According to folklore this perennial herb has wound-healing properties and is used to treat brain concussions.

All these effects are reinforced by experimental studies in animals or in humans, but as yet the active principles responsible for these effects have not been identified.

There is some evidence that Arnica root preparations are considerably more toxic than flower preparations. However, root preparations do not yet seem to be as popular.

Dose: Not recommended for internal use. The salve for external application was made by heating 1 ounce of flowers with equal amount of lard for several hours, then applied after cooling.

ARROWROOT
Maranta arundinacea

PARTS USED: Root
OTHER COMMON NAMES: Maranta

Botanical Description: The root of this plant is perennial, tuberous, fleshy, horizontal, nearly cylindrical, scaly, from 6 inches to a foot or more in length, and furnished with numerous long white fibers. The stems, of which several rise from the same root, are annual, slender, branched, jointed, leafy, and about 3 feet in height. The leaves are ovate lanceolate, about 4 inches

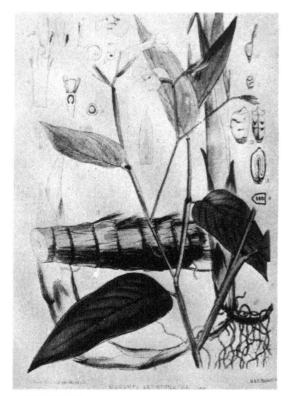

ARROWROOT: The mashed rhizomes were once used by Central and South American Indians as an antidote for arrow poisoning—hence the common name of this food plant.

39

long, alternate, and supported solitarily at the joints of the stem upon long, sheathing footstalks. The flowers are in a long, loose, spreading, terminal panicle, at each ramification of which is a solitary linear bract. The calyx consists of three small lanceolate leaves. The corolla is white and monopetalous, with a tube longer than the calyx, and a double border, of which the 3 outermost segments are smallest, and the two inner obovate, and slightly emarginate.

The Arrowroot plant is a native of South America and of the West Indies, where it is largely cultivated. It also grows in Florida, and has been cultivated in our southern states.

It is probable that other plants contribute to furnish the Arrowroot of commerce. It is procured in the West Indies from *Maranta allouya* and *M. nobilis*, besides *M. arundinacea*. Other species serve as sources of Arrowroot in the East Indies. (U.S.D.)

Medicinal Uses: The mashed rhizomes of Arrowroot were once used by Central and South American Indians as an antidote for arrow poisoning—hence the common name of the plant. Arrowroot is commonly utilized today in baked products, and is a superior carbohydrate as well as a source of digestible calcium, which makes it a valuable element in the diet of children after weaning and of delicate persons during convalescence. It may be prepared as a jell, gruel, blancmange, and beverage, and in baking.

It is recorded that the Mayas utilized the root in the making of poultices for smallpox and, when drunk as a beverage, as a remedy for pus in the urine. This latter usage is due to the root's demulcent properties, which made it valuable in bowel complaints as well as urinary problems.

When mixed with hot water, the root starch of this herbaceous perennial becomes gelatinous and serves as an effective demulcent to soothe irritated mucous membranes.

Dose: 1 tablespoon, boiled in a covered container of 1½ pints water for about ½ hour, at a slow boil. Liquid allowed to cool slowly in the *closed* container. Taken cold, 1 swallow or 1 tablespoon at a time, 1 to 2 cups per day.

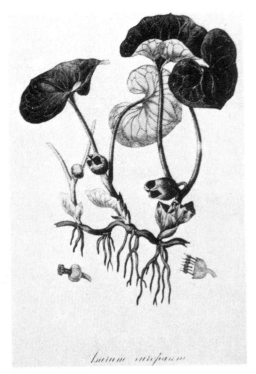

Asarum europaeum

ASARABACCA: The leaves contain a highly aromatic essential oil, which contains constituents that verify the reported value of extracts for promoting nasal secretion.

ASARABACCA
Asarum europaeum

PARTS USED: Rhizome, roots, and leaves
OTHER COMMON NAMES: European Snakeweed, Hazelwort, European Wild Ginger

Botanical Description: The Asarabacca has a perennial root, with a very short, round, simple, herbaceous, pubescent stem, which in general supports only 2 leaves and 1 flower. The leaves, which are opposite and stand on long footstalks, are kidney-shaped, entire, somewhat hairy, and of a shining deep-green color. The flower is large, of a dusky purple color, and placed upon a short terminal peduncle. The calyx, which takes the place of a corolla, is bell-shaped, greenish at the base, and divided at the mouth into 3 pointed purplish segments, which are erect, and turned inwards at their extremity. The filaments are 12, and prolonged beyond the anthers into a small hook. The style is surmounted by a 6-parted reddish stigma. The fruit is a 6-celled coriaceous capsule, crowned with the persistent calyx.

This species of *Asarum* is a native of Europe, growing between latitudes 60° and 37° N in woods and shady places, and flowering in May. All parts of the plant are acrid. The root is about as thick as a goose quill, of a grayish color, quadrangular, knotted and twisted, and sometimes furnished with radicles at each joint. It has a smell analogous to that of pepper, an acrid taste, and affords a grayish powder. The leaves are nearly inodorous, with a taste slightly aromatic, bitter, acrid, and nauseous. Their powder is yellowish-green. Both parts rapidly lose their activity by keeping, and ultimately become inert. Their virtues are imparted to alcohol and water, but are dissipated by decoction. (U.S.D.)

Medicinal Uses: This plant is mentioned for its emetic, diuretic, and cathartic properties. It has been used as a substitute for Ipecac for producing vomiting; the French use it for this purpose after drinking too much wine. However, it is violent in its action and its use in home practice is discouraged. In powder form and taken as a snuff, it causes a profuse discharge of mucus from the nasal membrances, and hence has been used to remedy headaches, drowsiness, giddiness, catarrhs, and other conditions caused by congestion. It has been a component in many popular commercial medicinal snuffs. There are numerous reports of the folkloric anticancer use of this plant.

Asarabacca has been extensively investigated, both chemically and pharmacologically. The leaves contain a highly aromatic essential oil which contains constituents that verify the value of extracts as an errhine (for promotion of nasal secretion).

Although the leaves are used as an emetic, human experiments have shown that the effect is not as pronounced as that of other, more effective drugs. On the other hand, the expectorant properties of infusions and decoctions of both the roots and leaves of *Asarum europaeum* are quite good, based on experiments on humans.

There is no experimental evidence in support of the use of any part of this plant as a cathartic, although, from the types of irritant chemical compounds known to be present in this plant, one would expect that catharsis would result from ingestion of extracts prepared from Asarabacca. Presumably, rather high doses would be required to obtain this effect.

Human experiments have been reported from Rumania, where infusions of *Asarum europaeum* were administered to humans suffering pulmonary insufficiency. The preparations were said to have a beneficial effect on the heart condition, including a diuretic effect.

Dose: CAUTION. Do not use as a cathartic. As a snuff, 0.065–0.13 gram is snuffed up the nostrils. (This plant is an ingredient of the European Schneeberger snuff.)

BALM
Melissa officinalis

PARTS USED: Whole plant
OTHER COMMON NAMES: Melissa, Lemon-Balm, Garden-Balm, Sweet-Balm

Botanical Description: Balm has a perennial root, which sends up annually several erect, quadrangular stems, usually branched toward the base, and a foot or two in height. The leaves are opposite, ovate or cordate, deeply serrate, pubescent, the lower on long footstalks, the uppermost nearly sessile. The flowers are white or yellowish, upon short peduncles, and in axillary whorls, surrounding only half the stem. The calyx is tubular, pentangular, and bilabiate, with the upper lip tridentate and flattened, the lower cut into two pointed teeth. The corolla is also tubular and bilabiate, the upper lip less convex and notched, the lower 3-cleft.

The plant is a native of the south of Europe. It has been introduced into this country, where it is cultivated in gardens, or grows wild along the fences of our roads and lanes. For medical use the herb should be cut before the appearance of the flowers, which begin to expand in July.

In the fresh state, it has a fragrant odor very similar to that of lemons; but is nearly inodorous when dried. The taste is slightly aromatic. The herb contains a minute proportion of a yellowish or reddish-yellow essential oil, which has its peculiar flavor in a very high degree. (U.S.D.)

Medicinal Uses: To break a fever, this plant has

been used for centuries. Taken as a strong infusion, using 2 teaspoonfuls of the dried herb per cup of boiling water, the desired effect (profuse sweating) is achieved without dangerous side effects. Lemon is often added to improve qualities of taste. Balm tea is a very useful home remedy for headache.

The essential oil extracted from this herb is known as lemon-balm and is also employed as a diaphoretic. This perennial herb is used throughout the Mediterranean for flavoring soups and salads, in egg dishes, and to make Tarragon vinegar.

Dose: 1–2 teaspoons of dried plant material per cup boiling water; steep for 3 to 5 minutes and drink hot, 1 to 2 cups per day, 1 tablespoon at a time. Make strong or weak as desired.

BALSAM OF PERU
Myroxylon Pereira

PARTS USED: Balsam

Botanical Description: *Myroxylon Pereira* is a handsome tree, with a straight, round, lofty stem, a smooth ash-colored bark, and spreading branches at the top. The leaves are alternate, petiolate, and unequally pinnate. The leaflets are from 5 to 11, shortly petiolate, oblong, oval-oblong, or ovate, about 3 inches long by somewhat less than 1½ inches in breadth, rounded at the base, and contracting abruptly at the top into an emarginate point. When held up to the light they exhibit, in lines parallel with the primary veins, beautiful rounded and linear pellucid spots. The common and partial petioles and midribs are smooth to the naked eye, but when examined with a microscope are found to be furnished with short hairs. The fruit, including the winged footstalks, varies from 2 to 4 inches in length. At its peduncular extremity it is rounded or slightly tapering; at the top enlarged, rounded, and swollen, with a small point at the side. The mesocarp, or main investment of the fruit, is fibrous, and contains in distinct receptacles a balsamic juice, which is most abundant in 2 long receptacles or vittae, one upon each side.

A gum resin is exuded in small quantities from the trunk of the tree, which, though containing, besides gum and resin, a small proportion of volatile oil, is distinct from the proper balsam, and yields no cinnamic

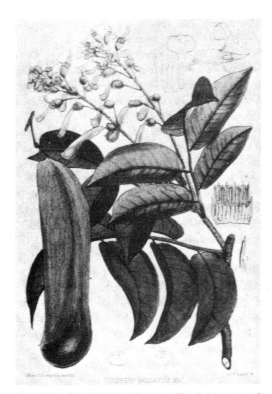

BALSAM OF PERU: Widely utilized in external ointments and salves for its healing effects, the gum from this species is created by the tree in response to stem wounds, to heal itself.

acid. The valuable wood of the tree resembles mahogany.

This tree grows in Central America, in El Salvador, upon the Pacific coast. It is found in the wild forests, singly or in groups. It is said it is never found at a greater height on the mountains than 1,000 feet, that it begins to be productive after 5 years, and continues to yield for 30 or more, and that the aroma of its flower may be perceived as far away as 100 yards. (U.S.D.)

Medicinal Uses: Balsam of Peru, "a thick, syrupy, dark reddish-brown substance," is widely used, in external ointments and salves, for its antiseptic and healing effect. The antiseptic action is due primarily to the high content of benzoic acid and related substances. The balsam is generally recognized by dermatologists as aiding in the healing process when applied externally.

When taken internally, the essential-oil portion of the balsam acts as an expectorant.

Interestingly, this healing substance is created

by the tree in response to stem wounds in order *to heal itself*.

Balsam of Peru has been used in medicine in asthma and chronic bronchitis. Externally, it has seen use in ulcers and "local tuberculosis of the skin, bone, larynx." The U.S. military was at one time aware of its values as a dressing for wounds, not only for its bactericidal effects but also because "it stimulates the local resistance of the tissues and . . . exercises a valuable protective action." (U.S.D.)

Dose: Internally, the gummy exudate was "administered suspended in water by the yolk of egg or Acacia." It was taken in a dose of from 0.3 to 3.9 milliliters. Externally, applied directly.

BARBERRY
Berberis vulgaris

PARTS USED: Root bark and berries
OTHER COMMON NAMES: Common Barberry

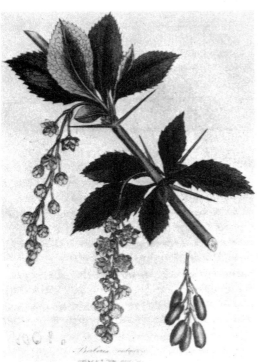

BARBERRY: The most credible medicinal uses of this handsome shrub are centered in the herb's strong purging effects, and in its utility as a gargle for sore throats.

Botanical Description: Root woody, creeping, branched, yellowish brown. Stems erect, 6 or 8 feet high. Branches diffuse, covered with a smooth greyish bark, and furnished at each joint with acute spines, generally 3 in number. Leaves inversely ovate, ciliato-serrate, smooth, arranged 4 or 5 together on the branches. Flowers in terminal pendulous racemes springing from the axils of the leaves. Calyx deciduous, greenish yellow, consisting of 6 ovate, concave, obtuse sepals, 3 of them alternately smaller with 3 bracts at the base. Corolla composed of 6 concave rounded petals, bright yellow, with 2 glands at the base of each. Stamens 6, opposite the petals, tipped with bifid anthers. Ovary simple, cylindrical, terminated by a large, sessile, depressed stigma. Fruit an ovoid, cylindrical berry, a little curved, orange-red, tipped with the black style, and containing 2 oblong seeds.

Distribution: Europe, temperate Asia, Northern Africa. In copses and hedges in many parts of England. Naturalized in Scotland and Ireland. Flowers May and June. (British Flora Medica [B.F.M.])

Medicinal Uses: The Barberry is noted throughout herb literature for its important economic and medicinal properties. The ripe fruit is eaten as a preserve; the roots yield a yellow dye which at one time was utilized in the dyeing of wool, cotton, and flax.

The most credible medicinal uses are centered in the herb's strong purging effects, and its utility as a gargle for sore throats. While the root bark, rich in berberine, is used for the former effect, the Barberry fruit itself is crushed for the latter; it also finds application as a mouthwash.

In ancient Egyptian medicine, syrup of Barberry combined with Fennel seed was reputedly of value in warding off the plague. This possibility is not to be laughed off, since the ancient Hebrews relied on Hops for the same purpose. Hops contain effective antibacterial principles, and were in fact valuable against the infectious agent *Yersinia pestis*, the plague bacillus. In exploring the possible validity of Barberry and Fennel seed for the same purpose we would have to evaluate potential antibacterial properties.

Throughout other traditional herbal literature we find patterns of usage surrounding the following ills: high fevers, jaundice, and chronic dysentery.

In fact, Barberry owes virtually all of its effects to the presence of the alkaloid berberine, which is present in all parts of the plant. Berberine, when applied externally, causes an astringent effect, and if placed in the eye will reduce the "bloodshot" appearance, since the blood vessels are constricted by the alkaloid. Thus, Barberry berries would be useful as a mouthwash and gargle for their astringent effect, and some local anesthetic effect due to the berberine.

Barberry roots have a high berberine content and, if the correct amount is used, will act as a purgative. Barberry root preparations are even more useful, however, to halt diarrhea. Such preparations are well established as effective in stopping diarrhea in cases of bacterial dysentery. The active compound is known to be berberine. Since berberine is not very well absorbed if taken by mouth, the risk of any possible toxic effects is reduced.

Dose: When used in medicine the dosage was 1 teaspoon of dried root bark per 1½ pints water, boiled in a covered container for about ½ hour, at a slow boil. Liquid allowed to cool slowly in the *closed* container. Drunk 1 cup at a time, twice daily. If the more potent *powdered* root bark was prepared as above, just 1 cup daily was considered sufficient.

BEARBERRY

Arctostaphylos uva-ursi

PARTS USED: Leaves

OTHER COMMON NAMES: Uva-Ursi, Mountain Box, Red Berry, Upland Cranberry, Bear's Grape, Whortberry, Arberry

Botanical Description: The Uva-Ursi, or Bearberry, is a low evergreen shrub, with trailing stems, the young branches of which rise obliquely upward for a few inches. The leaves are scattered, upon short petioles, obovate, acute at the base, entire, with green color on their upper surface, paler and covered with a network of veins beneath. The flowers, which stand on short reflexed peduncles, are collected in small clusters at the ends of the branches. The calyx is small, obscurely 5-toothed, reddish white, or white with a red lip, transparent at the base, contracted at the mouth, and divided at the margin into 5 short reflexed segments. The stamens are 10, with short filaments and bifid anthers; the germ round, with a style longer than the stamens, and a simple stigma. The fruit is a small, round, depressed, smooth, glossy, red berry, containing an insipid mealy pulp, and 5 cohering seeds.

This humble but hardy shrub inhabits the northern latitudes of Europe, Asia, and America. It is also found in the lofty mountains of southern Europe, such as the Pyrenees and the Alps; and, on the American continent, extends from Hudson's Bay as far southward as New Jersey, in some parts of which it grows in great abundance. It prefers a barren soil, flourishing on gravelly hills, and elevated sandy plains. The leaves are the only part used in medicine. They should be gathered in autumn, and the green leaves only selected.

In Europe the Uva-Ursi is often adulterated with the leaves of *Vaccinium vitis idaea*, which are wholly destitute of its peculiar properties and may be distinguished by their rounder shape, their revolute edges (which are sometimes slightly toothed), and the appearance of their under surface, which is dotted, instead of being reticulated as in the genuine leaves. (These distinguishing characteristics are noted because parcels of the drug may sometimes reach this country from abroad.) Leaves of *Chimaphila umbellata* may also sometimes be found among the Uva-Ursi as it exists in our own markets. They may be readily detected by their greater length, their cuneiform lanceolate shape, and their serrate edges. (U.S.D.)

Medicinal Uses: The strong astringent properties of the leaves have led to usage as diuretics and tonics. Inflammations of the urinary tract, especially in acute cystitis, were formerly treated with a decoction of these leaves. (Patients were forewarned to expect a sharp greenish color of their urine during treatment.)

Bearberry leaves, prior to the discovery of synthetic diuretic and urinary antiseptic drugs, were the major medicine available to physicians for these purposes. We have known for a number of years that the diuretic, astringent, and urinary antiseptic value of Bearberry leaves can be accounted for by the fact that they contain the active principles hydroquinone and arbutin. In the body, arbutin is rapidly converted to hydroquinone. Additionally, Bearberry leaves contain allantoin, a substance that is known to soothe and accelerate the repair of irritated tissues.

Dose: When made up by herbalists, the leaves were often soaked in brandy or alcohol for a few hours, then added to boiling water, using 1 teaspoon of the soaked leaves per cup of water. Two to three cups were taken per day, cold. An alternative preparation consisted of the dried leaves powdered and boiled in water without the alcohol soak.

BELLADONNA
Atropa belladonna

PARTS USED: Leaves

OTHER COMMON NAMES: Deadly Nightshade

Botanical Description: The Deadly Nightshade is an herbaceous perennial plant, with a thick and fleshy root, from which rise several erect, round, purplish, branching, annual stems, to the height of about 3 feet. The leaves, which are attached by short footstalks to the stem, are in pairs of unequal size, oval, pointed, entire, of a dusky green color on their upper surface, and paler beneath. The flowers are large, bell-shaped, pendent, of a dull reddish color; and are supported upon solitary peduncles, which rise from the axils of the leaves. The fruit is a roundish berry with a longitudinal furrow on each side, at first green, afterward red, ultimately of a deep purple color, bearing considerable resemblance to the cherry, and containing, in two distinct cells, numerous seeds, and a sweetish violet-colored juice. The calyx adheres to the base of the fruit.

This plant is a native of Europe, where it grows in shady places, along walls, and amidst rubbish, flowering in June and July, and ripening its fruit in September. (U.S.D.)

Medicinal Uses: Externally applied as a plaster or in ointment form, this poisonous plant has had long use as an effective painkiller. The highly toxic nature of Belladonna urges extreme caution in employing it internally.

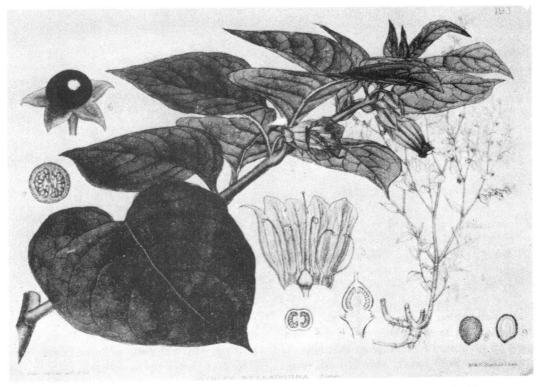

BELLADONNA: Externally applied as a plaster or in ointment form, this poisonous plant has had long use as an effective pain-killer. The plant has highly toxic properties when taken internally.

The alkaloid atropine obtained from Belladonna is used in medicine for five purposes: to check mucus secretion; to stimulate circulation; to overcome spasm of the involuntary muscles; locally to dilate the pupil of the eye and paralyze the muscles of visual accommodation; and externally, as a local anodyne.

As a circulatory stimulant, atropine is highly useful in such applications as countering the depressant effects of various compounds, including opium. Increasing heart rate by vagal inhibition, atropine is valuable in severe emergencies such as surgical shock.

Belladonna contains the potent alkaloids atropine (as already noted), hyoscyamine, and scopolamine, in all parts of the plant. These alkaloids are known to have an anodyne effect when applied to the skin. For example, Belladonna plasters have been used for decades, especially to alleviate back pain. When taken internally, the alkaloids are absorbed and produce a strong antispasmodic effect on the smooth muscle of the gut. These alkaloids block the nerve supply to the stomach and cause a relaxation that results in less pain, due to reduced stress on the organ. Both atropine and hyoscyamine have a depressing effect on higher nerve centers, which accounts for the energetic narcotic effect of Belladonna preparations. However, the scopolamine is most probably responsible for most of this effect, since it has a greater depressant action on the higher nerve centers than atropine or hyoscyamine.

A word of warning should be interjected here: Belladonna preparations are very potent and the greatest caution should attend their use. Even light overdosing will result in dilation of the pupils of the eyes, which results in a "blurry" vision and inability to see things clearly. An additional, very characteristic effect of Belladonna derivatives is a "drying up" of the mouth, which can be uncomfortable. Persons being treated for glaucoma should never take Belladonna preparations, or any of the alkaloids contained in this plant, since the usual treatment for glaucoma is with drugs that have an effect opposite to Belladona's. Should both drugs be used at the same time in a glaucoma patient, the effects of each would be nullified and the

patient would most likely suffer irreversible blindness, unless this self-negating treatment was discovered early and discontinued.

Dose: Tincture of Belladonna is occasionally employed by traditional physicians, in a dosage of 0.5 milliliter by mouth every 4 hours or as needed. When the plant itself is used, 1 teaspoonful of the leaves is steeped in 1 pint (3–5 minutes) of boiling water. The infusion is drunk cold, 1–2 teaspoonfuls 2 to 3 times daily.

CAUTION. Contains potent alkaloids. Heavy overdose can have very serious effects. Blindness, as noted, can occur if taken by people also using drugs for glaucoma.

BETEL NUT PALM
Areca catechu

PARTS USED: Nuts
OTHER COMMON NAMES: Areca Nut Palm

Botanical Description: The Areca Nut Palm is found cultivated throughout the tropical parts of Asia, the hotter parts of peninsular India, Ceylon, south China, the Philippines and other Eastern islands, and especially the Maylay Archipelago, where it is considered to be originally indigenous. It is a well-known tree in India, being the most elegant palm of that country. Like many other Palms, it flowers nearly all the year round. There is much variation in the form and size of the fruit; in one form the husk is white.

It is a tree with a straight, slender, unbranched stem reaching 40 or 50 feet in height, about 20 inches in circumference, cylindrical, smooth, gray, marked at not distant intervals with regular rings of scars left by the fallen leaves. (Bentley)

Medicinal Uses: This tall, elegant palm bears betel nuts, which are used by millions in Southeast Asia (Malaysia, New Guinea). The inside of the nut is powdered and chewed with lime enclosed in a fresh leaf from the *Piper betle* tree, while the red juice is spat out. There is a relief of tension, with a definite sedative effect. Normanby Islanders utilize these sedative nuts to "soothe a mad person."

The nuts contain the alkaloids arecoline and

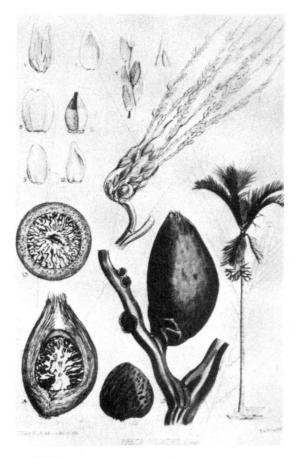

BETEL NUT PALM: Chewed by millions in South-east Asia for their sedative effects, the nuts contain potent alkaloids arecoline and arecaidine.

BITTERSWEET
Solanum dulcamara

PARTS USED: Twigs and leaves
OTHER COMMON NAMES: Woody Nightshade, Climbing Nightshade

Botanical Description: The Bittersweet, or Woody Nightshade, is a climbing shrub, with a slender, roundish, branching, woody stem, which, in favorable situations, rises 6 or 8 feet in height. The leaves are alternate, petiolate, ovate, pointed, veined, soft, smooth, and of a dull green color. Many near the top of the stem are furnished with lateral projections at their base, giving them a hastate form. Most of them are quite entire, some cordate at the base. The flowers are disposed in elegant clusters, somewhat analogous to cymes, and standing opposite to the leaves. The calyx is very small, purplish, and divided into 5 blunt persistent segments. The corolla is wheel-shaped, with 5 pointed reflected segments, which are of a violet-blue color, with a darker purple vein running longitudinally through their center, and 2 shining greenish spots at the base of each. The filaments are very short, and support large erect lemon-yellow anthers, which cohere in the form of a cone around the style. The berries are of an oval shape and a bright scarlet color, and continue to hang in beautiful bunches after the leaves have fallen.

This plant is common to Europe and North America. It flourishes most luxuriantly in damp and sheltered places, as on the banks of rivulets, and among the thickets which border our natural meadows. It is also found in higher and more exposed situations, and is frequently cultivated in gardens. In the United States it extends from New England to Ohio, and is in bloom from June to August. Bittersweet should be gathered in autumn, after the fall of the leaf; and the extreme twigs should be selected. That grown in high and dry situations is said to be the best. (U.S.D.)

arecaidine. Arecoline has known anthelmintic and tranquilizing properties. While habitual chewers of the nut have a high incidence of buccal cancer, attributed by some to the condensed tannins the nut contains (11-26 percent tannins), it is likely that other components of the nut or nutritional factors may also be involved. In fact, the very young unfolded leaves are even eaten as a vegetable.

The nuts, in addition to their sedative effects, are also used to increase perspiration (in colds), to kill worms, and in veterinary medicine as a laxative and worm remedy.

In Europe, ground nuts are used in some tooth powders.

Dose: The nuts are chewed as desired.

Medicinal Uses: Bittersweet was used extensively in treating a variety of diseases; internally, for example, it was reported to be beneficial in chronic rheumatism. However, its most usual application was external, for treating skin eruptions and irritations. A poultice of the leaves was

47

applied for this purpose, especially in injuries of the knee joint, and in hard and painful swellings of the female breast. Bittersweet was also reportedly helpful for bruises, promoting the absorption of blood from the swollen tissues.

This plant is one of 27 included in the March 1977 issue of the U.S. Food and Drug Administration (USFDA) Bulletin of Unsafe Herbs, "being a poisonous plant containing the toxic glycoalkaloid solanine, as well as solanidine and dulcamarin." However, some authorities report both the toxic and the medicinal properties of the plant to be rather insignificant, various investigators having administered considerable quantities without any noticeable medicinal or toxic effect.

We have been unable to document the rationale for the use of the root bark of Bittersweet in relieving skin irritation. The fruits of this plant, however, are commonly implicated in cases where children ingesting them are often poisoned. The severity of poisoning seems to depend on the stage of ripeness of the fruit.

Dose: When used in medicine the dose was 2 teaspoons of the root per pint of boiling water, drunk cold, 2 to 3 tablespoons, 6 times per day.

A fluidextract was once official in the National Formulary in doses of 2 to 3.9 grams.

Caution. See above.

BLOODROOT
Sanguinaria canadensis

PARTS USED: Root

OTHER COMMON NAMES: Red Puccoon, Indian Plant, Tetterwort, Sanguinaria

Botanical Description: The Bloodroot, or, as it is sometimes called, Puccoon, is an herbaceous perennial plant. The root is horizontal, abrupt, often contorted, about as thick as the finger, 2 or 3 inches long, fleshy, of a reddish-brown color on the outside, and brighter red within. It is furnished with numerous slender radicles, and makes offsets from the sides, which succeed the old plant. From the end of the root arise the scape and leafstalks, surrounded by the large sheaths of the bud. These spring up together, the folded leaf enveloping the flower-bud, and rolling back as the latter expands. The leaf, which stands upon a long channeled petiole, is

reniform, somewhat heart-shaped, deeply lobed, smooth, yellowish-green on the upper surface, paler or glaucous on the under, and strongly marked by orange-colored veins. The scape is erect, round and smooth, rising from 6 inches to a foot in height, and terminating in a single flower. The calyx is 2-leaved and deciduous. The petals, varying from 7 to 14, but usually about 8 in number, are spreading, ovate, obtuse, concave, mostly white, but sometimes slightly tinged with rose or purple. The stamens are numerous, with yellow filaments shorter than the corolla, and orange oblong anthers. The germ is oblong and compressed, and supports a sessile, persistent stigma. The capsule is oblong, acute at both ends, two-valved; and contains numerous oval, reddish-brown seeds. The whole plant **is pervaded by an orange-colored sap, which flows from**

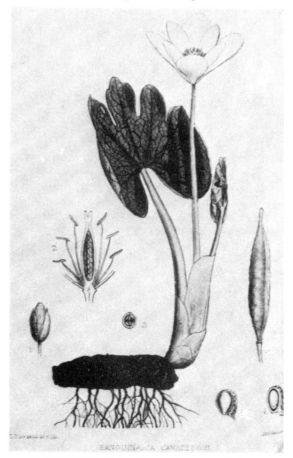

BLOODROOT: Owing its common name to the red juice (in the roots and stem) which was used as a facial dye by the Indians of North America, the plant is noted for its emetic and purgative effects.

48

every part when broken, but is of the deepest color in the root.

The Bloodroot is one of the earliest and most beautiful spring flowers of North America. It grows abundantly throughout the whole United States, delighting in rich loose soils, and shady situations, and flowering in March and April. After the fall of the flower, the leaves continue to increase in size, and by the middle of summer, have become so large as to give the plant an entirely different aspect. All parts of the plant are active, but the root only is officinal. (U.S.D.)

Medicinal Uses: The Bloodroot is named for the red juice in the roots and stem, which was used as a facial dye by the Indians of North America. The root is emetic and purgative in large doses; in smaller doses it is stimulant, diaphoretic, and expectorant. Bloodroot became popular in domestic American medicine for its ability to remove mucus from the respiratory mucous membranes, and was official in the *U.S. Pharmacopoeia* from 1820 to 1926. The plant was used by the Indians of the Mississippi region as a remedy for rheuma-

tism. An acro-narcotic poison in overdose, the plant has been reported to cause death. It is one of the 27 plants included in the USFDA unsafe herb list, published March 1977.

Experimentally, Bloodroot preparations are known to induce emesis, have expectorant properties, and be irritant. These activities are all due to the presence of the toxic alkaloid sanguinarine. Topically, sanguinarine and/or Bloodroot preparations have been helpful in the treatment of eczema, and most probably would give a mild local anesthetic effect. Mausert recommends an external application of the powder for nose polyps, ulcers, and bad sores, stating that it encourages new and healthy tissues.

Dose: For medicinal use, 1 level teaspoon of the ground root is steeped for ½ hour in 1½ pints of boiling water, then strained. Of the liquid thus produced, 1 teaspoon was taken 3 to 6 times per day. Avoid prolonged internal use.

BONESET
Eupatorium perfoliatum

PARTS USED: Tops and leaves
OTHER COMMON NAMES: Thoroughwort, Indian Sage, Fever Wort, Ague Weed, Crosswort, Eupatorium

Botanical Description: Of this numerous genus, comprising not less than 30 species within the limits of the United States, most of which probably possess analogous medical properties, 3 have found a place in the *Pharmacopoeia* of the United States—*E. perfoliatum*, *E. teucrifolium*, and *E. purpureum*—the first in the primary, the last two in the secondary list. *E. cannabinum* of Europe, the root of which was formerly used as a purgative, and *E. Aya-pana* of Brazil, the leaves of which at one time enjoyed a very high reputation as a remedy in numerous diseases, have fallen into entire neglect. The *Aya-pana* is an aromatic bitter, with the medical properties of *E. perfoliatum* in an inferior degree.

Eupatorium perfoliatum. The Thoroughwort, or, as it is perhaps more frequently called, Boneset, is an indigenous perennial plant, with numerous herbaceous stems, which are erect, round, hairy, from 2 to 5 feet high, simple below, and trichotomously branched near

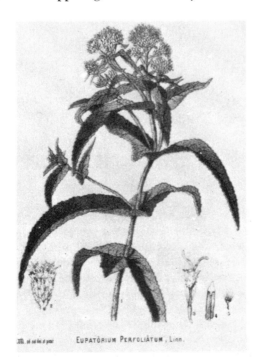

EUPATÓRIUM PERFOLIÁTUM, Linn.

BONESET: First employed by the Indians of North America, this remedy soon became very popular in domestic American medicine. A mild infusion has been found useful for inducing sweating in fevers.

49

the summit. The character of the leaves is peculiar, and serves to distinguish the species at the first glance. They may be considered either as perforated by the stem, *perfoliate*, or as consisting each of 2 leaves joined at the base, *connate*. Considered in the latter point of view, they are opposite and in pairs, which decussate each other at regular distances upon the stem; in other words, the direction of each pair is at right angles with that of the pair immediately above or beneath it. They are narrow in proportion to their length, broadest at the base where they coalesce, gradually tapering to a point, serrate, much wrinkled, paler on the under than the upper surface, and beset with whitish hairs which give them a grayish-green color. The uppermost pairs are sessile, not joined at the base. The flowers are white, numerous, supported on hairy peduncles, in dense corymbs, which form a flattened summit to the plant. The calyx, which is cylindrical and composed of imbricated, lanceolate, hairy scales, encloses from 12 to 15 tubular florets, having their border divided into 5 spreading segments. The anthers are 5 in number, black, and united into a tube, through which the bifid filiform style projects above the flower.

This species of *Eupatorium* inhabits meadows, the banks of streams, and other moist places, growing generally in bunches, and abounding in almost all parts of the United States. It flowers from the middle of summer to the latter end of October. All parts of it are active; but the herb only is officinal.

It has a faint odor, and a strongly bitter, somewhat peculiar taste. The bitterness and probably the medical

Medicinal Uses: Boneset was a favorite remedy of the Indians of North America, and it soon became a very popular remedy in American medicine. It is said to act as a mild tonic and diaphoretic in moderate doses and as an emetic and purgative in large doses. Drunk as hot as possible, it was given to induce vomiting and the evacuation of the bowels; when drunk at a warm temperature, the action was somewhat milder, producing increased perspiration and somewhat later a mild evacuation of the bowels. Boneset's ability to produce perspiration made it useful in catarrhal conditions, and especially influenza; the administration of a warm infusion would produce perspiration and sometimes vomiting, often arresting the complaint. The plant derives its common name from its usefulness in treating a kind of

influenza then prevalent in the United States known as "break-bone fever," which was characterized by pains as if all the bones of the body were broken. The plant has also been used in the treatment of intermittent fevers, although its action was acknowledged to be inferior to that of quinine. As a mild tonic, it was given in cases of dyspepsia and as an aid to indigestion in the elderly. The leaves contain several sesquiterpene lactones which stimulate the appetite. In sufficient amounts, they would have anthelmintac effects.

Dose: Not for broken bones (see above); but as a fever remedy Boneset is taken in the moderate dose described below.

Moderate dose: For drinking at room temperature, a mild infusion is brewed, 1 teaspoon of leaves per cup of boiling water, steeped 3–5 minutes. Drunk warm will produce perspiration and gentle vomiting. Drunk cold, effect is that of a simple tonic. One of the most valuable herbs in colds and fevers.

Strong dose: To be drunk as hot as the patient can tolerate, a strong decoction is brewed, using one ounce of plant material boiled with 3½ pints of water, boiled down to 1 pint and administered in doses of 4 ounces to ½ pint. This will produce vomiting rather rapidly.

BORAGE
Borago officinalis

PARTS USED: Whole plant
OTHER COMMON NAMES: Burrage, Common Bugloss

Botanical Description: Root long, whitish, divided, fibrous, mostly biennial. Stem much branched, erect, cylindrical, thick, succulent, clothed with stiff hairs; about 2 feet high. Leaves alternate, undulated, hispid, deep green; lower ones obovate, petiolate, and eared at the base; upper ovate, nearly sessile. Flowers large, in terminal drooping racemes, on long peduncles. Calyx divided into 5 deep, linear-lanceolate, persistent segments. Corolla brilliant blue, monopetalous, wheel-shaped; tube short; limb deeply divided into 5 acute segments; orifice closed with prominent teeth, which are obtuse and notched at the end. Stamens 5, very prominent; filaments tapering, converging; anthers oblong, connivent, fixed to the middle and inner sides of the filaments. Ovary 4-parted, with a cylindrical style, longer than the stamens. Fruit composed of 4 1-seeded carpels. Seeds irregular, ovate, wrinkled.

Distribution: Middle and southern Europe, Northern Africa. Introduced into America. Having been long cultivated in England, it has become naturalized there, and is sometimes found on rubbish and waste ground. Flowers June and July. Varieties are met with in gardens, with white or purple flowers and variegated leaves. (B.F.M.)

Medicinal Uses: Popular in salads and as a pot herb, Borage has also been credited with mild medicinal properties as a demulcent, refrigerant, gentle diaphoretic, cordial, and aperient. An infusion was drunk as a general tonic when one was feeling out of sorts. The plant has also been used to make other less palatable medicinals more agreeable.

Even though Borage is a widely used and

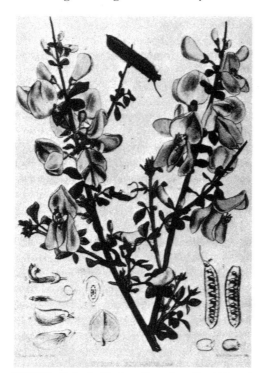

BROOM: Collected before flowering, the tops are especially valued in treating dropsical conditions, particularly those associated with heart disease, as they have been found efficacious in acting on the kidneys to produce urine flow.

popular herbal preparation and salad green, it should never be taken internally for any reason. Borage contains substances known as pyrrolizidine alkaloids (i.e. lasiocarpine), of the type that are known to cause liver damage (hepatotoxicity), and also to induce cancer in laboratory animals when fed to them over a long period of time.

Whether the amount of these liver poisons in Borage is sufficient to cause liver damage or cancer in humans has not yet been established. However, until this has been determined, we recommend that Borage not be taken orally by humans in any amount.

Dose: Not recommended.

BROOM
Sarothamnus scoparius

PARTS USED: Tops and seeds
OTHER COMMON NAMES: Scoparius, Spartium, Scotch Broom, Irish Broom

Botanical Description: This familiar and beautiful shrub is very common throughout England on heaths and open places, and in woods, often growing in great quantity and forming a marked feature in the vegetation of many sandy districts, especially noticeable in May and June, when covered with its brilliant, scented flowers. It is found in equal abundance throughout western Europe, but becomes rare in the central and eastern parts, and in the Mediterranean countries. It, however, occurs in Italy and in central and southern Russia, extending even into Siberia.

The 5 prominent winglike angles which give so striking a character to the young twigs are remarkably persistent, and can be traced on the very oldest stems; as the stem increases in thickness they become of course more widely separated, and at length appear as distant arching ridges, the summit of each arch marking the point of attachment of a leaf.

A pretty form with prostrate stems spreading in a circle is found on the cliffs of the west of France and England, where they are exposed to the winds and spray of the Atlantic Ocean.

A native of Europe, North Africa, and western Asia, this bush is 4 or 5 feet in height, with a short stem reaching about 1½ inches in diameter, breaking up into very numerous erect branches, bark yellowish green.

Twigs very long and wandlike, erect, tough, blunt at the ends, which are pubescent and grow till killed back by the frost, dark-green, angular, with 5 prominent wings of leaflike character originating from the sides of the attachment of each leaf and passing down between them. (Bentley)

Medicinal Uses: Broom is a plant of many uses. The seeds, dried and roasted, have been used as a coffee substitute, and the twigs have been employed as a fiber, to make brooms, and as a substitute for jute.

Collected before blooming, the flowering tops are a source of sparteine sulfate. The medicinal action of the plant, which has a most disagreeable taste in decoction, is diuretic and cathartic, while it is emetic in large doses. It has been especially valued in treating dropsical conditions, particularly those associated with heart disease, as it is efficacious in acting on the kidneys to produce urine flow. Because of its action on the kidneys it is contraindicated in acute renal disease.

Dose: A decoction is made from the leaves, 1 teaspoon of plant material per 1 cup of boiling water, drunk cold, 1 to 2 cups per day. The dose of the seeds, crushed and powdered, is ½ gram to 1 gram.

BUCKBEAN
Menyanthes trifoliata

PARTS USED: Leaves, root and rhizome
OTHER COMMON NAMES: Marsh Trefoil, Bogebean, Water Shamrock, Bog Bean

Botanical Description: The Buckbean, or Marsh Trefoil, has a perennial, long, round, jointed, horizontal, branching, dark-colored root, about as thick as the finger, and sending out numerous fibers from its under surface. The leaves are ternate, and stand upon long stalks, which proceed from the end of the root, and are furnished at their base with sheathing stipules. The leaflets are obovate, obtuse, entirely or bluntly denticulate, very smooth, beautifully green on their upper surface, and paler beneath. The scape or flower stalk is erect, round, smooth, from 6 to 12 inches high, longer than the leaves, and terminated by a conical raceme of

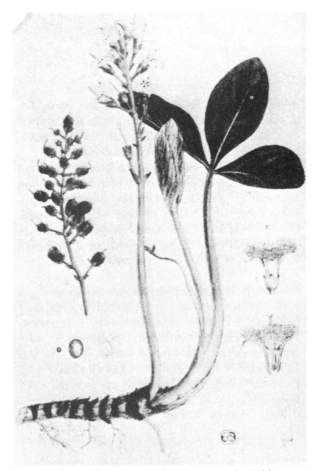

BUCKBEAN: This perennial herb contains a bitter glucoside, menyanthin, and is used for its tart taste in beer in Scandinavia and as a substitute for tea.

whitish somewhat rose-colored flowers. The calyx is 5-parted; the corolla funnel-shaped, with a short tube, and a 5-cleft, revolute border, covered on the upper side with numerous long, fleshy fibers. The anthers are red and sagittate; the germ ovate, supporting a slender style longer than the stamens, and terminating in a bifid stigma. The fruit is an ovate, 2-valved, 1-celled capsule containing numerous seeds.

This beautiful plant is a native both of Europe and North America, growing in boggy and marshy places which are always moist, and occasionally overflown with water. It prevails in the United States, from the northern boundary to Virginia. In this country the flowers appear in May, in England not till June or July. All parts of it are medicinal.

The taste of Buckbean is intensely bitter and somewhat nauseous; the odor of the leaves faint and disagreeable. The virtues of the plant depend on a bitter extractive matter which is dissolved by water and alcohol. (U.S.D.)

Medicinal Uses: Buckbean was formerly considered a medicinal of great value in Europe, and in some countries it was regarded as practically a panacea. According to strength and dosage, its action ranges from that of a bitter tonic and cathartic all the way to purgative and emetic effects. In earlier times, Buckbean was employed in the treatment of dropsy, catarrh, scabies and fever. Early modern physicians used the plant for rheumatic complaints, skin diseases, and also to reduce fever. Buckbean is also reportedly excellent for relieving gas and excess stomach acid.

This perennial herb contains a bitter glucoside, menyanthin, and is used for its tart taste in beer (Scandinavia) and as a substitute for tea.

Buckbean leaves contain a number of alkaloids, especially gentianine and gentianadine. In animals, gentianine shows analgesic and tranquilizing effects; gentianadine lowers blood pressure and has significant antiinflammatory activity.

Dose: The medicinal dosage is one teaspoon of root/rhizome/leaves, chopped fine, per cup of boiling water, drunk cold one mouthful at a time, during the course of the day.

BUCKTHORN
Rhamnus cathartica, R. frangula

PARTS USED: Bark and berries
OTHER COMMON NAMES: Alder Buckthorn, Purging Buckthorn

Botanical Description: *Rhamnus cathartica.* The Purging Buckthorn is a shrub 7 or 8 feet high, with branches terminating in a sharp spine. The leaves are in fascicles, on short footstalks, ovate, serrate, veined. The flowers are usually dioecious, in clusters, small, greenish, peduncled, with a 4-cleft calyx, and 4 very small scalelike petals, placed, in the male flower, behind the stamens, which equal them in number. The fruit is a 4-seeded berry.

The shrub is a native of Europe, and is said to have been found growing wild in this country. It flowers in May and June, and ripens its fruit in the latter part of September. The berries are the officinal portion. When ripe they are about the size of a pea, round, somewhat flattened on the summit, black, smooth, shining, with four seeds surrounded by a green, juicy parenchyma. Their odor is unpleasant, their taste bitterish, acrid, and nauseous. The expressed juice has the color, odor, and taste of the parenchyma. It is reddened by the acids, and from deep green is rendered light green by the alkalies. Upon standing it soon begins to ferment, and becomes red in consequence of the formation of acetic acid. (U.S.D.)

Medicinal Uses: Esteemed for its purgative powers, the freshly powdered bark of Buckthorn is highly irritating to the gastrointestinal mucous membrane, producing, when taken in sufficient quantity, violent catharsis coupled with vomiting and pain. The *dried* bark is much milder, resembling *Rheum* species (Rhubarb) in its action.

The berries of *Rhamnus cathartica* are known to contain anthraquinone glycosides that are responsible for the cathartic effect attributed to them. Similarly, Buckthorn bark (*R. frangula*) is used

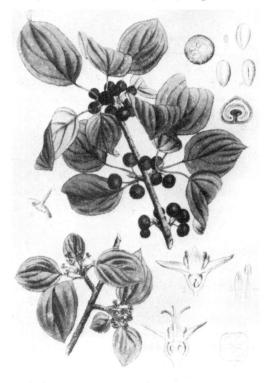

BUCKTHORN: The dried bark is considered an excellent purgative. Anthraquinone glycosides are responsible for the cathartic effect attributed to the berries.

widely in Europe as a cathartic, in the same way that *R. purshiana* (Cascara Sagrada) is used widely in North America. The active principles in Buckthorn bark and Cascara Sagrada bark are similar. For additional information see CASCARA SAGRADA.

Dose: 1 teaspoon of *dried* bark per 1½ pints of water, boiled in a covered container for about ½ hour, at a slow boil. Liquid allowed to cool slowly in the *closed* container. Administered cold, 1 tablespoon at a time, very carefully. (Note: bark must be at least two years old; fresh bark may cause vomiting.)

BURDOCK
Arctium lappa

PARTS USED: Root
OTHER COMMON NAMES: Clotburr, Bardana

Botanical Description: The Burdock is a biennial plant, with a simple spindle-shaped root, a foot or more in length, brown externally, white and spongy within, furnished with threadlike fibers, and having withered scales near the summit. The stem is succulent, pubescent, branching, and 3 or 4 feet in height, bearing very large cordate, denticulate leaves, which are green on their upper surface, whitish and downy on the under, and stand on long footstalks. The flowers are purple, globose, and arranged in terminal panicles. The calyx consists of imbricated scales, with hooked extremities, by which they adhere to clothes, and to the coats of animals. The seed-down is rough and prickly, and the seeds quandrangular.

This plant is a native of Europe, and is abundant in this country, where it grows on the road sides, among rubbish, and in cultivated grounds. The root, which should be collected in spring, loses four-fifths of its weight by drying.

The odor of the root is weak and unpleasant, the taste mucilaginous and sweetish, with a slight degree of bitterness and astringency. The seeds are aromatic, bitterish, and somewhat acrid. (U.S.D.)

Medicinal Uses: Burdock, which is widely eaten as a vegetable, has also been praised for its medicinal virtues since antiquity. A root decoction has been reported useful in the treatment of gout, rheumatism, and dropsy.

The leaves have been used externally on benign skin tumors as well as in the treatment of knee joint swellings unresponsive to other medicines. A poultice was made by boiling the leaves in urine and bran until most of the liquid was boiled off, then applying the hot, wet mass to the affected area. This same poultice was applied externally in the treatment of gout, in tandem with the drinking of the root decoction. Burdock poultices were also used to treat severe bloody bruises and burns.

According to Woodville, an eighteenth-century writer on medical botany, the plant is very useful as a diuretic, and it effects cure without increased irritation and nausea as side effects.

Burdock root extracts have been shown experimentally to produce diuresis and to inhibit tumors in animals. Extracts also lower blood sugar and have estrogenic activity. In test tube experiments, extracts show antibacterial and antifungal properties. The active antibacterial principle was isolated and partially characterized as a lactone.

These experiments indicate potential use of Burdock in female complaints, in diabetes, and for bacterial or fungal infection.

Dose: One teaspoon of root (only 1-year-old root should be used) to 1½ pints of boiling water, steeped ½ hour. Drunk at room temperature, 1 to 2 cups daily. (Mausert recommends that Burdock oil be rubbed into the scalp to prevent hair from falling out.)

BUTTERCUP
Ranunculus spp.

PARTS USED: Herb
OTHER COMMON NAMES: Pilewort, Crowfoot, Buttercup

Botanical Description: *Ranunculus bulbosus.* This species of Crowfoot is perennial, with a bulbous, solid, fleshy root, which sends up annually several erect, round, and branching stems, from 9 to 18 inches high. The radical leaves, which stand on long footstalks, are ternate or quinate, with lobed and dentate leaflets. The leaves of the stem are sessile, ternate; the upper more simple. Each stem supports several solitary, bright yellow, glossy flowers, upon furrowed, angular peduncles. The leaves of the calyx are reflexed or bent downwards against the flowerstalk. The petals are obcordate and arranged so as to represent a small cup in shape. At the inside of the claw of each petal is a small cavity, which is covered with a minute wedge-shaped emarginate scale. The fruit consists of numerous naked seeds, collected into a spherical head. The stem, leaves, peduncles, and calyx are hairy.

In the months of May and June our pastures are everywhere adorned with the rich yellow flowers of this species of *Ranunculus*. Somewhat later, *R. acris* and *R. repens* begin to bloom, and a succession of similar flowers is maintained till September. The two latter species prefer a moister ground, and are found most abundantly in meadows. *R. sceleratus* is found in ponds and ditches. (U.S.D.)

Medicinal Uses: The members of the *Ranunculus* genus are, from their close resemblance, often grouped under the common name of Buttercup. Most of the plants belonging to this genus have similar, extremely acrid properties; the alkaloids contained by the various species are violent irritants and active cardiac poisons, but are generally so volatile that their dangers can be reduced by drying or boiling.

Ranunculus species have been noted to produce severe blisters on the hand from the simple act of picking and carrying a specimen; their main use in folk medicine has been externally as vesicants, applied to the surface to draw out the deeper fluids in the form of a blister.

The Pilewort, *R. ficaria*, was recommended for the treatment of hemorrhoids because the tubers on the roots had a shape similar to that of hermorrhoids. According to the "doctrine of signatures," a plant with a part resembling a part of the human body was suitable for treating diseases of that body part ("like cures like").

The internal use of the *Ranunculus* species was less common, since the plants cause extreme irritation to the mucous membrane of the gastrointestinal tract.

A related species, *R. bulbosa*, was used as a counterirritant to skin irritations. That species was

held to be generally beneficial to the veins, and was believed to cure polyps of the nose.

The Cursed Crowfoot, *R. sceleratus*, was used only in homeopathic dilutions, since it was especially acrid and dangerous.

All species of Buttercup contain a principle known as anemonin. As soon as Buttercups are picked, a chemical reaction occurs that converts the inert anemonin into a powerful irritant and vesicant known as protoanemonin. It is protoanemonin that gives all of the effects attributed to the Buttercups.

Dose: Not recommended.

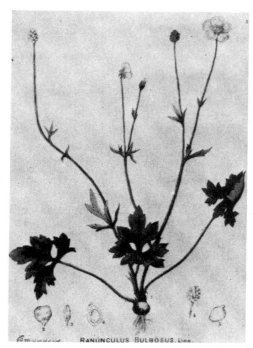

RANUNCULUS BULBOSUS. Linn.

BUTTERCUP: Most of the plants belonging to this genus have similar, extremely acrid properties; the alkaloids contained by the various species are violent irritants and active cardiac poisons.

BUTTERNUT; BLACK WALNUT
Juglans cinerea; Juglans nigra

PARTS USED: Inner bark
OTHER COMMON NAMES: White Walnut, Oilnut

Botanical Description: This is an indigenous forest

tree, known in different sections of this country by the various names of Butternut, Oilnut, and White Walnut. In favorable situations it attains a great size, rising sometimes 50 feet in height, with a trunk 3 or 4 feet in diameter at the distance of 5 feet from the ground. The stem divides, at a small distance from the ground, into numerous nearly horizontal branches, which spread widely, and form a large tufted head, giving to the tree a peculiar aspect. The young branches are smooth and of a graying color, which has given origin to the specific name of the plant. The leaves are very long, and consist of 7 or 8 pairs of sessile leaflets, and a single petiolate leaflet at the extremity. These are 2 or 3 inches in length, oblong-lanceolate, rounded at the base, acuminate, finely serrate, and somewhat downy. The male and female flowers are distinct upon the same tree. The former are in large aments, 4 or 5 inches long, hanging down from the sides of the shoots of the preceding year's growth near their extremity. The fertile flowers are at the end of the shoots of the same spring. The

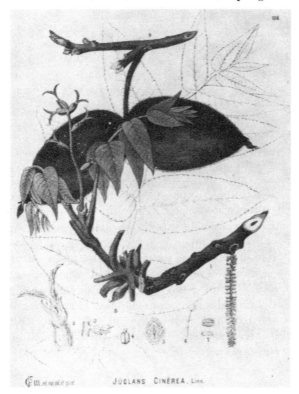

BUTTERNUT: The bark of this forest tree has been valued as one of the mildest and most certain laxatives given us by nature.

germ is surmounted by two large, feathery, rose-colored stigmas. The fruit is sometimes single, suspended by a thin pliable peduncle; sometimes several are attached to the sides and extremity of the same peduncle. The drupe is oblong-oval, with a terminal projection, hairy, viscid, green in the immature state, but brown when ripe. It contains a hard, dark-colored, oblong, pointed nut, with a rough deeply and irregularly furrowed surface. The kernel is thick, oily, and pleasant to the taste.

The Butternut grows in upper and lower Canada, and throughout the whole northern, eastern, and western sections of the United States. In the Midwest, the flowers appear in May, and the fruit ripens in September. The inner bark is the medicinal portion, and that of the root, being considered most efficient, was formerly recommended by the national *Pharmacopoeia*. It should be collected in May or June.

On the living tree, the inner bark when first uncovered is of a pure white, which becomes immediately on exposure a beautiful lemon color, and ultimately changes to deep brown. It has a fibrous texture, a feeble odor, and a peculiar bitter, somewhat acrid taste. Its medical virtues are entirely extracted by boiling water. (U.S.D)

Medicinal Uses: Butternut bark has been valued as one of the mildest and most certain laxatives given us by nature; it operates without causing nausea, irritation, or pain, and does not impair the digestive function. During the Revolutionary War it was commonly used as a habitual laxative and was also considered quite valuable in the treatment of liver disorders.

The common European Walnut, *J. regia,* is also used medicinally; the hull of the fruit has been used as a vermifuge and as a treatment for syphilis and ulcers, and the oil of the fruit has reportedly cured tapeworm as well as being employed as a laxative.

Butternut inner root bark owes all of its pharmacologic effect either to the presence of tannins or the simple quinone compound juglone. These have astringent, antiseptic, and vermifuge properties, especially juglone.

Information on the effectiveness of Butternut preparations for hepatic congestion has not been found in the scientific literature. However, folkloric use for liver complaints is reported. Gathered in the autumn, the bark contains resins, juglandin, juglone, juglandic acid, and essential oil.

The Black Walnut, *J. nigra*, contains the same active principles as the Butternut, and hence would have the same medicinal application.

Dose: 1 teaspoon of the inner bark, boiled in a covered container of 1½ pints of water for about ½ hour, at a slow boil. Liquid allowed to cool slowly in the *closed* container. Drunk cold, 1 swallow or 1 tablespoon at a time, 1 to 2 cups per day.

CASCARA SAGRADA
Rhamnus purshiana

PARTS USED: Bark

OTHER COMMON NAMES: Buckthorn, Coffee Tree, Sacred Bark, Chittembark

Botanical Description: *Rhamnus purshiana* is a small tree, attaining a height of 20 feet. Its leaves are rather thin, elliptic, for the most part briefly acutely pointed, finely serrated, at the base obtuse, somewhat pubescent beneath, from 2 to 7 inches long and from 1 to 3 wide. The rather large flowers are in somewhat umbellate cymes; the sepals 5; the minute cucullate petals bifid at the apex. The fruit is black, broadly obovoid, 3-lobed, and three-seeded. The seeds are convex on the back, with a lateral raphe. It is found in California, extending northward to Canada.

A number of species of *Rhamnus* have been described as growing in California, but according to the best authority there are only four species—*R. alnifolia, R. crocea, R. purshiana,* and *R. californica.* Of these species, *R. alnifolia* is too rare in the Cascara district to be important; while the spinescent twigs, the very thick oval or roundish leaves, and the small roundish red fruit of *R. corcea* make it so distinct that it cannot be confounded with the Cascara, whose bark, moreover, it does not resemble. On the other hand, *R. californica* appears to be very commonly confounded with the official species by collectors, and to have yielded some of the Cascara Sagrada bark of commerce. *R. californica* is rare in northern California, but abundant to the south and southeast, while *R. purshiana* is abundant in northern California, but scarce in the south, so that any bark collected in northern California is probably genuine. *R. californica* is chiefly distinguished from the official species by its leaves being thin, and, when not smooth, having a short close pubescence, and the primary veins of the under surface not nearly so numerous, straight, or fine as those of *R. purshiana.* One writer thinks that its leaves are especially distinguished by the channel of the midrib of *R. californica* being altogether absent, or shallow, or inconspicuous. Nevertheless, the species so run into one another that many competent botanists believe them identical. (U.S.D.)

Medicinal Uses: The bark of Cascara Sagrada has been called the most widely used cathartic on earth. Traditionally employed as a remedy by the North American Indians, the bark became known to the settlers and eventually passed into use by the medical profession. The pharmaceutical house of Parke, Davis and Co. first marketed Cascara Sagrada in 1877, although the plant did not become official in the *U. S. Pharmacopoeia* until 1890. No synthetic substance can equal the mild and speedy action of the "holy bark"; it is marketed in pills, powders, and fluidextracts by many pharmaceutical companies.

The basis for Cascara's effect is the presence of a mixture of anthraquinones, either free (i.e., aloe-emodin) or as sugar derivatives (glycosides). The free anthraquinones remain in the intestine and cause catharsis by irritating the intestinal wall. Those anthraquinones present in the plant as sugar derivatives are largely absorbed from the intestine, circulate through the bloodstream, and eventually stimulate a nerve center in the lower part of the intestine, which causes a laxative effect.

Cascara bark should always be aged for at least one year before being used as a laxative. During this period of time certain chemical changes occur in the bark that reduce the "griping" effect that often accompanies the use of a laxative preparation of this type.

Dose: 1 teaspoon of bark, boiled, covered, in a container of 1½ pints of water for about ½ hour, at a slow boil. Liquid allowed to cool slowly in the *closed* container. Drunk cold, 1 swallow or 1 tablespoon at a time, 1 to 2 cups per day.

57

CASTOR BEAN
Ricinus communis

PARTS USED: Seeds

OTHER COMMON NAMES: Castor Oil Plant, Palma Christi, Bofareira

Botanical Description: The Castor Oil Plant attains in the East Indies and Africa the character of a tree; and rises sometimes 30 or 40 feet in height. In the temperate latitudes of North America and Europe it is an annual plant. The following description applies to the plant as cultivated in cool latitudes. Its general aspect is very peculiar, and not inelegant. The stem is of vigorous growth, erect, round, hollow, smooth, glaucous, somewhat purplish toward the top, branching, and from 3 to 8 feet or more in height. The leaves are alternate; peltate or supported upon footstalks inserted into their lower disk; palmate, with 7 or 9 pointed serrate lobes; smooth on both sides; and of a bluish-green color. The flowers are monoecious, stand upon jointed peduncles, and form a pyramidal terminal raceme, of which the lower portion is occupied by the male flowers, the upper by the female. Both are destitute of corolla. In the male flowers the calyx is divided into 5 oval, concave, pointed, reflected, purplish segments, and encloses numerous stamens, which are united into fasciculi at their base. In the female, the calyx has 3 or 5 narrow lanceolate segments; and the ovary, which is roundish and 3-sided, supports 3 linear, reddish stigmas, forked at their apex. The fruit is a roundish glaucous capsule, with 3 projecting sides, covered with tough spines, and divided into 3 cells, each containing one seed, which is expelled by the bursting of the capsule.

This species of *Ricinus* is a native of the East Indies and Northern Africa; has become naturalized in the West Indies; and is cultivated in various parts of the world, in no country perhaps more largely than in the United States. The flowers appear in July, and the seeds ripen successively in August and September. The part employed in medicine is the fixed oil extracted from the seeds. (U.S.D.)

Medicinal Uses: All parts of the plant, and especially the seeds, or beans, are poisonous to humans and animals. The toxic action is due to ricin, a severe irritant that produces nausea, vomiting, gastric pain, diarrhea, thirst, and dimness of vision.

Castor oil, expressed from the Castor bean (seed), has an unpleasant, acrid taste, and is highly valued as a safe and reliable cathartic and purgative, useful in irritable conditions of the gastrointestinal tract and the genito-urinary system, particularly in infants and young children. Often attempts are made to mask the unpleasant taste with the addition of aromatic and essential oils, but the dominant Castor taste is difficult to subdue.

Although the Castor Bean seed yields an oil that is well established to be an effective cathartic, it also contains one of the most poisonous substances known to man. In the preparation of castor oil, the seeds are usually pressed and the oil that exudes is collected and purified. The toxic components of the seeds are completely insoluble in oil and therefore are not found in castor oil. However, one should *never* eat the seed by itself; there are documented cases in which a single bean has been lethal when eaten.

As stated, the poisonous principle in Castor bean is known as *ricin;* recently scientists have found that ricin is not a single substance, but a complex mixture of toxic materials that are very difficult to separate and purify. Ricin causes red blood cells to hemolyze (dissolve), and also disturbs the immune system in the body.

However, if castor *oil* is to be used as a cathartic, one should be confident that it will not be poisonous. Only the seeds are poisonous if ingested.

Dose: CAUTION. Highly poisonous. Use only manufactured products.

CATNIP
Nepeta cataria

PARTS USED: Leaves

OTHER COMMON NAMES: Catmint

Botanical Description: Root perennial, long, woody, with numerous slender blackish fibrils. Stems numerous, branched, quadrangular, pubescent, 2 to 3 feet high. Leaves opposite, cordate, petiolate, green above,

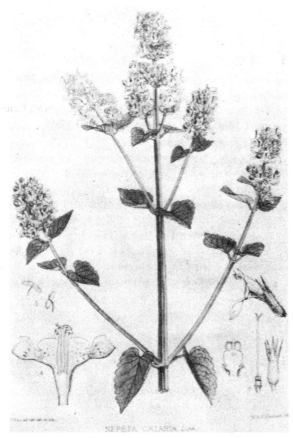

CATNIP: Reportedly efficacious in the treatment of iron-deficiency anemia, menstrual and uterine disorders, and dyspepsia, and as a gentle calmative, this perennial herb has been known to cause cats to exhibit extreme mania.

whitish beneath, with large acute serratures. Flowers in spiked, somewhat pedunculate whorls. Calyx monophyllous, tubular, many-ribbed, 5-toothed. Corolla large, white, or purplish, with deep rose-colored spots; tube long, cylindrical; upper lip emarginate, lower with 3 lobes, central one large, rounded, concave and notched, lateral ones reflexed. Stamens didynamous, approximating, shorter than the upper lip of the corolla, with reddish anthers. Ovary superior, 4-lobed, supporting a filiform curved style, terminated by a bifid stigma.

Distribution: Europe, Siberia, western Asia to the Himalayas. Introduced in North America. The plant is found in hedgebanks and waste places in some parts of England and Ireland, but very local in Scotland. Flowers July and September. (B.F.M.)

Medicinal Uses: Surely a plant which has such a powerful impact on our feline friends, causing them to "roll upon, chew, and tear to bits any withered leaf till nothing remains," could not be destitute of medicinal value in humans.

Catnip has been reported efficacious in the treatment of iron-deficiency anemia, menstrual and uterine disorders, and dyspepsia, and as a gentle calmative. It has been administered in a variety of forms, including infusion, injection, lavement, and in the bath. It has been drunk as a treatment for chronic cough, and chewed for relief of toothache. Containing a bitter principle, this perennial herb has also been useful for infantile colic.

Dose: Approximately ½ ounce of leaves to 1 pint of water. Water boiled separately and poured over the plant material and steeped 5–10 minutes, depending on the desired effect. Drunk hot or warm, 1 to 2 cups per day, at bedtime and upon awakening.

CAYENNE PEPPER
Capsicum annuum

PARTS USED: Seeds
OTHER COMMON NAMES: Red Pepper

Botanical Description: Numerous species of *Capsicum*, inhabiting the East Indies and tropical America, are enumerated by botanists, the fruit of which, differing simply in the degree of pungency, may be indiscriminately employed. *C. baccatum*, or the Bird Pepper, and *C. frutescens* are said to yield most of the cayenne pepper brought from the West Indies and South America. The species most extensively cultivated in Europe and this country is *C. annuum*.

Capsicum annuum. The stem of the annual Capsicum is thick, roundish, smooth, and branching; rises 2 or 3 feet in height; and supports ovate, pointed, smooth, entire leaves, which are placed without regular order on long footstalks. The flowers are solitary, white, and stand on long peduncles at the axils of the leaves. The calyx is persistent, tubular, and 5-cleft; the corolla, monopetalous and wheel-shaped, with the limb divided into 5 spreading, pointed, and plaited segments; the filaments, short, tapering, and furnished with oblong anthers; the germ ovate, supporting a slender style which is no longer than the filaments, and terminates in a blunt stigma. The fruit is a pendulous, podlike berry, light, smooth, and shining, of a bright scarlet, orange, or sometimes yellow color, with 2 or 3 cells, containing a dry loose pulp, and numerous flat, kidney-shaped, whitish seeds.

The plant is a native of the warmer regions of Asia and America, and is cultivated in almost all parts of the world. It is abundantly produced in this country, both for culinary and medicinal purposes. The flowers appear in July and August, and the fruit ripens in October. Several varieties are cultivated in our gardens, differing in the shape of the fruit. The most abundant is probably that with a large irregularly ovate berry, depressed at the extremity, which is much used in the green state for pickling. The medicinal variety is that with long, conical, generally pointed, recurved fruit, usually not thicker than the finger. Sometimes we meet with small, spherical, slightly compressed berries, not greatly exceeding a large cherry in size. When perfectly ripe and dry, the fruit is ground into powder, and brought into market under the name of red or cayenne pepper. Our markets are also partly supplied by importation from the West Indies. A variety of *Capsicum*, consisting of very small conical, exceedingly pungent berries, has been imported from Liberia. (U.S.D.)

Medicinal Uses: The stimulant effect of the seeds is reflected in their use as a condiment in foods, with a resulting promotion of digestion. As a medicine, cayenne pepper is a general stimulant, and has been reported of value in the treatment of dyspepsia, diarrhea, and prostration. It has been used as a remedy for scarlet fever and for nausea from seasickness. As a gargle, the seeds are valued as a treatment for sore throat and hoarseness. In the treatment of ague (painful swelling of the face due to decayed or ulcerated teeth or a cold), inhalation of the steam of Cayenne and vinegar, coupled with a small mouth poultice containing one teaspoon of cayenne pepper, will reportedly afford relief by producing a free discharge of saliva.

Cayenne pepper acts as a rubefacient when applied externally, and as a stimulant internally, due to the presence of capsaicin, which is the "hot principle" in the fruits of this plant. Oleoresin of *Capsicum* is still used in the preparation of a number of popular proprietary products to be applied locally for the relief of sore muscles, and

produces the desired effect by mildly irritating the surface of the skin, which causes an increased blood flow to the area of application. The increased blood flow results in reduced inflammation of the affected area.

Internally, both cayenne pepper preparations and the active principle capsaicin have been shown in humans and in animals to stimulate the production of gastric juices, resulting in improved digestion.

One must remember that in concentrated form, cayenne pepper preparations left on the skin too long will result in the formation of blisters.

Dose: ¼ to 1 whole teaspoon per cup of hot water.

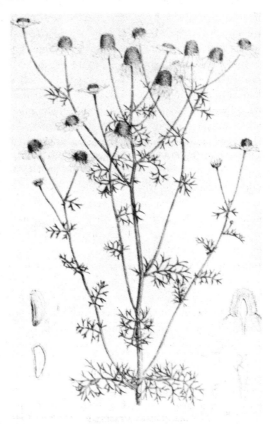

GERMAN CHAMOMILE: Here is a usually safe sedative from nature's garden. Animal experiments have shown that extracts relax the smooth muscle of the intestine. With the exception of an occasional allergic response, there have been no reported cases of adverse effects.

CHAMOMILE, GERMAN
Matricaria chamomilla

PARTS USED: Flower heads

Botanical Description: *Matricaria chamomilla* is a weed of waste and cultivated ground throughout Europe except the extreme north, extending through temperate and northern Asia to peninsular India.

The Greek name signifies "ground-apple" and is appropriate, the whole plant when bruised affording a pleasant aromatic smell very similar to that of apples; by this character *M. chamomilla* can be easily distinguished from *M. inodora*, to which it bears a strong resemblance, but which is scentless. This latter has also large flower heads, a flatter receptacle, and the fruit, which is twice as large, has 3 very strong ribs on one side and 2 deep pits on the other. *Anthemis nobilis* (Roman Chamomile), another plant likely to be confounded with this, has a very disagreeable fetid odor, and is also characterized by having the receptable provided with long setaceous scales, and the ray flowers usually barren.

The German Chamomile is an annual herb, stem erect, 1–2 feet high, much branched, solid, smooth and shining, strongly striate, pale green, branches long, slender. Leaves numerous, alternate, sessile, with a dilated base embracing half the stem, oblong-oval in outline, obtuse, bi- or tripinnatisect, the ultimate segments narrow, setaceous, acute, spreading and curved, quite smooth, bright green. Flower heads numerous, terminating the slender branches and forming a more or less corymbose inflorescence, small, about ⅝ inch wide; involucre flat, composed of a single or 2 or 3 rows of very small, equal, linear, smooth, blunt scales with scarious brownish ends and transparent margins; receptacle at first ovoid and hollow, smooth, without scales. Disk-flowers bisexual, very small and numerous, corolla deeply 5-toothed, pale greenish-yellow, brighter before expansion, with a few small glands on the outside; anthers with a large terminal appendage, not tailed at the base. Ray-flowers female, rather numerous (15–25), crowded and overlapping, limb scarcely ¼ inch long, oval-oblong, faintly and bluntly 2- or 3-lobed at the apex, white, involute and erect in the bud, spreading in flower, afterwards quickly deflexed, styles spreading. Fruit is very small, oblong-ovoid, somewhat curved, with 5 ribs on the concave side, quite smooth, pale grey, crowned with a very slight raised border, no pappus. (U.S.D.)

Medicinal Uses: There are two major types of Chamomile; they should not be confused. Roman Chamomile is derived from the flowers of *Anthemis nobilis*, whereas German, or Hungarian, Chamomile makes use of the flowers of *Matricaria chamomilla*.

The latter, a showy annual, cultivated in Europe, has long been taken in home remedies for anthelmintic and antispasmodic effects. The dried flower heads are known to stimulate the digestive process and are equally well established for the mild relaxing properties. (The flowers are even useful as a rinse to keep the hair golden.) This Chamomile species is also used for flavoring liqueurs and in perfumes, shampoos, and special tobaccos.

In 1973, a study was carried out in the United States, in which 12 hospitalized patients having various types of heart disease, were administered Chamomille tea in order to determine its effect. Each patient was given a 6 ounce cup of hot tea prepared from 2 commercial Chamomille tea bags. Approximately 10 minutes after the ingestion of the tea, ten of the patients fell into a deep sleep. They could be aroused, but immediately fell again into a deep sleep. The sleep lasted approximately 90 minutes. The only other effect seen in the patients was a small but significant increase in arterial blood pressure.

Experimentally in animals, the volatile oil from Chamomille flowers was given orally to rabbits with impaired kidney function, so that the amount of urea in the blood was increased. In all cases, the uremic condition in the rabbits normalized.

Another study in animals, using a flavonoid found in Chamomille flowers (apigenin), showed that this substance had antihistaminic effects. Chamomille essential oil, when administered orally to rats with experimental arthritis, reduced the inflammation markedly. It was further shown that the constituent in the oil responsible for most of this effect was a substance known as alpha-bisabolol.

Chamomille oil has also been shown to relax the

61

smooth muscle of the intestine, in test-tube experiments.

With the exception of an occasional allergic response, there have been no adverse effects reported in the literature in humans for Chamomile. Thus, here is another safe sedative from nature's garden.

CHAMOMILE, ROMAN
Anthemis nobilis

PARTS USED: Flowers and their oil
OTHER COMMON NAMES: English Chamomile

Botanical Description: This is an herbaceous plant with a perennial root. The stems are from 6 inches to a foot long, round, slender, downy, trailing, and divided into branches, which turn upward at their extremities. The

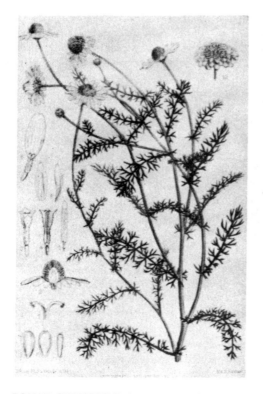

ROMAN CHAMOMILE: In moderate doses these flowers are an excellent stomachic in indigestion, flatulent colic, gout, and headaches. A strong infusion reportedly acts as an efficient emetic.

leaves are bipinnate; the leaflets small, threadlike, somewhat pubescent, acute, and generally divided into 3 segments. The flowers are solitary, with a yellow convex disc, and white rays. The calyx is common to all the florets, of a hemispherical form, and composed of several small imbricated hairy scales. The receptacle is convex, prominent, and furnished with rigid bristle-like paleae. The florets of the radius are numerous, narrow, and terminated with 3 small teeth. The whole herb has a peculiar fragrant odor, and a bitter aromatic taste. The flowers only are official.

This plant is a native of Europe, and grows wild in all the temperate parts of that continent. It is also widely cultivated for medicinal purposes. In France, Germany, and Italy, it is generally known by the name of Roman Chamomile. The flowers become double by cultivation, and in this state are usually preferred; though, as the sensible properties are found in the greatest degree in the disc, which is not fully developed in the double flowers, the single are the most powerful. It is rather, however, in aromatic flavor, than in bitterness, that the radial florets are surpassed by those of the disc. If not well and quickly dried, the flowers lose their beautiful white color, and are less efficient as a medicine. Those which are whitest should be preferred.

Though not a native of America, Chamomile grows wild in some parts of this country, and is occasionally cultivated in our gardens for family use, the whole herb being employed. The medicine, as found in our shops, consists chiefly of the double flowers, and is imported from Germany and England. From the former country are also occasionally imported, under the name of German Chamomile, the flowers of *Matricaria chamomilla*, a plant belonging to the same family as *Anthemis*, and closely allied to it in sensible as well as medicinal properties. The flowers of *Matricaria* are, however, less pleasant to the smell, and are considerably weaker than the true Chamomile's. As they reach us they are also much smaller, and differ, moreover, in exhibiting a much larger proportion of the disc florets, compared with those of the ray. They are much used in Germany. (U.S.D.)

Medicinal Uses: In moderate doses, the flowers are an excellent stomachic in indigestion, flatulent colic, gout, and headaches. A strong infusion acts as an efficient emetic (try it combined with ginger!). The oil has stimulant and antispasmodic properties; it is useful in treating flatulence, and is added to purgatives to prevent griping pain in the bowels.

A related species, *A. cotula*, Stinking Chamomile, or May Weed, was once widely used in the United States to promote sweating in chronic rheumatism, and was recommended by Tragus, a sixteenth-century herbalist, in the form of a decoction as a remedy for hysteria.

Dose: Approximately ½ ounce of flowers to 1 pint of water. Water boiled separately and poured over the plant material and steeped for 5 to 20 minutes, depending on the desired effect. Drunk hot or warm, 1 to 2 cups or more per day. (Used as a hair wash, it will brighten the hair.)

CHERRY LAUREL
Prunus laurocerasus

PARTS USED: Leaves

Botanical Description: This is a small evergreen tree, rising 15 or 20 feet in height, with long spreading branches, which, as well as the trunk, are covered with a smooth blackish bark. The leaves, which stand alternately on short strong footstalks, are oval oblong, from 5 to 7 inches in length, acute, finely toothed, firm, coriaceous, smooth, beautifully green and shining, with oblique nerves, and yellowish glands at the base. The flowers are small, white, strongly odorous, and disposed in simple axillary racemes. The fruit consists of oval drupes, very similar to small black cherries, both in their shape and internal structure.

The Cherry Laurel is a native of Asia Minor, but has been introduced into Europe, throughout which it is cultivated, both for medical use and for the beauty of its shining evergreen foliage. Almost all parts of it are more or less impregnated with the odor supposed to indicate the presence of hydrocyanic acid. (U.S.D.)

Medicinal Uses: The leaves contain hydrocyanic acid (HCN), which gives them a somewhat astringent and strongly bitter taste, with the flavor of the peach kernel.

Water distilled from Cherry Laurel leaves was often employed in Europe for the same illnesses in which hydrocyanic acid was applied; dilute

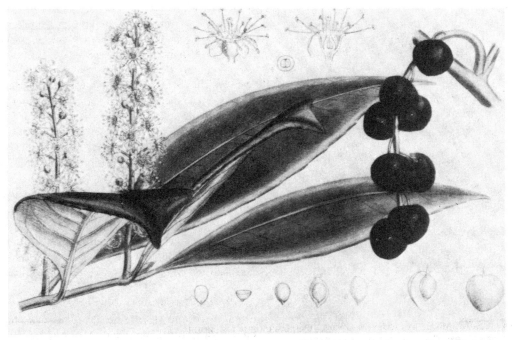

CHERRY LAUREL: The leaves contain hydrocyanic acid, which gives them a somewhat astringent and strongly bitter taste, with the flavor of the peach kernel.

HCN was used in respiratory ailments and to calm coughs, as a sedative, as a tonic for stomach upset of nervous origins, and externally as a cure for severe itching.

Hydrocyanic acid is an extremely fast-acting poison; overdoses can kill within minutes. Extreme caution should therefore be employed when using the distillate of Cherry Laurel leaves, since HCN content varies widely and too high a content can prove fatal. The Bitter Almond is preferred as a source of HCN when more uniform HCN content is desired in order to avoid accidental overdose.

Most *Prunus* species are much alike in chemical composition. Therefore all remarks indicated for Wild Cherry (*P. virginiana:* see article) apply to Cherry Laurel as well.

Dose: "The proportion of HCN in the leaves varies according to the season, the age of the plant and the character of the soil and of the weather . . . . [the] consequence of this variability . . . has prevented the general introduction of so variable a remedy." (U.S.D.)

No recommended home usage.

CHESTNUT, SPANISH
Castanea sativa, and other *Castanea* species

PARTS USED: Leaves and bark

Botanical Description: Trees or shrubs, with simple, alternate, straight-veined leaves; flowers appearing after the leaves.

Staminate flowers in slender, elongate, axillary catkins, several together in the axil of a minute, early deciduous bract. Calyx campanulate, 6-parted. Stamens 12-20. Pistillate flowers borne on the base of the staminate catkins or from separate axils, within an ovoid prickly involucre. Calyx adnate to the ovary, 6-lobed. Ovary usually 6-celled, 12-ovuled; styled slender, as many as the cell. Fruit a 1-seeded nut, solitary or 2–3 (rarely more) together within the accrescent, long-spined, 2–4-valved involucre.

About 10 species of the Northern Hemisphere. (B&B)

Medicinal Uses: Being astringent, the bark and leaves were used to make a tonic which was also

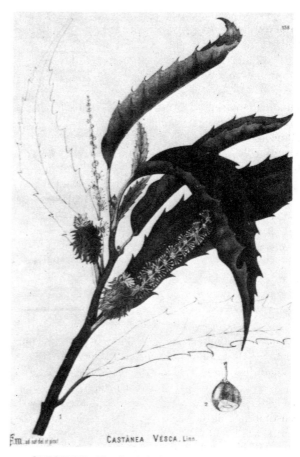

CASTÀNEA VESCA, Linn.

CHESTNUT: The bark is known to contain high concentrations of tannins, which explain the astringent effect claimed when water extracts of this plant are applied externally.

reportedly useful in the treatment of upper respiratory ailments such as coughs, and particularly whooping cough.

Chestnuts are, of course, better known for their edibility, traditionally being ground into flour in order to make breads and cakes, for thickening soups, as well as being eaten roasted or boiled. Eating too many can result in constipation.

The bark of Spanish Chestnut is known to contain high concentrations of tannins, which explain the astringent effect claimed when water extracts of this plant are applied externally.

Although there is no direct experimental evidence to corroborate claims that the leaves of this plant have value in treating whooping cough, they are rich in polysaccharides, which, if taken orally in a water infusion, would produce a demulcent and soothing effect on the irritated mucous membranes, and hence have a tendency to lessen the symptoms of whooping cough.

Dose: 1 teaspoon of leaves and bark, chopped fine, boiled in a covered container with 1 pint of water for about ½ hour, at a slow boil. Liquid allowed to cool slowly in the *closed* container. Drunk cold, 1 swallow or 1 tablespoon at a time, 1 to 2 cups per day.

CINCHONA
Cinchona ledgeriana, C. calisaya, C. succirubra, C. officinalis

PARTS USED: Bark
OTHER COMMON NAMES: Jesuit's Powder, Peruvian Bark

Botanical Description: A vast number of plants belonging to the Linnaean genus *Cinchona* were in the course of time discovered; and the list became at length so unwieldy and heterogeneous that botanists were compelled to distribute the species into several groups, each constituting a distinct genus, and all associated in the natural family of Rubiaceae.

C. calisaya is tall, usually surpassing those about it, the trunk often more than 2 feet in diameter. Leaves petiolate, the blade ovate-oblong to slightly obovate, 7 to 17.5 centimeters long by 2.5 to 7 centimeters broad, obtuse, the base acute or slightly attenuated, very thin, smooth, and, especially below, with a satiny luster, above dark green, below emerald-green or deep purple-green, scrobiculate, the glands scarcely visible above. Stipules oblong, about equalling the petioles, very smooth, very obtuse. Panicles ovate to subcorymbose. Calyx pubescent, with a cup-shaped limb and short triangular teeth. Corolla rose-colored (in cultivation often white or nearly so), the tube cylindrical and about 8 millimeters long, the laciniaae more deeply colored, the edges white-hairy. Stamens included. Capsule ovate, scarcely as long as the flowers. Seeds elliptical lanceolate, the margin irregularly fimbriate-toothed. Bolivia and southern Peru, 4,000 to 6,000 feet. Source of the Calisaya or yellow-bark. The species presents many forms, and two varieties are recognized.

C. ledgeriana, formerly recognized as a variety of *C. calisaya,* differs from the type chiefly in its thicker, narrower, oblong leaves, with attenuate base, often bluish-green below. It yields a thick and remarkably rich bark, and is probably the most valued of all the cinchonas. This species was named in honor of Ledger, who first brought seed of this species from Bolivia.

C. succirubra. Extreme size even greater than that of last. Branches silvery. Petiole pubescent, leaf ovate to oval, acute with a very short point, the base more or less narrowing, often 6 by 9 inches, dark green and smooth above, below paler and pubescent to a variable degree, especially on the veins, not scrobiculate, the maring slightly revolute. Stipules entire, oblong, obtuse, sub-amplexicaul. Flowers much as in the last, but rather smaller. Fruit lanceolate. Western slopes of Mt. Chimborazo (Ecuador). The source of the Red Bark.

C. officinalis. Petioles smooth, cylindrical, and, like the veins, reddish; blade 10 to 12.5 centimeters long, varying from broadly oval to lanceolate, acute at both ends, the margins usually recurved, smooth and deep green above, paler, but bright green below, scrobiculate, the principal veins pubescent. Stipules equalling the petioles, ovate, acute, entire, pubescent. Flowers and fruit much as in *C. calisaya.* Widely distributed in the equatorial Andes, at an elevation of 5,000 to 7,500 feet. The source of the barks known as pale, crown, Loxa, Cuneca, and Huanuco. This is the original species, upon which the genus *Quinquina* or *Cinchona* was founded. All things considered, it is, perhaps, to be regarded as the principal species of the genus and its variability is extreme.

The genuine Cinchona trees are natives exclusively of South America. In that continent, however, they are widely diffused, extending from latitude 19°S considerably south of La Paz, in Bolivia, northward to the mountains of Santa Maria, or, according to one writer, to the vicinity of Caracas, on the northern coast, at about latitude 10°N. (U.S.D.)

Medicinal Uses: The alkaloid quinine is derived from Cinchona bark and is well known for its antimalarial properties. The bark was brought to Europe in 1640 through the auspices of the Countess of Chinchon, of Peru, but it was not until 97 years later that a French naturalist identified the tree from which the bark was obtained while journeying in the Loxa province of Peru.

Once Cinchona became popular as a cure for intermittent fevers, it was distributed and sold by the Jesuit fathers, who maintained missions in the area; in the latter eighteenth century, other sources of the bark were discovered in Colombia, central Peru, and Bolivia. Quinine has been recognized as one of nature's most important medicinal gifts to the human race, for it has been instrumental in relieving great suffering from malaria and other intermittent fevers.

Besides its antiperiodic action against intermittent fevers, Cinchona bark has tonic, antiseptic, and astringent properties. However, excessive doses of Cinchona can lead to a condition known as cinchonism or quinism, marked by buzzing in the ears, deafness, headache, vertigo, and nausea. While these effects generally pass off within a few hours, they are a warning signal regarding dosage.

Although quinine and preparations containing quinine are relatively safe, one must be cautious of the amounts used. Nature, as in many cases, has provided a built-in warning to notify us when the safe limit of these preparations is approaching. When one experiences a ringing in the ears, the amount being taken should be reduced, and the sounds will disappear.

During the Vietnam War, a strain of malarial parasite developed which was highly resistant to both well-established and new synthetic anti-malarial drugs. It was soon found, however, that most cases of malaria caused by the new parasite could be effectively treated with the centuries-proven drug, quinine.

Dose: If available, the compound tincture is taken in doses of 0.65-3.9 grams. However, commercially available drugs are more reliable.

CLUB MOSS
Lycopodium clavatum, L. cernuum

PARTS USED: Spores and moss

OTHER COMMON NAMES: Stag's Horn; Vegetable Sulphur

Botanical Description: *Lycopodium cernuum.* This far-creeping, evergreen, mosslike plant, which roots at intervals and has successively 2 forked branches on stiff,

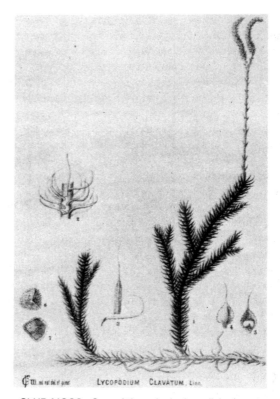

LYCOPODIUM CLAVATUM, Linn.

CLUB MOSS: One of the principal medicinal uses of the spores is as a dusting powder, both for rashes of babies and also for eczematous skin conditions in adults.

erect, cylindrical stems that may grow 1 to 5 feet tall, often develops luxuriantly along the edges of woods. Narrow, awl-like leaves about 0.17 inch long thickly clothe stems and branches, those on the branches being curved. Eventually each branch is tipped with a nodding, conelike spike 0.25 to nearly 1 inch long, closely covered with ovate, 8-ranked bracts. Each bract is 0.08 inch long and overlaps a round, 1-chambered case that contains countless yellow spores, resembling pollen in general appearance but functioning as seeds. This Club Moss is widespread in tropical parts of the world.

In the mainland United States, a few Club Mosses are called by the name Ground Pine. Club Mosses of today are descendants of giant treelike Club Mosses, which were dominant in ancient geological times and contributed largely to our coal supply. (Neal)

Medicinal Uses: The spores consitute a light yellow, very mobile powder, which is not wetted

66

by water but floats on it. Consequently, one of the principal medicinal uses of *Lycopodium* spores is as a dusting powder, both for rashes of babies in the genital area and eczematous skin conditions in adults. The spores are also utilized to keep pills and suppositories from adhering to each other.

Both the spores and the whole herb were considered diuretic and antispasmodic, and decoctions were used in rheumatism and diseases of the lungs and kidneys.

This primitive plant has been useful in other ways as well. In Sweden, the stems are made into matting, while the spores were formerly used to create articial lightning on the stage.

Dose: For internal use: 1 teaspoon of spores and/or moss, boiled in a covered container of 1½ pints of water for about ½ hour, at a slow boil. Liquid allowed to cool slowly in the *closed* container. Drunk cold, 1 swallow or 1 tablespoon at a time, 1 to 2 cups per day.

External use: spores applied directly.

COCA
Erythroxylon coca

PARTS USED: Leaves

Botanical Description: The Coca is cultivated to a very large extent in the Andes of Peru and in Bolivia and Colombia, especially in the very moist mild climate met with at 2,000 to 5,000 feet above sea level or higher.

It is scarcely possible to mistake the leaves of the Coca for those of any other plant, the two longitudinal arched lines on the under surface being characteristic. (Bentley)

It is conjectured that the original habitat was in the Peruvian mountains, between latitudes 7° and 10° N, but either spontaneously or through cultivation the Coca shrubs have spread until they are found in the whole eastern curve of the Andes, from the Strait of Magellan to the borders of the Caribbean Sea, growing on the moist sides of the mountains at elevations between 1,500 and 6,000 feet, the climatic requisites being moisture and equable temperature, with a mean of about 17.7°C (64°F). The wild Coca shrub commonly reaches the height of 2 feet—as high as 18 feet—but the cultivated Coca is usually kept down to about 6 feet.

The leaves are gathered three times a year; the first harvest, or preliminary picking, is taken at the time of the trimming of the bushes, from the cut-off twigs. Then about the end of June, a scanty crop is gathered, while the last crop of the season is gathered in October or November. Harvesting must always take place in dry weather, so that the fresh leaves when spread out in layers 2 or 3 inches thick on the drying pavement can be collected in 6 or 8 hours.

The Coca plant, which is propagated from the seed in nurseries, begins to yield in 18 months, and continues productive for half a century. The leaves when mature, are carefully picked by hand so as to avoid breaking them or injuring the young buds, are slowly dried in the sun, and are then packed in bags *(cestos)* holding from 25 to 150 pounds each. They were in general use among the natives of Peru at the time of the conquest, and have continued to be much employed to the present time. (U.S.D.)

Medicinal Uses: So much has been written about this famous medicinal plant in recent years that it may be appropriate to see how medical writers viewed Coca in the heydey of plant therapeutics in the United States. The following is from the twentieth edition of the *U.S. Dispensatory* (1918):

Systemically it is a stimulant to all parts of the central nervous system including the brain, the spinal cord, and the medulla. Its effects upon the brain are shown by an exaltation of the intellectual faculties similar to that which is produced by caffeine. In overdose it produces a delirium somewhat suggesting that of atropine to which it is chemically related. Its action upon the spinal cord is shown by increased activity of the reflexes but the convulsions which are seen in cocaine poisoning both in the lower animals and in man seem to be due to an action upon the motor area of the brain, rather than to its effect on the cord. The effects of the medullary centers are shown by an increased rapidity of the respiration and sometimes also of its depth. After toxic doses the primary stimulation is followed by a depression of the respiratory center. The blood pressure is elevated chiefly through an action upon the vasomotor center, although there is some evidence that it also stimulates the heart. Concerning the changes in the pulse rate there is difference of opinion. . . . Cocaine in moderate quantities also stimulates both the voluntary and involuntary muscle fibers. It appears also to have some effect upon the nutritive processes since it causes a marked rise in the bodily temperature. . . . When instilled into the eye it causes dilatation of the pupil, usually without paralysis of accommodation. The widening of the pupil seems to be the result of an action upon the peripheral ends of the sympathetic nerve and can be further increased by the instillation of atropine.

Cocaine is used in medicine both as a local and a systemic remedy. Internally it is of value as a circulatory and respiratory stimulant and is occasionally of use as a cerebral stimulant or as a tonic. Its employment, however, in any condition which requires prolonged administration of the drug is fraught with so great danger of formation of a habit that it is rarely justifiable. In *narcotic poisonings* the simultaneous stimulation of the respiration, circulation, and cerebrum makes it a remedy of particular value.

The most important use of cocaine is as a local application to mucous membranes either for the purpose of contracting the blood vessels or lessening sensation. For the former reason it is useful to relieve congestion such as *hayfever, coryza,* or *laryngitis,* and to control or prevent *hemorrhage* from the nose and throat. There are two great drawbacks to cocaine in this use, the first that the primary contraction of the blood vessels is liable to be followed by a reactive relaxation, and the second is the ever present peril of habit-formation. As a local anesthetic it is useful in operations on the eye, nose, throat, etc., in painful *hemorrhoids, fissure in ano, vomiting, gastralgia,* and other painful diseases of the mucous membranes. While cocaine passes through mucous membranes with greater or less ease, the unbroken skin offers a practically impassable barrier. Nevertheless, the drug is often used as a local anesthetic, especially for operative purposes, in all parts of the body. . . . There is a widespread belief among both pharmacists and physicians that solutions of cocaine cannot be sterilized by heat without danger of decomposition, but a number of chemists have shown that if the solution is not allowed to become alkaline the degree of hydrolysis is insignificant.

Dose: "Of the salts of cocaine, 0.016–0.03 gm."

The habitual use of cocaine as a narcotic stimulant seems to be approaching an extent of sociological importance. In the United States the conditions under which it may be prescribed or dispensed are strictly limited both by Federal, and in many states, by state laws. Koch . . . estimates that there is 130,000 ounces of cocaine used annually by its victims. The cocaine habit is not only one of the most seductive but also one of the most rapidly injurious and difficult of eradication of all drug habits. The characteristic symptoms are changes in the mental and moral qualities, especially characterized by alternate periods of exaltation and depression, loss of appetite and of weight, peculiar pallor of the skin, insomnia, and general failure of health. A symptom which is seen in many cases and is said to be characteristic of chronic cocaine poisoning, is a sensory hallucination, as of some foreign body under the skin or of insects crawling over the person.

COHOSH, BLACK
Cimicifuga racemosa

PARTS USED: Root
OTHER COMMON NAMES: Black Snakeroot, Squaw Root, Rattleroot

Botanical Description: This is a tall, stately plant,

having a perennial root, and a simple herbaceous stem, which rises from 4 to 8 feet in height. The leaves are large, and ternately decomposed, consisting of oblong ovate leaflets, incised and toothed at their edges. The flowers are small, white, and disposed in a long, terminal, wandlike raceme, with occasionally 1 or 2 shorter racemes near its base. The calyx is white, 4-leaved, and deciduous; the petals are minute, and shorter than the stamens; the pistil consists of an oval germ and a sessile stigma. The fruit is an ovate capsule containing numerous flat seeds.

The Black Snakeroot, or Black Cohosh, is a native of the United States, growing in shady and rocky woods, from Canada to Florida, and flowering in June and July. The root is the part employed.

This, as found in the shops, consists of a thick, irregularly bent or contorted body or caudex, from ⅓ inch to an inch in thickness, often several inches in length, furnished with many slender radicles, and rendered exceedingly rough and jagged in appearance by the remains of the stem of successive years, which to the length of 1 inch or more are frequently attached to the root. The color is externally dark brown, almost black, internally whitish; the odor is feeble; the taste bitter, herbaceous, and somewhat astringent, leaving a slight sense of acrimony. The root yields its virtues to boiling water. (U.S.D.)

Medicinal Uses: Collected in the autumn, particularly in the Blue Ridge mountains, this interesting root has been used as a relaxant, antispasmodic, and sedative. In the course of its employment as a treatment for chorea, or St. Vitus' dance, it was reported to have the undesirable side effects of inducing vomiting, giddiness, headache, and prostration. Black Cohosh has also been employed in acute and chronic rheumatism, neuralgias, and painful menstruation.

Extracts of Black Cohosh rhizomes and roots have been shown to decrease experimental inflammation by one third in laboratory animals, although the constituents responsible for this effect have not yet been identified. Thus, it appears that the use of this plant for neuralgia and rheumatism has a rational basis.

Extracts of Black Cohosh also have been tested for estrogenic effects in mice and are devoid of this

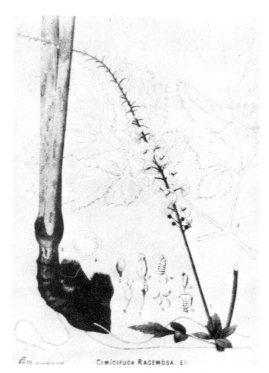

CIMICIFUGA RACEMOSA. EII

BLACK COHOSH; Collected in the autumn, particularly in the Blue Ridge Mountains, this interesting root has been used as a relaxant, antispasmodic, and sedative. Experimentally, extracts of the roots have been shown to decrease inflammation.

activity. Since this type of biological test is most always predictive for humans, it must be presumed that the use of Black Cohosh for dysmenorrhea cannot be based on an estrogenic effect. Nevertheless, folklore rarely carries useless information through time, and we must acknowledge the stated benefits of Squaw Root in female complaints.

Dose: When used in medicine, the usual dose is 2 teaspoon of powdered root per 1½ pint of boiling water, boiled in a covered container for about ½ hour, at a slow boil. Liquid allowed to cool slowly in the *closed* container. Drunk cold, 2 to 3 tablespoons 6 times a day.

COHOSH, BLUE
Caulophyllum thalictroides

PARTS USED: Root

OTHER COMMON NAMES: Papoose Root, Squaw Root

Botanical Description: Flowers late March-May.

Occurs in rich woods of valleys, ravines, north-facing wooded slopes and bluffs, and moist banks at the base of bluffs. Ranges from New Brunswick to Manitoba, south to South Carolina, Alabama, Tennessee, and Missouri; also in eastern Asia.

The unusual ultramarine blue spherical fruits are actually naked seeds surrounded by their fleshy coat. They are generally mature in summer, and are consid-

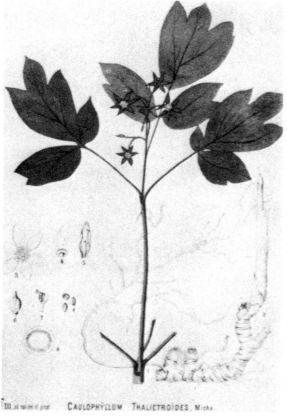

CAULOPHYLLUM THALICTROIDES, Michx.

BLUE COHOSH: The most common use of this root is to promote menstruation and to speed childbirth.

ered as poisonous if eaten by children especially.

Like the May-Apple, this plant is quite bitter, and is therefore avoided by grazing animals. The thickened rootstocks have been used in medicine. Some persons are susceptible to handling the plant and develop a dermatitis. (Missouri, Steyermark)

Medicinal Uses: The main use of the root of this perennial herb was to precipitate and promote the menstrual discharge; also to speed childbirth. Reportedly, Blue Cohosh has also been employed to purge the intestinal tract of infestations of worms. The root is a diuretic as well, promoting urination; it has also been used medicinally for its ability to produce sweating.

Dose: The medicinal preparation consists of 1 teaspoon of granulated root boiled with 1½ pints of slowly boiling water for ½ hour, in a covered container. This is drunk cold, a mouthful at a time, a total of 1 cupful per day.

COLTSFOOT
Tussilago farfara

PARTS USED: Leaves

OTHER COMMON NAMES: Coughwort, Foal's Foot, Horse Hoof, Horse Foot, Bull's Foot

Botanical Description: Coltsfoot is a perennial herb, with a creeping root, which early in the spring sends up several leafless, erect, simple, unifloral scapes or flower-stems, 5 to 6 inches high, and furnished with appressed scalelike bracts of a brownish-pink color. The flower, which stands singly at the end of the scape, is large, yellow, compound, with hermaphrodite florets in the disk, and female florets in the ray. The latter are numerous, linear, and twice the length of the former. The leaves do not make their appearance until after the flowers have blown. They are radical, petiolate, large, cordate, angular and toothed at the margin, bright green upon their upper surface, white and downy beneath.

The plant grows spontaneously both in Europe and North America. In this country it is found upon the banks of streams in the Midwest and North, and flowers in April. The leaves are most frequently employed.

They should be gathered after their full expansion, but before they have attained their greatest magnitude.

The flowers have an agreeable odor, which they retain after desiccation. The dried root and leaves are inodorous, but have a rough bitterish mucilaginous taste. Boiling water extracts all their virtues. (U.S.D)

Medicinal Uses: Coltsfoot has been recognized as a remedy for coughs and respiratory ailments since antiquity; Hippocrates recommended the root mixed with honey for ulcerations of the lungs, while other classical Greek physicians reported that the smoke of the leaves was helpful in coughs and difficult breathing. An external emollient and internal demulcent, Coltsfoot has been considered very helpful in relieving the coughs of colds, and was applied externally as a poultice for relief of chest congestion. Reportedly the fumes of the burning leaves relieved toothache.

Containing an acrid essential oil, a bitter glucoside, a resin, and gallic acid, the leaves are often used as a tobacco substitute and are sometimes smoked in an herbal blend for asthma.

Dose: CAUTION. See articles on Borage and on Comfrey. Coltsfoot preparations should be approached cautiously for the same reasons.

COMFREY
Symphytum officinale

PARTS USED: Root
OTHER COMMON NAMES: Blackwort, Bruisewort, Wallwort, Sumplant, Healing Herb

Botanical Description: Root perennial, thick, tapering, somewhat branched, fibrous, brownish black externally, white within. Stems succulent, erect, branched, rough, with strong hairs, somewhat angular, slightly membranous at the angles, about 2 feet high. Leaves alternate, large, attenuate, acute, deep green, rough, and fringed with short hairs; lower ones ovate, petiolate; upper nearly sessile, ovate-lanceolate, very decurrent, so as to form winged appendages to the stem. Flowers in a short, drooping raceme, somewhat incurved toward the summit, and generally turned toward the same side; they vary from a yellowish white to a purplish or reddish hue. Calyx divided into 5 lanceolate segments, which

are rough, erect, pointed, about the length of the tube of the corolla. Corolla cylindrical, swollen upwards, with a short tube, and divided at the limb into 5 short recurved segments, the throat closed with 5 subulate scales converging into a cone. Stamens 5, filaments short, inserted into the corolla. Anthers yellow, erect, sagittate, concealed by the scales. Ovary 4-parted, style longer than the corolla, stigma small, obtuse. Fruit consists of 4 angular, dark, shining achenia, or small nuts, situated in the bottom of the persistent calyx.

Distribution: Europe, western Siberia. In England by river banks, and in moist or watery places. Flowers May and June. (B.F.M.)

Medicinal Uses: This popular herb has been widely used for a variety of medical problems. The juice of the crushed root, mixed with wine, was drunk to stop internal bleeding, particularly uterine hermorrhaging; similarly, powdered root was snuffed up the nostrils to prevent or allay nosebleeds. External applications in the form of plasters made from decoctions of the glutinaceous root reportedly aided the knitting of tissues cut during surgery or torn apart from injury. Comfrey has also been recommended as a direct application to aid the union of fractured bones. The root, crushed and boiled, has been drunk to relieve chest congestion.

Comfrey is another example of a popular herbal preparation that should not be taken regularly by humans, for the same reason that Borage should not be used, i.e., they both contain chemical compounds that are known to be potentially toxic and/or carcinogenic (see article on Borage). While the plant may be safe in small doses, it is advisable to restrict its use until the controversy surrounding its toxicity is resolved.

On the other hand, many herbal manuals allude to the fact that Comfrey promotes the growth of healthy cells, both externally and in mucous membranes, owing to its component allantoin. While we have stated our caution, it may be reasonable to suggest that *external* applications of the leaves are still useful to heal wounds and broken bones, and to diminish various skin growths.

Dose: Avoid internally. Externally, apply freshly crushed leaves, changing twice daily.

71

CORN POPPY
Papaver rhoeas

PARTS USED: Flower petals

OTHER COMMON NAMES: Red Poppy, Corn Rose, Wind rose, Cup Rose, Canker Rose, Head-Wark

Botanical Description: The Red or Corn Poppy is distinguished by its hairy stem, which is branched and rises about a foot in height, by its incised pinnatifid leaves, by its urn-shaped capsule, and by the full, bright, scarlet color of its petals. It is a native of Europe, where it grows wild in great abundance, adorning especially the fields of grain with its brilliant flower. It has been introduced and naturalized in this country.

Its capsules contain the same kind of milky juice as that found in *P. Somniferum*, and an extract has been prepared from them having the properties of opium; but the quantity is too small to repay the trouble of its preparation. The petals are the officinal portion. They

have a narcotic smell, and a mucilaginous, slightly bitter taste. (U.S.D.)

Medicinal Uses: Although the capsules and herb of the Corn Poppy have been found to contain the same kind of milky juice as that found in the Opium poppy (*P. somniferum*), which possesses distinct narcotic and sedative properties, the quantity of active principle in this juice is too small, in proportion to the amount required to produce an effect, to warrant its extraction. The principal value of the Corn Poppy rather lies in the ability of its petals to impart their beautiful scarlet color to water, and the plant is more useful as a dye than as a medicine.

Dose: Per cup of brewed tea, use in proportions of about ¼ petals, the balance of ¾ plant materials being the medically active constituents (i.e., the petals are added for coloration effects).

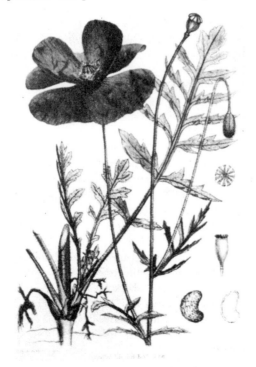

CORN POPPY: The principal value of the corn poppy lies in the ability of the petals to impart their beautiful scarlet color to water; the plant is more useful as a dye than a medicine.

COTTON
Gossypium herbaceum

PARTS USED: Root bark (inner)

Botanical Description: *Gossypium herbaceum* is a biennial or triennial plant, with a branching stem from 2 to 6 feet high, and palmate hoary leaves, the lobes of which are somewhat lanceolate and acute. The flowers possess yellow petals, having a purple spot near the claw. The leaves of the involucre or outer calyx are serrate. The capsule opens when ripe, and displays a loose white tuft of long slender filaments, which surround the seeds and adhere firmly to the outer coating. The plant is a native of Asia, but is cultivated in most tropical countries. It requires a certain duration of warm weather to perfect its seeds, and, in the United States, does not mature north of Virginia.

In consequence of changes produced in the plants of this genus by cultivation, botanists have found great difficulty in determining which are distinct species and which are merely varieties. By some taxonomists more than 50 species of *Gossypium* are recognized. There are only 5 or 6 species which yield useful products and the bulk of the cotton is the product of two species: *G. herbaceum*, which furnishes the Upland or short staple cotton, and *G. barbadense*, the source of the Sea Island or long staple cotton. All of the species are of tropical origin. The Upland cotton has been cultivated in eastern India and Arabia since ancient times. The Sea Island cotton is indigenous to America and is of the type observed by Columbus. (U.S.D.)

Medicinal Uses: The inner root bark of the Cotton plant, the most common crop in the southern United States, was used in that region instead of Ergot of rye to promote uterine contractions. It was reputed to act as a stimulant for menstruation and to arrest uterine hemorrhage. The slaves in the South used the root bark to produce abortion; and it was employed during labor, childbirth, and delivery of the placenta. Southern practitioners used the plant from 1840 well into the twentieth century; in unskilled hands, however, it was considered a dangerous

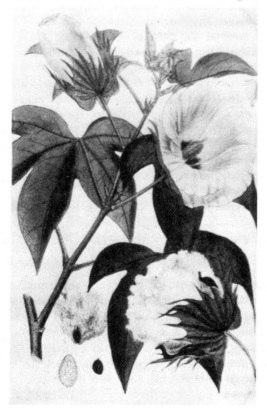

COTTON: Experimentally, extracts of the root bark have been well established as causing contractions of the uterus, not only in test tube experiments, but by administration to animals as well.

remedy, causing nausea and vomiting when taken in large doses.

Experimentally, extracts of Cotton root bark have been well established as causing contractions of the uterus, not only in test tube experiments, but by administration to animals as well. This effect, if similar in humans, would result in abortions, and would also constrict blood vessels in the vaginal tract, thus resulting in a diminution of blood flow in cases of menorrhagia. These findings support such folkloric claims.

(In India the petals are a source of a brown and yellow dye, while a mild honey is derived from the flowers in unsprayed fields.)

Dose: Not recommended. Very strong. A decoction was prepared using 1 teaspoon of the root bark per 1½ pints of water, boiled in a covered container, at a slow boil, for about ½ hour. Liquid was allowed to cool slowly in the closed container and was drunk cold, 1 swallow or 1 tablespoon at a time, 1 to 2 cups per day.

COUCH GRASS
Agropyron repens

PARTS USED: Rhizomes and roots
OTHER COMMON NAMES: Creeping Twitch, Quackgrass

Botanical Description: Culms erect from long horizontal rhizomes, usually 5–10 decimeters tall. Leaf-blades flat, soft, 5–10 millimeters wide, with numerous slender nerves about 0.2 millimeter apart. Spike 6–17 centimeters long, with numerous ascending, overlapping spikelets; rachisjoints usually flat on one side, rounded on the other. Spikelets 10–18 millimeters long, 4–8 flowered; glumes narrowly oblong to lanceolate, 8-14 millimeters long, sharply nerved, acuminate or short-awned; lemmas similar in size and shape, less sharply nerved, acuminate or with an awn up to 10 millimeters long.

Found in meadows, fields, roadsides, sea shores, and waste places, northward to Alaska, south to North Carolina, New Mexico, and California, abundant and often a noxious weed northward, chiefly introduced from Europe but apparently indigenous along the North Atlantic coast. Highly variable in color from green to glaucous, in pubescence of sheaths, blades, and rachis,

73

in shape of glumes, and in presence and length of awns. On the basis of these variations, a number of varieties have been recognized, which are so intergradient and in the field so intermingled that they probably have little taxonomic significance. (B&B)

Medicinal Uses: Dogs and cats, when they are ill, will seek out and eat this plant in preference to any other field grasses. The roots possess both diuretic and demulcent properties, and have been used by herbalists for centuries to treat inflammation of the bladder, frequent or painful urination, blood in the urine, and other urinary-tract diseases.

An old home remedy for coughing, the roasted rootstocks have also long been used as a coffee substitute and as a source of bread in times of famine.

Couch Grass roots are known to contain high concentrations of mucilage, which gives the plant its demulcent and soothing effect on mucous membranes. Water extracts of the roots of *A. repens* have been studied in laboratory animals and when administered orally give rise to pronounced diuretic effects. In addition, the extracts are known to have antibiotic effects against a variety of bacteria and molds.

Dose: 1 teaspoon of root, boiled in a covered container with 1½ pints of water for about ½ hour, at a slow boil. Liquid allowed to cool slowly in the *closed* container. Drunk cold, 1 swallow or 1 tablespoon at a time, as much as desired.

In the form of a fluidextract, 3.8 milliliters every 3 hours in 5 or 6 ounces of water.

COWSLIP
Primula veris, P. officinalis

PARTS USED: Flowers, Roots, and Leaves

Strew, strew the glad and smiling ground
With every flower, yet not confound
The primrose drop—the Spring's own
    spouse,
Bright days-eyes, and the *lips-of-cows.*
       —Ben Jonson

The Cowslips tall her pensioners be,
In their gold coats spots you see,
These be rubies, fairy favours.

Where the bee sucks there suck I,
In a Cowslip's bell I lie,
There I couch when owls do cry.
       —Shakespeare

Botanical Description: Root perennial, consisting of a fleshy rhizome, beset with several small tubercles, furnished with numerous long, nearly simple fibers. Leaves ovate-oblong, wrinkled, toothed, obtuse, more or less pubescent, bright green above, lighter beneath, and tapering into a petiole at the base, proceeding immediately from the root. From the middle of the leaves rise 1 or 2 upright scapes, naked, cylindrical, somewhat pubescent, about 4 or 5 inches high, terminated by an umbel of sweet-smelling flowers, which are pedicellate, drooping, and furnished with a short subulate bract at the base of each pedicel. Calyx pale yellowish green, permanent, tubular, with 5 angles, and 5 short obtuse teeth. Tube of the corolla as long as the calyx; limb concave, with 5 short lobes, yellow, marked near the orifice with 5 orange-colored spots. Stamens 5; filaments very short; anthers erect, acute, included in the tube. Ovary globose, surmounted by a filiform style and a globose stigma. Capsule glabrous, ovate-oblong, 1-celled, opening at the, with 10 acute teeth. Seeds numerous, brown, wrinkled, attached to a free central placenta.

Distribution: Europe, Siberia, western Asia, Northern Africa. In meadows and pastures in many parts of England. Flowers April and May. (B.F.M.)

Medicinal Uses: Once highly renowned as a narcotic and sedative, by 1837 Cowslip had ceased to be much more than a rustic remedy. Linnaeus deemed it useful as an analgesic and as a sleep inducer, as did many of the old herbalists, and at one time it was the chief plant used to treat paralysis and headache. All parts of the plant were used, but the dried flowers were believed to be most potent.

In some countries fermented beverages are made from the flowers with sugar, honey, and lemon juice, while the roots are also put into casks of wine or beer to enhance the strength and flavor of those beverages.

From all accounts it appears that Cowslip was an extremely gentle pain reliever and sleep inducer, which caused none of the undesirable side effects that are encountered in some other such remedies.

Containing primulin and cyclamin, the leaves are a good substitute for tea used to improve various nervous conditions.

Dose: Approximately ½ ounce of leaves or flowers to 1 pint of water. Water boiled separately and poured over the plant material and steeped for 5–20 minutes, depending on the desired effect. Drunk hot or warm, 1 to 2 cups or more per day, at bedtime and upon awakening.

DAMIANA
Turnera aphrodisiaca, T. diffusa

PARTS USED: Leaves
OTHER COMMON NAMES: Mexican Damiana, Pastorata, Hierba del Venado

Botanical Description: About 60 species mainly in tropical and subtropical America.

Damiana is a shrub, to 2 meters tall, usually much smaller, the herbage aromatic; leaves alternate, petiolate, oblong-elliptic to elliptic-oblanceolate, to 35 millimeters long and 15 millimeters wide, usually much smaller, cuneate at base, obtuse to subacute at apex, coarsely crenate-dentate to serrate, tomentose or merely pilose beneath, often glabrate above; flowers usually solitary, sessile, 8–12 millimeters long; peduncle often adnate to the petiole; calyx with 5 narrow lobes, tomentose; petals yellow, obovate to spatulate, thin; capsule thin-walled, 4–5 millimeters long; seeds with a membranaceous aril. On dry brushy hillsides along the Rio Grande in south Texas, throughout the year; from throughout most of tropical America. (Texas, Correll & Johnston)

Medicinal Uses: The two *Turnera* species which yield Damiana are small shrubs indigenous to southern California, Mexico, and the Antilles. The leaves are reputedly aphrodisiac, and have also been utilized for tonic, stimulant, and laxative purposes.

Damiana acquired a reputation for curing sexual impotence; however, in these treatments it was generally administered in conjunction with a more powerful stimulant such as strychnine or phosphorus, and so it is difficult to assess the degree to which Damiana alone contributed to the results.

In Mexico, the leaves are used as a substitute for Chinese tea and also to flavor liqueurs.

Damiana is one of the most popular and safest of all plants claimed to have an aphrodisiac effect. Although some sources claim that caffeine is present in this plant, we have been unable to substantiate this claim from an exhaustive search of the literature. In fact, there are no animal experiments that have been reported which would lead one to believe that Damiana has an aphrodisiac effect, and no chemical compounds have been found in this plant that would be expected to cause such an effect. Clearly, this is a plant that needs and deserves a careful chemical and pharmacological study.

Dose: 2–4 grams of the leaves in the form of an infusion or fluidextract.

DANDELION
Taraxacum officinale

PARTS USED: Leaves and root
OTHER COMMON NAMES: Puff-Ball

Botanical Description: The Dandelion is an herbaceous plant, with a perennial, fusiform root. The leaves, which spring immediately from the root, are long, pinnatifid, generally runcinate, with the divisions toothed, smooth, and of a fine green color. The common name of the plant was derived from the fancied resemblance of its leaves to the teeth of a lion. The flower-stem rises from the midst of the leaves, 6 inches or more in height. It is erect, simple, naked, smooth, hollow, fragile, and terminated by a large golden-colored flower, which closes in the evening, and expands with the returning light of the sun. The calyx is smooth and double, with the outer scales bent downwards. The florets are very numerous, ligulate, and toothed at their extremities. The receptacle is convex and punctured. The seed-

75

down is stipitate, and at the period of maturity, is disposed in a spherical form, and is so light and feathery as to be easily borne away by the wind, with the seeds attached.

This species grows spontaneously in most parts of the globe. It is abundant in this country, adorning our grass plots and pasture grounds with its bright yellow flowers, which, in moist places, show themselves with the first opening of spring, and continue to appear till near the close of summer. All parts of the plant contain a milky bitterish juice, which exudes when they are broken or wounded.

The fresh full-grown root of the Dandelion is several inches in length, about as thick as the little finger, round and tapering, somewhat branched, of a light brownish color externally, whitish within, having a yellowish ligneous cord running through its center, and abounding in a milky juice. In the dried state it is much shrunk, wrinkled longitudinally, brittle, and when broken presents a shining somewhat resinous fracture. It is without smell, but has a sweetish, mucilaginous, bitterish, herbaceous taste. Its active properties are yielded to water by boiling, and do not appear to be injured in the process. (U.S.D.)

Medicinal Uses: A mild laxative and tonic medicine, Dandelion is commonly administered as a home remedy for mild constipation and stomach ache. Dandelion leaf tea, drunk often, is recommended as an aid for promoting digestive regularity. The plant was noted to have an almost specific affinity for the liver, modifying and increasing its secretions; hence it has been used in chronic diseases of the digestive organs, especially hepatic disorders, including jaundice and chronic inflammation and enlargement of the liver.

The young leaves of Dandelion, collected in the spring, make a healthful and tasty addition to salads. The root, dried and powdered, may be added to coffee for its medicinal value or used as a coffee substitute.

Experimentally, extracts of Dandelion rhizomes and roots have been shown to increase the bile flow in animals when administered orally, and thus might have beneficial effects in hepatic disorders. The specific substance responsible for this reported cholagogue effect has not yet been identified, but it is known that the roots contain inulin, an essential oil and a bitter compound.

Although some herbalists have claimed that the plant has diuretic effects, we are unable to confirm that Dandelion has such properties on the basis of laboratory research.

Dose: Leaves: Approximately 1 ounce of leaves to 1 pint of water. Water boiled separately and poured over the plant material and steeped for 5 to 20 minutes, depending on the desired effect. Drunk hot or warm, 1 to 2 cups per day, at bedtime and upon awakening.

Root: 1 teaspoon, boiled in a covered container of 1½ pints of water for about ½ hour, at a slow boil. Liquid allowed to cool slowly in the *closed* container. Drunk cold, 1 swallow or 1 tablespoon at a time, 1 to 2 cups per day.

DEVIL'S CLAW
Harpagophytum procumbens

PARTS USED: Tuber

OTHER COMMON NAMES: Grapple Plant, Devil's Craw Root

Botanical Description: Calyx campanulate, 5-partite. Corolla 5-lobed; tube funnel-shaped, equal or slightly gibbous; lobes orbicular, sub-equal. Stamens 4, didynamous, fixed below the middle of the corolla-tube, included; anther-thecae parallel, pendulous from the apex of the connective. Disc fleshy, filated. Ovary 2-chambered, with the chambers undivided and having many ovules in 2 series attached to the septum. Fruit an ovoid or oblong 2-locular tardily dehiscent capsule, flattened at right angles to the septum, armed along the edges with 2 rows of long horny arms bearing recurved spines. Seeds numerous, obovate, horizontal.

Perennial herbs; rootstock stout; stems long, trailing; leaves shortly petioled, opposite or alternate, divided; flowers solitary on short pedicels in the axils of the leaves.

Species 3, all Africa; 2 species in South Africa, found in the Transvaal, and Griqualand West. (Phillips)

Medicinal Uses: Devil's Claw root has been introduced into North America as an herbal remedy during recent years. It is also currently very popular in Europe. For more than 250 years decoctions of the roots of this plant were popularly embraced by various cultures in South Africa, including the Hottentots, Bantus, and Bushmen. The claims for Devil's Claw root are as a tonic and for arthritis and rheumatism.

This plant has been found to contain at least three bitter principles, the main one being an iridoid glucoside named harpagide. Extracts of the plant have been evaluated in recent times in clinical trials involving human subjects with arthritis. It was claimed that the extract had a beneficial effect.

In animal studies, harpagide has shown anti-inflammatory activity in a number of different types of animal models in which inflammation was induced by the injection of various types of agents.

There have been no adverse effects published **for extracts of Devil's Claw root; thus the folkloric** claims seem to be justified. To reduce fevers an infusion of the roots is employed, while an ointment is applied to ulcers, sores, and boils.

Dose: Unknown.

DOGWOOD
Cornus florida, and other *Cornus* species

PARTS USED: Bark
OTHER COMMON NAMES: Box Wood, Flowering Cornel, Green Ozier

Botanical Description: We have ten indigenous species of *Cornus*, all of which are supposed to possess similar medicinal properties; and three—*C. florida*, *C. circinata*, and *C. sericea*—were formerly official in the *Pharmacopoeia* of the United States.

Cornus florida. This is a small indigenous tree,

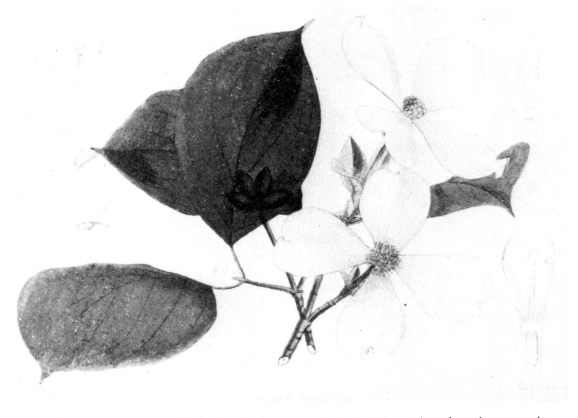

DOGWOOD: The bark possesses astringent, stimulant, and tonic properties, and was formerly very popular as a fever remedy.

usually about 15 to 20 feet in height, though sometimes not less than 30 or 35 feet. It is of slow growth; and the stem, which generally attains a diameter of 4 or 5 inches, is compact, and covered with a brownish bark, the epidermis of which is minutely divided by numerous superficial cracks or fissures. The branches are spreading, and regularly disposed, sometimes opposite, sometimes in fours nearly in the form of crosses. The leaves are opposite, oval, about 3 inches long, pointed, dark green, and sulcated on the upper surface, glaucous or whitish beneath, and marked with strong parallel veins. Toward the close of summer they are speckled with black spots, and on the approach of cold weather assume a red color. The proper flowers are small, yellowish, and collected in heads, which are surrounded by a very large conspicuous involucre, consisting of 4 white obcordate leaves, having the notch at their summit tinged with red or purple. It is this involucre that constitutes the chief beauty of the tree at the period of flowering. The calyx is 4-toothed, and the corolla composed of 4 obtuse reflexed petals. The fruit is an oval drupe of a vivid glossy red color, containing a 2-celled and 2-seeded nucleus. The drupes are usually collected together to the number of 3 or 4, and remain on the tree till after the early frosts. They ripen in September.

The Dogwood is found in all parts of the United States from Massachustts to the Mississippi and the Gulf of Mexico; but it's most abundant in the Midwest. In the month of May it is clothed with a profusion of large white blossoms, which render it one of the most conspicuous ornaments of the American forests. The bark is the officinal portion, and is derived for use both from the stem and branches, and from the root. The bark of the root is preferred. It is brought into market in pieces, of various sizes, usually more or less rolled, sometimes invested with a fawn colored epidermis, sometimes partially or wholly deprived of it, of a reddish-gray color, very brittle, and affording, when pulverized, a grayish powder tinged with red. (U.S.D.)

Medicinal Uses: The bark of the Dogwood tree possesses astringent, stimulant, and tonic properties. The bark was used in the treatment of intermittent fevers (as in malaria), and when Cinchona bark, from Peru, was unavailable, Dogwood bark was often substituted. When the al-

kaloid quinine was successfully isolated from the Peruvian bark and administered as a sulfate, the use of both Cinchona and Dogwood bark for intermittent fevers ceased almost completely. Up until that time Dogwood bark had also been given for typhoid fevers and other disorders in which the Peruvian bark was also employed.

In folk medicine the Dogwoods are esteemed for their tonic properties. Chemically the bark contains cornin, a bitter principle, and high concentrations of tannin, which explains their astringent effect.

Dose: ½ ounce of the dried powdered bark; or 1.8-3.8 milliliters of the fluidextract.

ELDER
Sambucus canadensis

PARTS USED: Flowers, berries, root, and inner bark
OTHER COMMON NAMES: Sambucus, American Elder, Sweet Elder

Botanical Description: Our indigenous common Elder is a shrub from 6 to 10 feet high, with a branching stem, which is covered with a rough gray bark, and contains a large spongy pith. The small branches and the leafstalks are very smooth. The leaves are opposite, pinnate, sometimes bipinnate, and composed usually of 3 or 4 pairs of oblong oval, acuminate, smooth, shining, deep-green leaflets, the midribs of which are somewhat pubescent. The flowers are small, white, and disposed in loose cymes, having about 5 divisions. The berries are small, globular, and when ripe of a deep purple color.

The shrub grows in low moist grounds, along fences, and on the borders of small streams, in all parts of the United States, from Canada to Carolina. It flowers from May to June, and ripens its berries early in the autumn. (U.S.D.)

Medicinal Uses: The medicinal properties of the Elder have been recognized since the time of the ancient Greeks; Hippocrates mentions its employment as a purgative. One ounce of pure juice squeezed from the berries will strongly purge. A tea made from the root of the Elder, taken daily in

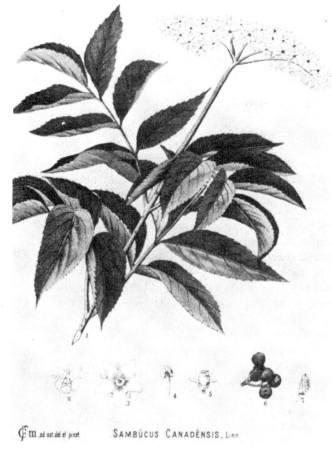

SAMBÚCUS CANADÉNSIS, Linn.

ELDER: The inner bark and young leaf buds of this shrub promote the watery evacuation of the bowels. However, the young leaf buds are so violent in their purgative action that they are considered particularly unsafe.

half-ounce doses, will perform as a gentle laxative. The juice from the berries was also used as a remedy for rheumatism, gout, external skin eruptions, and syphilis. The berries are also the source of the popular elderberry wine, as well as a jam.

The inner bark and the young leaf buds, as well as the juice of the root, are all considered active hydragogue cathartics, promoting the watery evacuation of the bowels. The plant was therefore used to treat dropsical affections. The inner bark was considered emetic in strong doses. The young leaf buds are so violent in their purgative action that they are considered unsafe.

The flowers were utilized in the form of poultices, fomentations, and ointments for topical application to lesions, tumors, and rheumatic limbs. They were considered gently excitant and sudorific, although they were rarely taken internally. Today, however, they are utilized in eye washes.

Dose: Those who use this herb begin with a mild dosage, and then increase gradually if necessary.

Flowers: External use—macerated with olive oil and applied topically. For eyewash, infusion consisting of approximately 1 ounce of flowers to 1 pint of sterile water. Water boiled separately and poured over the plant material and steeped for 5-20 minutes.

Leaf buds: UNSAFE. Do not use.

Berries: Fresh juice, 1 ounce, is a strong purgative.

Inner bark and root juice: Mild decoction of 1 teaspoon of plant material boiled in a covered container with 1 pint of water for only 5 minutes, cooled slowly in closed container and drunk cold, 1 swallow or 1 tablespoon at a time, 1 to 2 cups per day.

Dried root: 1 teaspoon of root, boiled in covered container with 1½ pints of water for about ½ hour, at a slow boil. Liquid allowed to cool slowly in the *closed* container. Drunk cold, 1 swallow or 1 tablespoon at a time, no more than ½ ounce dose daily.

ELECAMPANE
Inula helenium

PARTS USED: Root
OTHER COMMON NAMES: Scabwort

Botanical Description: Elecampane has a perennial root, and an annual stem which is round, furrowed, villous, leafy, from 3 to 6 feet high, and branched near the top. The leaves are large, ovate, serrate, crowded with reticular veins, smooth and deep green upon the upper surface, downy on the under, and furnished with a fleshy midrib. Those which spring directly from the root are petiolate, those of the stem sessile and embracing. The flowers are large, of a golden yellow color, and stand singly at the ends of the stem and branches. The calyx exhibits several rows of imbricated ovate scales. The florets of the ray are numerous, spreading, linear, and tridentate at the apex. The seeds are striated, quadrangular, and furnished with a simple, somewhat chaffy pappus.

79

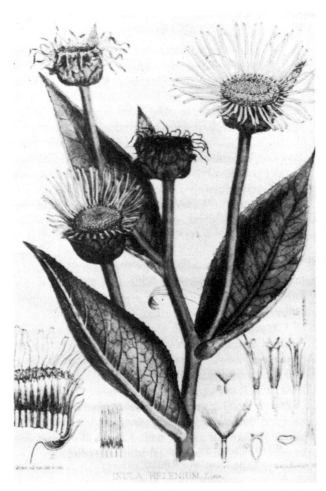

ELECAMPANE: This large and handsome plant has been used in medicine for thousands of years. Its tonic properties are confirmed by the lactones contained in the rhizomes and roots.

This large and handsome plant is a native of Europe, where it is also cultivated for medical use. It has been introduced into our gardens, and has become naturalized in some parts of the country, growing in low meadows, and on the roadsides, from New England to Pennsylvania. It flowers in July and August. The roots, which are the officinal part, should be dug up in autumn, and in the second year of their growth. When older they are apt to be stringy and woody.

The fresh root of Elecampane is very thick and branched, having whitish cylindrical ramifications which are furnished with threadlike fibers. It is externally brown, internally whitish and fleshy; and the transverse sections present radiating lines. The dried root, as found in the shops, is usually in longitudinal or transverse slices, and of a graying color internally. The smell is slightly camphorous, and, especially in the dried root, agreeably aromatic. The taste, at first glutinous and said to resemble that of rancid soap, be-

comes, upon chewing, warm, aromatic, and bitter. Its medical virtues are extracted by alcohol and water, the former becoming most strongly impregnated with its bitterness and pungency. (U.S.D.)

Medicinal Uses: Elecampane has been used in folk medicine for thousands of years, and was well known to the ancient Greeks. It was valued for its ability to promote menstruation, as a tonic and a gentle stimulant, and as a means of promoting perspiration, particularly in relieving the common cold. As a diuretic the root was employed in cases of dropsy, or water retention. The root was also used as an expectorant, aiding the discharge of matter from the lungs; it was particularly valued in chronic conditions in which lung problems were accompanied by gastric complaints, since it was the one medicine which was applicable for both conditions. Elecampane was applied externally as well as taken internally for a variety of skin eruptions. After its use in medicine declined, it remained popular in veterinary practice.

The rhizomes and roots of Elecampane are known to contain several sesquiterpene lactones, many of which have varying degrees of antiseptic properties. They are also all bitter substances, and thus would produce a tonic effect if extracts of this plant were taken orally.

Dose: 1 teaspoon of root, boiled in a covered container of 1½ pints water for about ½ hour, at a slow boil. Liquid allowed to cool slowly in the *closed* container. Drunk cold, 1 swallow or 1 tablespoon at a time, 1 to 2 cups per day.

EPHEDRA
Ephedra trifurca, and other *Ephedra* species

PARTS USED: Branches
OTHER COMMON NAMES: Ma Huang, Mormon Tea

Botanical Description: *Ephedra trifurca* is an erect shrub to 2 meters high; branches rigid, hard, terete, to 3.5 millimeters thick, solitary or whorled at the nodes; internodes 3-9 centimeters long; young stems pale green, almost smooth, with numerous small longitudinal furrows, becoming yellow, then gray-green; bark of

80

older stems cinereous, cracked and somewhat irregularly fissured longitudinally; terminal buds 1 centimeter long, spinose; leaves ternately whorled, 5-13 millimeters long, subspinosely tipped from a dorsomedian thickening, connate for one-half to three-fourths their total length; sheath at first membranaceous, later fibrous, shredded and grayish, persistent; cones sessile or shortly scaly-pedunculate, solitary or numerous in a whorl at the nodes of the young branches, elliptic to obovate; staminate cones 6-9 millimeters long; staminate bracts ternate, in 8 to 12 whorls, obovate, slightly clawed, 3-4 millimeters long, 2-3 millimeters broad, membranaceous, reddish-brown, the lower whorls empty; perianth almost equaling the subtending bract, staminal column 4-5 millimeters long, one-fourth exserted, with 4 to 5 short-stipitate anthers; ovulate cones 10-14 millimeters long; ovulate bracts ternate, in 6 to 9 whorls, orbicular, clawed, 8-12 millimeters long and broad, translucent except for the reddish-brown center and basal portion, margins entire; seed solitary or (occasionally) two or three, usually tetragonal, light-brown, smooth, 9-14 millimeters long, 1.5-3 millimeters wide, equalling the bracts; tubillus straight, twisted, about 1 millimeter long, conspicuously exserted. Sandy and gravelly soils on hills and plains, along dry creek beds in arroyos and in desert scrub areas in west Texas east to Loving, Ward, and Pecos counties; from west Texas and southern New Mexico, west to California and adjacent Mexico.

This species is easily recognized by its yellowed and spinosely tipped branches and the frayed but persistent spinose leaves of the older stems. (Texas)

Medicinal Uses: Ephedra, of which there are approximately 40 species, is one of the most valuable contributions of the Chinese to Western medicine. The plant has been in use in Chinese medicine for over five thousand years; in that country it has been employed to relieve cough and reduce fevers.

Ephedrine, the alkaloid derived from the branches of the plant, is employed as a vasoconstrictor and cardiac stimulant, and as a bronchodilator in the treatment of hay fever and asthma. Topically, Ephedra has been used as an eyewash.

Most Ephedra species contain the alkaloid ephedrine in all parts of the plant. Ephedrine produces many effects when taken orally by humans, the most important being dilation of the bronchioles of the lungs and increase in blood pressure. The major use of Ephedra, therefore, is to relieve the symptoms of bronchial asthma.

Dose: For both internal and external use, an infusion is prepared using approximately ½ ounce of the branches to 1 pint of water. Water boiled separately and poured over the plant material and steeped for 5 to 20 minutes, depending on the desired effect. When taken internally, it is drunk hot or warm, 1 to 2 cups per day.

ERGOT
Claviceps purpurea

PARTS USED: Sclerotium of fungus

Botanical Description: Ergot is the sclerotium of the fungus *Claviceps purpurea*, originating in the ovary of *Secale cereale*, the rye plant.

In all the Gramineae, or grass family, and in some of the Cyperaceae, the place of the grains or fruits is sometimes occupied by a morbid growth which, from its resemblance to the spur of a cock, has received the name Ergot (adapted from the French). This product is most frequent in the rye, *Secale cereale*, and from that grain it was adopted in the first edition of the *U.S. Pharmacopoeia*, under the name of *Secale cornutum*, or Spurred Rye.

Investigations have shown that Ergot is not the diseased grain of the rye, but the sclerotium of a fungus, the *Claviceps purpurea*. This fungus has three stages in its life history. (U.S.D.)

Medicinal Uses: When the fungus *Claviceps purpurea* parasitizes the rye embryo (*Secale cereale*), a dark-brown or purple hardened mass forms, which is called a sclerotium. This is more commonly known as Ergot, or *Secale cornutum*. Other fungi are known to parasitize a number of grasses to form such sclerotia, and in some cases the product has the same or similar biological effects as Ergot.

In the Middle Ages epidemics of ergotism from eating contaminated rye flour were characterized by both gangrenous and convulsive symptoms.

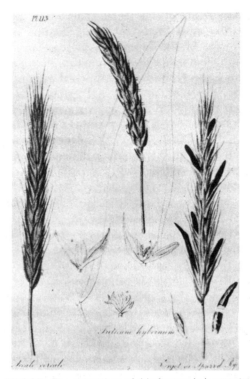

ERGOT: The sclerotium of this fungus is known to contain a number of complex and potent alkaloids, some of which have the lysergic acid (LSD-like) basic skeleton.

The principal uses of Ergot are as a uterine stimulant and as a vasoconstrictor. It was long used by midwives to promote contraction of the uterus during labor, particularly at the end of the second stage, to speed childbirth and prevent possible postpartum hermorrhage. Ergot was also used in the nonpregnant uterus to check excessive menstrual bleeding or other uterine hermorrhaging. Ergot alkaloids also have important applications in the treatment of migraine. This medicinal fungus also stimulates other involuntary muscle fibers, including the heart and the arteries.

The sclerotium of Ergot is known to contain a number of complex and potent alkaloids, some of which have the lysergic acid (LSD-like) basic skeleton. The two major indole alkaloids are ergonovine, which acts primarily to contract uterine muscle and to constrict blood vessels of the endometrium of the uterus, and ergotamine. Ergotamine acts primarily on the blood vessels of the brain, with minimal effects indicated here for ergonovine. Thus, Ergot (or ergonovine) has been an indispensable drug for centuries for use in obstetrics. It initiates contractions of the pregnant uterus, primarily at the time of delivery, and is used to aid difficult deliveries. Of greater importance is the fact that Ergot constricts blood vessels of the endometrium, and prevents the hemorrhaging that often accompanies childbirth.

A common belief is that Ergot extracts are useful, when taken *orally*, to induce abortion. There is no evidence that supports this belief, since Ergot only acts in the terminal stages of pregnancy, when abortion is not desired (abortion being the expulsion of fetus). Thus Ergot preparations do not usually induce abortion, but are extremely useful to aid in term delivery of the fetus, to expel the placenta, and to prevent hermorrhage after delivery.

Maximum labor-induction effect is attained only by injection of Ergot extract or ergonovine.

The other useful alkaloid of Ergot, ergotamine, is used extensively to relieve the symptoms of migraine headaches. Ergot itself is not used for this purpose, because of the predominant effects of this drug in the crude form on the uterus.

It must be pointed out that regular use of Ergot preparations must be avoided, since the blood vessels of the extremities, i.e., fingers and toes, will be constricted. This constriction restricts the blood supply to the extremities, and the end result is gangrene.

As with any drug plant, when used properly and in the correct amount, its virtues are an asset. When misused, the attributes are changed to the detriment of the health and well-being of the user.

Dose: CAUTION. Only prepared pharmaceutical preparations are advised. Avoid self-medication.

EUCALYPTUS
Eucalyptus globulus

PARTS USED: Leaves; also oil distilled therefrom
OTHER COMMON NAMES: Blue Gum Tree, Australian Fever-Tree

Botanical Description: About 300 species of trees and a

few shrubs belonging to the genus *Eucalyptus* are natives of Australia and Malaysia. All species of *Eucalyptus* commonly have alternate, thick, entire leaves; those on young shoots sometimes opposite, stemless, wide to heart-shaped, or even united around the stem (for example, *E. globulus*). White to yellow or red flowers form clusters or heads of 3 or more, or rarely are solitary. The calyx tube is bell-shaped and edged with 4 teeth or none, the petals joined to the calyx and forming a lid, which on opening falls off and leaves the numerous stamens. The fruiting capsule opens at the top by 3 to 6 valves and contains numerous angled seeds. (Neal)

Medicinal Uses: Eucalyptus had applications in the treatment of respiratory ailments, both through the smoking of the leaves for relief of bronchitis and asthma, and through the inhalation of the steam of a mixture of a few drops of the oil to a gallon of boiling water, as a stimulating expectorant to treat chronic bronchitis and tuberculosis as well as asthma.

The volatile oil, distilled from the leaves, has also been used as a germicide and has been applied locally as an antiseptic; in this connection it has been employed to treat both skin diseases and upper respiratory infections.

Eucalyptus oil was sometimes used as a substitute for quinine in the treatment of malaria and other intermittent fevers. The leaves have a characteristic aromatic odor that is due to an essential oil made up almost entirely of a monoterpene compound known as eucalyptol. Eucalyptus essential oil and eucalyptol are both known by animal and human testing to dilate the bronchioles in the lungs, and to have antiseptic effects against a variety of microorganisms. Experiments have also shown that Eucalyptus preparations have stimulating expectorant properties.

Dose: 0.65-2 grams of the leaves to 1 pint of water. Water boiled separately and poured over the plant material and steeped for 5-20 minutes, depending on the desired effect. Drunk hot or warm, 1 to 2 cups per day.

The oil may be used in the amount of 0.3-0.6 milliliter in water.

EYEBRIGHT
Euphrasia officinalis

PARTS USED: Herb
OTHER COMMON NAMES: Eyewort

Botanical Description: Root annual, twisted, dark brown, slender, with several minute, whitish fibers. Stems 3 or 4 inches high, branched from the base, purplish, occasionally simple, nearly square, slightly pubescent. Leaves small, in pairs, nearly sessile, tending upwards, somewhat concave, smooth, ovate, deeply toothed, light green, deeper at the margin, and tinged with purple; veins branching, prominent beneath. Flowers solitary and sub-sessile in the axils of the upper leaves, which they rather exceed in length. Calyx tubular, angular, pubescent, light green with purplish ribs, and divided at the margin into 4 deep, erect, nearly equal, emarginate lobes. Stamens didynamous, with thread-shaped filaments; anthers 2-celled, purple, spurred at the base. Ovary ovate, 4-parted, rather hairy, surmounted by a filiform, downy style, and an obtuse, bifid stigma, fringed with minute glands. Capsule ovate-oblong, compressed, emarginate, 2-valved, and 2-celled, containing several whitish, striated seeds.

Distribution: Europe (Arctic), northern Asia, western Asia to the Himalayas, North America. Common in meadows and heaths in England. Flowers May to September. (B.F.M.)

Medicinal Uses: Eyebright has been mentioned as a medicinal plant since it appeared in an herbal in 1305. It is a very old and revered folk medicine for all sorts of eye troubles. The powers of the herb are even recorded by the poet Milton:

Michael from Adam's eye the film removed,
Which the false fruit, that promised clearer sight,
Had bred; then purged with "euphrasy" and rue
The visual nerve, for he had much to see.
    —*Paradise Lost*, Book xi, line 412

Eyebright had the reputation of being able to restore sight to persons over seventy years of age; it was used to treat cataract, inflammation, and

83

irritation. The expressed juice of the plant was used in Iceland to treat all sorts of eye complaints, and in Scotland the Highlanders mixed the juice with milk and applied the lotion to the eyes with a feather.

Besides its widespread employment in eye problems, the herb was also occasionally used to treat jaundice, loss of memory, and vertigo.

And Shenstone exclaims:

Famed *euphrasy* may not be left unsung,
That gives dim eyes to wander leagues
    around.

Dose: Approximately ½ ounce of herb to 1 pint of water. Water boiled separately and poured over the plant material and steeped for 5-20 minutes, depending on the desired effect. Drunk hot or warm, 1 to 2 cups per day, at bedtime and upon awakening. As an eyewash (when cool) its action is healing and strengthening (one part of the herb to 6 parts of water).

FENNEL
Foeniculum vulgare, F. officinale

PARTS USED: Fruit, stem, and root
OTHER COMMON NAMES: Finkel

Botanical Description: Fennel has a perennial, tapering root, and an annual, erect, round, striated, smooth, glaucous, jointed, and branching stem, which usually rises 3 or 4 feet in height. The leaves, which stand alternately at the joints of the stem, upon membranous striated sheaths, are many times pinnate, with long, linear, pointed, smooth, deep green leaflets. The flowers are yellow, and form large, many-rayed umbels, destitute both of general and partial involucres. The corolla consists of 5 ovate, emarginate leaflets, with their points turned inwards. The flower is succeeded by 2 ovate seeds.

There are several varieties of this plant; but the Sweet Fennel, derived originally from the south of Europe, and cultivated in our gardens, is the one which furnishes the seeds of the shops. The whole plant has an aromatic odor and taste, dependent on a volatile oil by which it is pervaded.

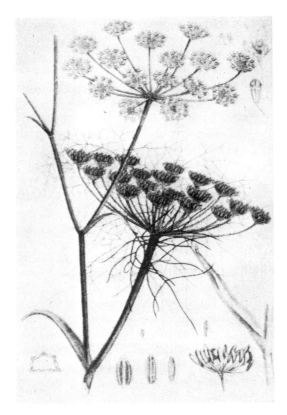

FENNEL: A decoction of the dried seeds is highly valued in preventing colic in infants. Hippocrates and Dioscorides employed the plant to increase the secretion of milk in nursing mothers.

Fennel seeds are oblong oval, flat on one side, convex on the other, not unfrequently connected by their flat surfaces, straight or slightly curved, of a graying-green color, with longitudinal yellowish ridges on the convex surface. Their odor is fragrant, their taste warm, sweet, and agreeably aromatic. The seeds of domestic growth are usually smaller and darker, but sweeter than the imported. They impart their virtues to hot water, but more abundantly to alcohol. Their essential oil may be separated by distillation with water. (U.S.D.)

Medicinal Uses: Fennel was employed by the ancient physicians Hippocrates and Dioscorides to increase the secretion of milk in nursing mothers. Pliny recommended that it be used in visual problems, including blindness, on the basis of the old observation that serpents, when they shed their skins, eat the plant to restore their sight.

The entire plant has a fragrant, aromatic odor; it has been widely employed in foods both for flavoring and as a vegetable, both raw and cooked. Fennel is used to flavor absinthe and other liquors.

Topically, the gum-resin from the cut stems was applied to treat indolent tumors and chronic swellings. The juice expressed from the root was considered a diuretic and was given for intermittent fever. Externally it was popular as a remedy for toothache and earache.

The main applications of the plant are as an aromatic, stimulant, and carminative, and especially to prevent colic in infants. It is often combined with Senna or Rhubarb to make these stronger-tasting medicinals more palatable as well as more tolerable to the upset gastrointestinal tract. An infusion of Fennel seeds was administered as an enema to infants to aid expulsion of flatus.

Fennel remained an important element of veterinary medicine long after its use in human ailments declined.

Oil of Fennel is known to contain 50 to 60 percent anethol, and 20 percent fenchose, chavicol, and anisic aldehyde.

Dose: In its fresh state, the drug is too irritant. A decoction is prepared, using ½ ounce of crushed dried plant material (at least 1 year old) to 1 pint of water, boiled in a covered container for about ½ hour, at a slow boil. Liquid allowed to cool slowly in the *closed* container. Drunk cold, 1 swallow or 1 tablespoon at a time, 1 to 2 cups per day.

FEVERFEW, EUROPEAN
Chrysanthemum parthenium (Matricaria parthenium)

PARTS USED: Flowering tops, sometimes whole herb

OTHER COMMON NAMES: Wild Quinine

Botanical Description: Root perennial, thick, much branched, with numerous long tufted fibers. Stem erect, firm, smooth, striated, branched, about 2 feet high. Leaves alternate, petiolate, light ash-colored green, pinnated; pinnules more or less ovate, decurrent, pinnatifid, with incised, somewhat obtuse lobes. Flowers large, pedunculate, disposed in a corymbose manner at the extremity of the stem and branches. Involucre hemispherical, imbricated with membranous scales, somewhat villous at the margin. Florets of the disk numerous, perfect, tubular, and 5-toothed, yellow; those of the ray pistilliferous, short, oblong, nearly round, with three small terminal teeth, white. Filaments 5, very short; anthers forming a hollow cylinder. Ovary angular, abrupt, with a short filiform style, and a bifid, obtuse, spreading stigma. Receptacle naked, slightly conical, brownish black, dotted. Fruit oblong, truncate at the base, smooth, furrowed, whitish, destitute of pappus, crowned with a shallow, slightly toothed, membranous border.

Distribution: Middle and southern Europe, introduced into many parts; a garden escape in England. Flowers July to September. (B.F.M.)

Medicinal Uses: Feverfew smells, tastes, and looks like Roman Chamomile (*Anthemis nobilis*). In France the two plants were at one time used interchangeably. A Cuban variety of the plant was used by local practitioners as a febrifuge and antiperiodic to treat intermittent fevers; an American variety was used in the southwest United States as a tonic and antiperiodic. The plant's action against fevers earned it its name, Feverfew.

Since ancient times, physicians dating back to Dioscorides have considered the herb to be especially valuable for its action on the uterus. It was thought to promote menstrual evacuation, as well as the lochial discharge after childbirth; it was used during difficult parturitions as an aid in the expulsion of the placenta.

The plant has also been used as an antispasmodic, stomachic, diuretic, and treatment for ague. In foods, this perennial herb is sometimes added in wine making and certain pastries, for its flavor, which is similar to that of Roman Chamomile.

Dose: Approximately ½ ounce of flowering tops or whole herb to 1 pint of water. Water boiled separately and poured over the plant material and steeped for 5-20 minutes, depending on the desired effect. Drunk hot or warm, 1 to 2 cups per day, at bedtime and upon wakening.

FLAX
Linum usitatissimum

PARTS USED: Seeds
OTHER COMMON NAMES: Linseed, Lint Bells

Botanical Description: Common Flax is an annual plant with an erect, slender, round stem, about two feet in height, branching at top, and, like all other parts of the plant, entirely smooth. The leaves are small, lanceolate, acute, entire, of a pale-green color, sessile, and scattered alternately over the stem and branches. The flowers are terminal and of a delicate blue color. The calyx is persistent, and composed of 5 ovate, sharp-pointed, 3 nerved leaflets, which are membranous on their border. The petals are 5, obovate, striated, minutely scalloped at their extremities, and spread into funnel-shaped blossoms. The filaments are also 5, united at the base; and the germ, which is ovate, supports 5 slender styles, terminating in obtuse stigmas. The fruit is a globular capsule, about the size of a small pea, having the persistent calyx at the base, crowned with a sharp spine, and containing ten seeds in distinct cells.

This highly valuable plant, now almost everywhere cultivated, is said by some to have been originally derived from Egypt, by others from the great elevated plain of central Asia. It flowers in June and July, and ripens its seeds in August. Both the seeds, and an oil expressed from them, are officinal.

The seeds are oval, oblong, flattened on the sides with acute edges, somewhat pointed at one end, smooth, glossy, of a brown color externally, and yellowish-white within. They are without smell, and have an oily mucilaginous taste. Their cuticle abounds in a peculiar gummy matter, which is readily imparted to hot water, forming a thick viscid mucilaginous fluid, bearing some resemblance to the solution of Gum Arabic, but differing from it in several respects. (U.S.D.)

Medicinal Uses: It is estimated that Flax has been grown as a fiber crop, for weaving into fabric, since the twenty-third century B.C. The seed is a valuable demulcent and emollient, with soothing qualities both internally for coughs and externally for skin irritations. The soothing mucilage is obtained by infusing the seeds in water. This infusion is valuable in treating irritations and inflammations of the mucous membranes, particularly of the lungs, intestines, and urinary passages; it has therefore been used for pulmonary catarrhs, dysentery, diarrhea, urinary infections, kidney diseases, and urinary stones. A laxative enema is derived from the decoction.

The meal, from the pressed seeds, mixed with hot water, makes an excellent emollient poultice. Linseed oil, expressed from the seeds, also has emollient properties and is applied externally for burns and scalds, mixed with lime water or oil or turpentine; this treatment is said to reduce the pain considerably and prevent undue blistering.

Flax seeds have a thick outer coating of mucilage cells. When water comes in contact with these cells they swell and give rise to a soothing, demulcent and/or emollient protective effect. When the skin or mucous membranes are coated with this mucilage, this effect becomes evident.

The seeds also contain a high concentration of fixed oil, which explains the laxative effect when taken internally.

Dose: Infusion of seeds—½ ounce of seeds to 1 pint of water. Water boiled separately and poured over the seeds and steeped for 5 to 20 minutes. Drunk hot or warm, 1 to 2 cups per day.

As a laxative, 1 tablespoon of the seeds is taken orally.

FOXGLOVE
Digitalis purpurea

PARTS USED: Leaves
OTHER COMMON NAMES: Fairy Bells, Lady's Glove, Cottagers, Digitale

Botanical Description: Foxglove is a beautiful plant, with a biennial or perennial, fibrous root, which sends forth large tufted leaves, and a single, erect, downy, and leafy stem, rising from 2 to 5 feet in height, and terminating in an elegant spike of purple flowers. The lower leaves are ovate, pointed, about 8 inches in length, and 3 in breadth, and stand upon short winged footstalks; the upper are alternate, sparse, and lanceolate; both are obtusely serrated at their edges, and have wrinkled velvety surfaces, of which the upper is of a fine deep-green color, and the under paler and more downy. The flowers are numerous, and attached to the upper part of the stem by short peduncles, in such a manner as generally to hang down upon one side. At the base of each peduncle is a floral leaf, which is sessile, ovate, and pointed. The calyx is divided into 5 segments, of which the uppermost is narrower than the others. the corolla is monopetalous, bell-form, swelling on the lower side, irregularly divided at the margin into short obtuse lobes, and in shape and size bearing some resemblance to the end of the finger of a glove, a circumstance which has suggested most of the names by which the plant is designated in different languages. The mouth of the corolla is guarded by long, soft hairs. Its general color is bright purple; but sometimes the flowers are whitish. The internal surface is sprinkled with black spots upon a white ground. The filaments are white, curved, and surmounted by large yellow anthers. The style, which is simple, supports a bifid stigma. The seeds are very small, numerous, of a dark color, and contained in a pyramidal, 2-celled capsule.

The foxglove grows wild in most of the temperate countries of Europe, where it flowers in the middle of the summer. In this country it is cultivated both as an ornamental garden plant, and for medicinal purposes. (U.S.D.)

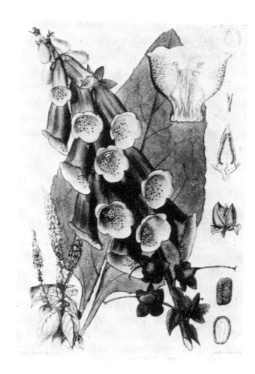

FOXGLOVE: Probably the best example of an herbal remedy that eventually became a drug indispensable to the medical profession are the leaves of this spectacular plant, which yield digitalis.

Medicinal Uses: Probably the best example of an herbal remedy that eventually became an indispensable drug to the medical profession are the leaves of Foxglove *(D. purpurea)*. The point of departure was that Foxglove was being used by a Welsh woman as one of several plants in a tea for the treatment of dropsy. (Dropsy is a symptom of a poorly operating heart, with a resulting accumulation of fluid in the body, particularly in the legs and ankles.) The English botanist Dr. William Withering observed this use in 1775, and by experimentation found that the major plant in the mixture responsible for this effect was *Digitalis purpurea* leaves. Withering then used an infusion of the leaves of this plant in his medical practice for the treatment of dropsy, a symptom of congestive heart failure.

Digitalis, the active principle of Foxglove, came to be used as a stimulant in acute circulatory failure, as a diuretic, and as a cardiac tonic in chronic heart disorders.

Prior to the discovery of its cardiac applications in 1775, Foxglove was used as an expectorant, in epilepsy, and to reduce glandular swellings. The juice obtained by bruising the leaves was mixed with honey and drunk to purge the gastrointestinal tract in both directions. Culpepper recommended that Foxglove be used in treating obstructions of the liver and spleen, as well as externally for scabies. The plant was used externally in Italy to heal wounds and reduce swellings.

The cardiotonic and diuretic effects of digitalis make Foxglove very useful in cases of dropsy associated with heart disease; the drug reduces the force and velocity of the circulation and helps to regulate irregular heartbeats.

Both powdered Foxglove leaves and the major active principle, digitoxin, are currently widely used for the treatment of congestive heart failure.

87

A symptom of overdose is vomiting, but when taken in proper amounts Foxglove causes the heart to beat slower and stronger, which then causes fluids to be excreted from the body more efficiently, resulting in a secondary diuretic effect.

Dose: Digitalis preparations are very powerful medicines, and should only be used cautiously, under proper medical supervision. An overdose could be fatal.

GENTIAN, YELLOW
Gentiana lutea

PARTS USED: Root and rhizome
OTHER COMMON NAMES: Bitter Root, Fel Root

Botanical Description: Yellow Gentian is among the most remarkable of the species which compose the *Gentiana* genus, both for its beauty, and its great comparative size. From its thick, long, branching, perennial root, an erect, round stem rises to the height of 3 or 4 feet, bearing opposite, sessile, oval, acute, 5-nerved leaves, of a bright green color, and somewhat glaucous. The lower leaves, which spring from the root, are narrowed at their base into the form of a petiole. The flowers are large and beautiful, of a yellow color, peduncled, and placed in whorls at the axils of the upper leaves. The calyx is a membranous deciduous spathe; the corolla is rotate, and deeply divided into 5 lanceolate, acute segments.

This plant grows among the Appenines, the Alps, the Pyrenees, and in other mountainous or elevated regions of Europe. Its root and rhizomes are the only parts used in medicine. (U.S.D.)

Medicinal Uses: Gentian has been used medicinally since ancient times; it is said to have derived its name from Gentius, a king of Illyria. It is a constituent of many of the complex medicinal preparations handed down from the Greeks and Arabs.

It is an excellent bitter, stimulating gastric digestion. It has been given to treat problems arising from weakened muscular tone of the digestive organs, and as an appetite stimulant it is useful for convalescing and weak patients. At one time Gentian was used as a remedy for intermit-

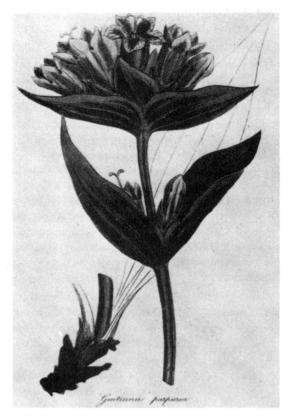

Gentiana purpurea

GENTIAN: Used medicinally since ancient times, this beautiful species is used as a bitter tonic to stimulate the appetite. It is a frequent constitutent of many of the complex medicinal preparations handed down from the Greeks and Arabs.

tent (malarial) fevers, and for gout. Overdosing may produce nausea and vomiting.

Yellow Gentian contains a complex mixture of chemical substances of the xanthone, iridoid, and monoterpenoid alkaloid type. All of these are extremely bitter substances. Thus, it is clear that Gentian preparations owe their bitter tonic effect to one or more of these substances.

Collected in late summer or autumn, the roots must be cured prior to use.

Dose: 1 teaspoon of the root, powdered, boiled in a covered container of 1½ pints of water for about ½ hour, at a slow boil. Liquid allowed to cool slowly in the *closed* container. Drunk cold, 1 swallow or 1 tablespoon at a time, 1 to 2 cups per day. (To reduce the desire for cigarettes chew the root.)

GINGER
Zingiber officinale

PARTS USED: Rhizome

Botanical Description: The Ginger plant has a perennial, creeping, tuberous root, and an annual stem, which rises 2 or 3 feet in height, is solid, round, erect, and enclosed in an imbricated membranous sheathing. The leaves are lanceolate, acute, smooth, 5 or 6 inches long by about an inch in breadth, and stand alternately on the sheaths of the stem. The scape or flowerstalk rises by the side of the stem from 6 inches to a foot high, like it is clothed with oval acuminate sheaths, but is without leaves, and terminates in an oval, obtuse, bracteal, imbricated spike. The flowers are of a dingy yellow color, and appear 2 or 3 at a time between the bracteal scales.

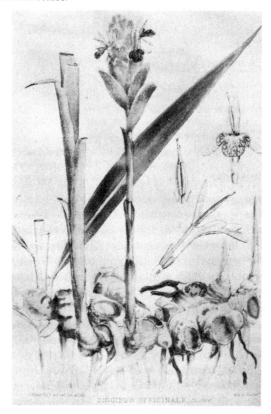

GINGER: This widely used condiment is also employed in gastrointestinal upsets, including flatulence. Applied externally, the root has been known to relieve headache and toothache.

The plant is a native of India, and is cultivated in all parts of that country. The flowers have an aromatic smell, and the stems, when bruised, are slightly fragrant; but the root is the portion in which the virtues of the plant reside. This is fit to be dug up when a year old.

The recent root is an inch or more in length, somewhat flattened on its upper and under surface, knotty, obtusely and irregularly branched or lobed, externally of a light ash color, and marked with circular rugae, internally fleshy, and yellowish-white. It sometimes germinates when kept in the shops. (U.S.D.)

Medicinal Uses: This widely used condiment has also had important medicinal applications. It is mainly employed in gastrointestinal upsets; as a stimulant and carminative (removing gas from the gastrointestinal tract) it is used to treat indigestion and flatulence. Because of these properties, as well as its aromatic qualities, it is often combined with bitters to make them more palatable; Ginger adds an agreeable, warming feeling.

Ginger tea has become a popular remedy for colds, producing perspiration and also helping to bring on menstruation if suppressed by a cold. Externally, Ginger is a rubefacient, and has been credited in this connection with relieving headache and toothache.

The flavor is due to the presence of borneol, while gingerol imparts its pungency.

Dose: Approximately 1 ounce of rhizome to 1 pint of water. Water boiled separately and poured over the plant material and steeped for 5 to 20 minutes, depending on the desired effect. Drunk hot or warm, 1 to 2 cups per day.

GINSENG
Panax quinquefolium, P. ginseng,
Eleutherococcus senticosus

PARTS USED: Root
OTHER COMMON NAMES: American Ginseng, Korean Ginseng, Siberian Ginseng

Botanical Description: The Ginseng has a perennial root, which sends up annually a smooth, round stem, about a foot in height, dividing at the summit into 3 leafstalks, each of which supports a compound leaf,

89

consisting of 5, or more rarely of 3 or 7 petiolate, oblong obovate, acuminate, serrate leaflets. The flowers are small, greenish, and arranged in a simple umbel, supported by a peduncle, which rises from the top of the stem in the center of the petioles. The fruit consists of kidney-shaped, scarlet berries, crowned with the styles and calyx, and containing 2, and sometimes 3 seeds.

The plant is indigenous, growing in the hilly regions of the northern, middle, and western states, and preferring the shelter of thick, shady woods. It is also a native of China. The root is the part employed.

The root is fleshy, somewhat spindleshaped, from one to three inches long, about as thick as the little finger, and terminated by several slender fibers. Frequently there are 2 portions, sometimes 3 or more, connected at their upper extremity, and bearing a supposed though very remote resemblance to the human figure, from which circumstance it is said that the Chinese name *ginseng* originated. When dried, the root is yellowish-white and wrinkled externally, and within consists usually of a hard central portion, surrounded by a soft whitish bark. It has a feeble odor, and a sweet, slightly aromatic taste, somewhat analogous to that of licorice root. It is sometimes submitted, before being dried, to a process of clarification, which renders it semi-transparent and horny. (U.S.D.)

Medicinal Uses: Ginseng is employed in Oriental medicine for its abilities to preserve health, invigorate the system, and prolong life. It is furthermore held to be a cure for many diseases, too numerous to mention. But its main use in Chinese medicine, as elsewhere, is as a preventive measure, taken as a daily tonic.

American Ginseng was an important export up to World War I. A number of North American Indian tribes used Ginseng as an ingredient in love potions, reinforcing its international reputation as an aphrodisiac.

Currently, there are three major types of Ginseng available in North America. Since the names of these are often confusing as they appear in the market place, a few remarks should be made to clarify the situation.

Any mention of "Ginseng" prior to about 1965, relative to human use, could be presumed to mean *Panax ginseng* (family Araliaceae). This spe-

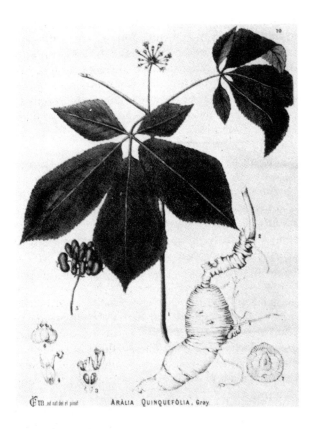

ARÀLIA QUINQUEFÒLIA, Gray.

cies is primarily found in the Orient, and it does not grow naturally in North America. Thus, "Korean Ginseng" is *Panax ginseng*, "Chinese Ginseng" is *Panax ginseng*, and so on.

There are two species of *Panax* normally found growing in North America, only one of which is found in relative abundance, and this is *Panax quinquefolius* (also family Araliaceae). Until just recently, 90-95 percent of all *Panax quinquefolius* (American Ginseng) collected from wild-growing plants, or cultivated in the United States and Canada, was exported to the Orient. Undoubtedly, "American Ginseng" sold in the Orient was simply sold as "Ginseng," and thus a great deal of confusion has resulted, since much of the scientific research in support of certain effects of "Ginseng" was carried out in the Orient, and the evidence required to substantiate whatever species was used in these experiments was never given in the scientific reports. Hence, prior to about 1965, we really cannot say whether "Ginseng" scientific

90

studies were conducted with extracts of *Panax ginseng* or *Panax quinquefolius*. As the situation exists today, there is not a single definitive report existing in the scientific literature concerning the pharmacologic testing of authentic *Panax quinquefolius*. Chemical evidence, however, seems to point out that these two species are very similar. Hence, their pharmacologic effects would be expected to be very similar.

During the past decade, a new "Ginseng" has appeared in the marketplace in North America; indeed, it is being widely used throughout Europe also. This is the so-called "Siberian Ginseng," or *Eleutherococcus senticosus*, sometimes erroneously named *Acanthopanax senticosus*. Since the family Araliaceae is known popularly as the Ginseng family, many different species of this family are referred to as Ginsengs. Since the habitat for *Eleutherococcus senticosus* is primarily in Siberia, this vernacular name was given to the plant from Siberia. Indeed, because of the amazing similarity of pharmacologic effects of the *Panax* species, with comparison to *Eleutherococcus senticosus*, it seems that the name Siberian Ginseng is appropriate.

Confusion results when manufacturers of the Ginseng line of products fail to clearly indicate on the label the exact Latin name for the product being sold. As one can see, the name Ginseng on a bottle tells us very little about the content. One often finds labels such as Manchurian Ginseng, Swiss Ginseng, Korean Ginseng, Oriental Ginseng, and the like, with no further elaboration. Indeed, we have examined a large number of these products and find that they contain neither *Eleutherococcus senticosus*, nor any of the common *Panax* species. Here are the results, in four categories.

1. *Panax ginseng*. Clearly, the biological effects of *Panax ginseng* root extracts are fairly well defined, as are the chemical constituents present in this plant that are responsible for most of these effects. The chemical substances are complex glycosides known as "ginsenosides."

All of the Ginsengs are used primarily as so-called adaptogens, or substances which produce nonspecific resistance in the body. By definition, an adaptogen usually exerts no specific biological effects, but it tends to normalize adverse conditions of the body; at least this is the claim of Russian scientists, who have contributed immensely to this field of research. Thus, a person with mild high blood pressure, after taking an adaptogen, will usually have a normal blood pressure. Conversely, a person with low blood pressure, will also have a normal blood pressure.

A great deal of evidence from animal studies, as well as data from dozens of human experiments, seems to verify the adaptogenic effects of *Panax ginseng*. However, the major use for *Panax ginseng* seems to be as a preventive medicine against various forms of stress, the common cold, and similar conditions. A popular belief is that *Panax ginseng* has aphrodisiac properties, but there is no evidence, in animals or humans, to verify such an action.

There are no reports in the scientific literature (and there have been more than 1,400 scientific papers published on this subject) that indicate any adverse effects for *Panax ginseng*. However, there are indications that regular use of this plant may cause a mild insomnia in some people. Thus, it should not be taken in the early evening or at bedtime.

2. *Panax quinquefolius*. As indicated previously, American Ginseng has not been studied for its pharmacological effects, and only preliminary studies have been carried out to identify its chemical constituents. These chemical constituents seem to be quite similar to those in *Panax ginseng*, and several of the ginsenosides are common to both species. Thus, at this point, and until further studies are reported, we can only presume that the biological effect of *Panax quinquefolius* is similar to that of *Panax ginseng*.

3. *Eleutherococcus senticosus*. Even though the chemical constituents, which are referred to as "eleutherosides," are completely different from those of *Panax* species, the pharmacological effects of Siberian Ginseng are quite similar to those of *Panax ginseng*. This plant has been studied more rigorously by the Russians than *Panax ginseng*; they have studied both species, in fact. Extracts of Siberian Ginseng have been shown to relieve stress, lower the toxicity of some common drugs that tend to produce side effects in humans,

increase mental alertness, improve resistance to colds and mild infections, and be beneficial in cases where a person is continuously in contact with environmental stresses.

Unlike *Panax ginseng*, *Eleutherococcus senticosus* does not seem to cause insomnia, and like *Panax ginseng*, there do not appear to be any adverse effects in humans from the use of Siberian Ginseng.

It is not likely that any of the eleutherosides or ginsenosides will ever be used as adaptogens by themselves, since they are only present in their respective plants in small amounts. Similarly, they are too complex to expect a commercially feasible synthesis. Indeed, Professor I. I. Brekhman of the Soviet Union, who has conducted numerous animal and human experiments with both *Panax ginseng* and *Eleutherococcus senticosus*, claims that the adaptogenic effect requires the total mixture of eleutherosides, in the case of Siberian Ginseng at least, and that the full effects cannot be obtained with any one of the pure eleutherosides.

In recent years, a flood of products claiming to contain Siberian Ginseng have appeared on the market. We have found that most of these contain no *Eleutherococcus senticosus* root. The substitute products most frequently are offered for sale in capsule form. We have found that most of the substitute products have an intense bitter taste, which is not true of the authentic material, and that the substitute products also have a characteristic "vanillan-like" odor, but it is not the typical pleasant odor of vanillin.

4. Red American "Ginseng"—*Rumex hymenosepalus* (family Polygonaceae). The root of this plant, native to the southwestern part of the United States, but introduced in other parts of the country, has been sold very recently under the name of Red American Ginseng. Indeed, it has also been used as an adulterant for Ginseng. Previously, it has been used in American herbal medicine, primarily in Texas, as an astringent for colds, loose teeth, sore throats, and to heal sores.

Originally utilized by the Hopi and Papago Indians to treat colds and sore throats, the plant soon found its way into early American medicine. The tuberous roots, which resemble those of the Dahlias, contain a yellow dye which the Navahos

use to dye wool. As a food the leaf stalks are used in pie making.

Recent purveyors of this plant allege effects similar to those of *Panax ginseng*, especially as regards its aphrodisiac properties. Needless to say, there is no evidence for any Ginseng-like activity for this plant. The roots contain reasonable amounts of anthraquinone derivatives that would predictably result in a laxative effect if ingested. Thus, if any of our readers purchase Ginseng products, and the use results in loose bowel movements, it can be suspected that the product did not contain Ginseng, but rather was replaced with *Rumex hymenosepalus*.

Dose: Ginseng: Of the powder, ½ teaspoon to 1 cup of hot water. Drink in the morning, at lunch, at bedtime (add Lemon Grass, if you find the flavor wanting).

Of the root, chew as desired.

Of the extract, 5 milliliters in 1 cup of any liquid, after meals.

GOLDENSEAL
Hydrastis canadensis

PARTS USED: Rhizome and root

OTHER COMMON NAMES: Yellow Root, Yellow Puccoon, Jaundice Root, Hydrastis, Orange Root, Indian Dye, Indian Turmeric, Indian Paint, Eye Root, Eye Balm, Yellow Eye

Botanical Description: *Hydrastis canadensis* is a small, herbaceous, perennial plant, with a thick, fleshy, yellow rhizome, from which numerous long roots arise, and an erect, simple, pubescent stem, from 6 inches to 1 foot in height. There are usually but 2 leaves, which are unequal, one sessile at the top of the stem, the other attached to the stem a short distance below by a thick roundish footstalk, causing the stem to appear as if bifurcate near the summit. The leaves are pubescent, roundish-cordate, with from 3 to 7, but generally 5, lobes, which are pointed and unequally serrate. A solitary flower stands upon a peduncle rising from the basis of the upper leaf. It is without corolla, but with a greenish-white calyx, the sepals of which closely resemble petals, and are very caducous, falling very soon after the flower has expanded. The fruit is a globose, com-

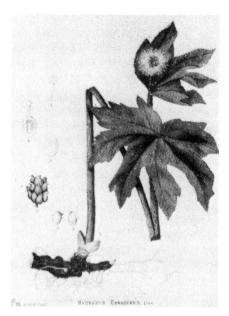

GOLDENSEAL: This plant drug has been found useful in treating various inflammations of the mucous membranes as well as vaginitis and urethritis. The alkaloids it contains are excreted quite slowly from the body, and experience has shown it is inadvisable to take it for extended periods of time.

pound, red or crimson berry, ½ inch or more in diameter, composed of many fleshy carpels, each tipped with a short curved beak, and containing 1 or rarely 2 seeds. The plant grows in moist, rich woodlands in most parts of the United States, and at one time abundantly in the North and West. The fruit bears a close resemblance to the raspberry, but is not edible. The root is the part used. There is but one other species of *Hydrastis* known—viz., *H. jezoensis,* which is found in northern Japan. (U.S.D.)

Medicinal Uses: Goldenseal enjoys a tremendous reputation for its medicinal virtuosity. It has been recommended in the treatment of dozens of ailments; the more reliable reported virtues are listed herein.

As a specific for uterine complaints it was given to arrest uterine hemorrhage, as well as to check excessive menstrual evacuation. In very small dosage it was advocated to cure morning sickness; however, it is critical to note that in large doses Goldenseal *may produce abortion,* and in fact has been used deliberately as an abortifacient.

Moreover, taken in too large a dose, Goldenseal can dangerously overstimulate the nervous system. It is inadvisable to continue even limited usage for extended periods of time since the alkaloids are eliminated quite slowly from the body.

Goldenseal is a potent drug that owes its effect primarily to the alkaloids hydrastine and hydrastinine, in addition to berberine. These alkaloids produce a strong astringent effect on mucous membranes, reduce inflammation and have antiseptic effects.

Recommended in the treatment of various inflammations of the mucous membranes, the plant has been utilized to treat vaginitis, gastritis, rhinitis, and urethritis. It has even been recommended as a cure for gonorrhea. Anal complaints, such as chronic or subacute inflammations of the rectum and colon and chronic constipation, were soothed by Goldenseal enemas.

Applied topically, Goldenseal has been used to treat eczema and other skin irritations and eye inflammations.

Recent research has shown that Goldenseal can be used as an external application to the arms and legs in the treatment of disorders of the blood vessels and lymphatics. Berberine, one of the alkaloids in Goldenseal, was found to have anticonvulsive effect on the intestines and uterus, and was also very effective against the bacteria *Staphylococcus aureus*.

Dose: ½ teaspoon of ground, dried and powdered root, boiled in a covered container in 1 pint of water for about ½ hour, at a slow boil. Liquid allowed to cool slowly in the *closed* container. Drunk cold, 1 swallow or 1 tablespoon at a time, a maximum of 1 cup per day for a length of time not to exceed 1 week.

GOTU KOLA
Centella asiatica (Hydrocotyl asiatica)

PARTS USED: Herb
OTHER COMMON NAMES: Thickleaved
   Pennywort, Indian or Asiatic Pennywort

Botanical Description: A weed widely distributed in

many tropical regions, it is common between sea level and an altitude of 1,000 feet or more. It grows in fields and gardens and crowds out other plants. New individuals are produced both by seeds and by runners. The plant resembles the March Pennywort. It is small, has a creeping stem bearing rosettes of long-stemmed, rounded, scalloped leaves, 0.75 to 2 inches in diameter, deeply indented at the base, and resembling those of the Violet. But the flowers are quite different from Violets, being small, white, inconspicuous, and 3 or 4 together in a short-stemmed umbel at leaf bases close to the ground. In Java and Ceylon it has been planted to prevent soil erosion. (Neal)

Medicinal Uses: Gotu Kola is used primarily as a sedative, diuretic, tonic and to accelerate healing of wounds. It is claimed to strengthen and energize the brain. In large doses it is said to act as a narcotic, causing stupor, headache, and sometimes coma.

It has been employed to alleviate bowel complaints and to treat syphilis and tubercular inflammation of the cervical lymph nodes. Its ability to aid in these and urinary-tract disorders has been attributed to its demulcent properties.

Recent pharmacological studies have shown that extracts of Gotu Kola exhibit a sedative activity similar to that of meprobamate and chlorpromazine. The mode of action appears to be mainly on the cholinergic mechanism in the central nervous system.

The major active principle in this plant is most probably the triterpene glycoside asiaticoside. Asiaticoside is well tolerated when given by mouth to mice and rabbits at a single dose of 1.0 gram. This would imply that it is a relatively safe substance. When asiaticoside is implanted under the skin, or injected subcutaneously in mice, rats, guinea pigs, or rabbits, improved blood supply of connective tissue occurs. A rapid thickening of the skin is also noted in the treated animals, as well as an accelerated growth of hair and nails.

There is some evidence in humans, because of the sum total of these effects, that asiaticoside, and hence extracts of *Centella asiatica,* are useful to accelerate healing of wounds, and some infectious diseases such as tuberculosis and leprosy. The microbes that cause both of these diseases are well known to have a waxy coating that most other disease-producing organisms lack. This waxy coating prevents the body's own defense mechanisms from killing the organisms, hence it is difficult to cure both of these diseases. It is thought that asiaticoside acts to dissolve the waxy covering on the organisms, which then allows the normal defense mechanisms of the body to destroy the causative organisms of leprosy and/or tuberculosis.

It must be pointed out that the foregoing is indicated only as a reasonable explanation for part of the useful action of *C. asiatica* preparations. Further work must be carried out in animals and in humans to determine whether or not this is the case.

It has also been shown that asiaticoside-pretreated rats (12.5 mg/kg/day/3 days, subcutaneously), who were subjected to cold conditions, did not develop gastric ulcers. Control animals in the experiment did develop gastric ulcers under these conditions.

Because of the pronounced effect of asiaticoside on skin, a study was carried out in 1972 to determine if repeated applications would produce cancer. A 0.10 percent solution of asiaticoside was applied to the back of hairless mice twice weekly for the lifetime of the animals (about 18 months). It was found that sarcomas (cancers) were produced on the skin of 2.5 percent of the treated mice. These findings probably have little significance, since the test is not specific, and is recognized as invalid for weak carcinogens. The results of the experiment described above would indicate that in that test, asiaticoside would be classified as a weak carcinogen.

Despite these minor pharmacological problems, Gotu Kola awaits discovery and possible wide adoption by the medical establishment. Fijian healers have long known of the values of this plant; it is the most frequently utilized medicinal plant in their pharmacopoeia. It has long been known in India, and its use was probably brought to Fiji by Indian settlers.

Dose: Small doses of ½ teaspoon of the dried herb per cup of boiling water are recommended by those who use the plant. They say that the dose is sometimes increased, as needed, for sedative and anticonvulsive action. (Headache and stupor are a natural warning sign that the dose is too strong.)

GRINDELIA
Grindelia spp.

PARTS USED: Leaves and flowering tops
OTHER COMMON NAMES: California Gum Plant, Shore Grindelia, Curly Cup

Botanical Description: The genus *Grindelia* includes some 25 species, 6 or 8 of which are found in South America, the remainder occurring in the United States west of the Mississippi. They are coarse perennial or biennial herbs, being occasionally shrublike. Most, if not all, of the species produce a resinous exudation on the stem and leaves and especially on the flower heads. The leaves are alternate, sessile or clasping and spinulose-dentate. The flowers occur in large terminal heads composed of both discoid and radiate yellow flowers. The ray flowers are pistillate and the involucre is more or less hemispherical, the bracts being imbricated, in several series, being usually subulate, tipped. The drug of the market appears to be derived in large part from *G. camporum*, which is the common Gum Plant of California. It occurs abundantly in the inner coast ranges, where it has been collected in quantity in Lake and Napa Counties. It is also common in the foothills of the Sierra Nevada and is almost the only plant found on the plains in certain regions of the Sacramento Valley. The leaves are oblong or spatulate, sessile or clasping, coarsely serrate and of a pale-green color. The flower heads are yellow and the involucre consists of several rows of lanceolate acuminate recurved bracts. The achenes are distinctive in this species and are usually biauriculate or more rarely unidentate at the summit.

G. squarrosa is a common plant on the prairies and dry banks of the West. It has been reported as occurring from the Saskatchewan to Minnesota, Texas, and California. It is a glabrous, erect, branching herb having linear-oblong or spatulate leaves, which are more or less clasping at the base and sharply spinulose-dentate. It is especially characterized by the bracts of the involucre being linear-lanceolate, subulate tipped and spreading or squarrose at the summit, giving the species its name.

The achenes are truncate, those of the outer flowers being usually thicker. The pappus consists of two or three awns.

It was formerly supposed that the drug of commerce was derived from *G. robusta*. This is not the case. *G. robusta* is apparently not a very common plant and is distinguished by having cordate-oblong, amplexicaul, coarsely serrate leaves. The involucre is squarrose and leafy at the base. The pappus consists of 2 awns. At one time both *G. cuneifolia* and *G. camporum* were considered merely varieties of *G. robusta*. (U.S.D.)

Medicinal Uses: The principal use of *G. camporum* (Gum Plant) in traditional medicine was in the treatment of bronchial catarrh, or inflammation of the bronchial mucous membranes, particularly in cases of asthma. It is thought to act as a stimulating expectorant and antispasmodic. The herb contains an essential oil, over 20 percent resin, grindelol, saponin, tannin, and robustic acid.

Combined with Stramonium, Grindelia was used in "asthma powders," which were also given for whooping cough and hay fever.

A fluidextract of the aerial parts of *Grindelia squarrosa* has been tested in guinea pigs, rabbits, and cats for expectorant activity. The fluidextract was administered orally. Expectorant effects were shown in the cat experiments, but not in the rabbit and guinea pig experiments. Species variation in drug testing is not uncommon and thus it appears that this herbal use for Grindelia has been verified.

In the form of topical poultices and solutions, Grindelia has been reported to be useful in treating burns, vaginitis, and genitourinary membrane infections and inflammations. *G. squarrosa* (Curly Cup) is beneficial in the treatment of poison ivy and other skin irritations and rashes. It contains a resinous substance and an essential oil, grindelol.

Dose: Approximately ½ oz. of leaves or flowering tops to 1 pint of water. Water boiled separately and poured over the plant material and steeped for 5-20 minutes, depending on the desired effect. Drunk hot or warm, 1 to 2 cupfuls per day, at bedtime and upon awakening. For poison ivy or poison oak *boil* 1 oz. of plant material in a pint of water for about 10 minutes. Let cool, strain, and apply cold to affected parts on saturated cloth.

GROUNDSEL
Senecio vulgaris

PARTS USED: Herb

OTHER COMMON NAMES: Life Root, Golden Ragwort, Squaw Weed, False Valerian, Golden Senecio, Female Regulator, Fireweed

Botanical Description: The members of this genus are herbs or subshrubs; leaves alternate, often pinnatifid; involucre usually campanulate or obconic-campanulate (or urceolate at anthesis); phyllaries usually in 2 size-classes; longer (inner) phyllaries 12 to 25, equal in length, in a double row, linear, often acute, with a herbaceous median area and usually thin margins; outer phyllaries much shorter, subulate-setaceous, forming a calyculum or in many species entirely absent; receptacle slightly convex, essentially naked; ray flowers present, pistillate, fertile; rays linear or elliptic-linear, yellow, terminally 3-toothed; disk flowers numerous, perfect, fertile; corolla equally 5-toothed, yellow; achenes columnar, nearly terete, several-nerved, alike in ray and disk; pappus of numerous capillary bristles.

An enormous worldwide genus of between 2,000 and 3,000 species, reputed to be among the several largest seed-plant genera. (Texas)

Medicinal Uses: Groundsel was used to stimulate menstruation and to ease painful menstruation, both by European and American domestic practitioners. American Indians used the plant to speed childbirth. All these functions recall the applications of Ergot, and Groundsel was employed at various times as a substitute for that fungus, for example, in controlling pulmonary hemorrhage. In general the plant has been used as a diaphoretic, diuretic, and tonic. In dentistry, the herb is employed for bleeding gums.

Dose: Approximately ½ ounce of the herb to 1 pint of water. Water boiled separately and poured over the plant material and steeped for 5 to 20 minutes, depending on the desired effect. Drunk hot or warm, 1 to 2 cups per day.

96

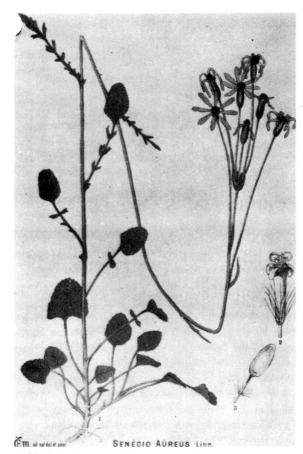

SENÉCIO AÙREUS Linn.

GROUNDSEL: An infusion of the ground herb has been used to stimulate menstruation and to ease painful menstruation, both by European and American domestic practitioners.

GUARANÁ
Paullinia cupana var. *sorbilis*

PARTS USED: Seeds

OTHER COMMON NAMES: Paullinia, Brazilian Cocoa, Guaraná Bread

Botanical Description: A native of tropical America, this woody climber has an erect angular smooth stem. Leaves alternate, on long stalks, pinnate, with 2 pairs of leaflets and a terminal one, stipulate, petioles angular, glabrous, leaflets oblong-oval, 5 or 6 inches long by 2½–3 inches broad, rather coriaceous, shortly stalked, the lateral ones rounded at the base, the terminal one tapering, all suddenly contracted into a shortly attenuated blunt point, the margin distantly, coarsely, and irregularly sinuate-dentate, smooth on both surfaces, rather strongly veined beneath. Inflorescence is erect, spicate, narrow panicles, 4 inches or more in length, from the axils of the leaves, pubescent, the flowers shortly stalked in small clusters, laxly arranged on the thick rachis, small. Sepals 5 (or 4), rounded, concave, imbricate. Petals 4, alternate with the sepals, ovate-spathulate, each with a large appendage attached to the upper surface near the base, pubescent on the front, and doubled over in the form of a claw at the apex. Stamens and pistil elevated on the summit of a wide column (gynophore), which projects into the upper part of the flower; in front of this, in the lower part of the flower, are 2 large, oval, compressed glands, and behind it 2 much smaller ones. Stamens 8, inserted on the top of the gynophore round the base of the ovary; filaments thick, tapering, hairy, anthers attached by their back, bluntly pointed at apex, wide and rounded below. Ovary cylindrical, thick, short, 3-celled, ovules one in each cell, style none; stigma sessile on the ovary, 3-lobed. Fruit about the size of a grape, ovoid or pyriform, on a stalk about half its length (the gynophore), and with a short strong beak, glabrous, marked with 6 longitudinal ribs; pericarp thin, tough, strongly hairy within, 3-valved. Seed usually solitary (rarely 2 or 3), not quite filling the fruit, attached to the base, about the size of a small hazelnut, roundish, usually slightly pointed at the apex, shining, purplish-brown, surrounded at the flattened base by a tough membranous white arillus; testa thin, brittle; embryo without endosperm, cotyledons thick and firm, unequal, large.

The Guaraná plant grows in the northern and western portions of Brazil. Its seeds ripen in October and November; they have just the appearance of Horse-chestnuts in miniature. The flowers of many species of this genus are imperfectly bisexual. (Bentley)

Medicinal Uses: A traditional beverage of the Brazilian Indians, Guaraná is prepared from the dried seeds which are powdered, sometimes mixed with cassava flour, then kneaded into dough and formed into cylindrical or globular masses which are found in the native marketplaces. It may also be mixed with chocolate. Besides having refreshing and nutritive value, Guaraná has been used medicinally by natives in Brazil for bowel complaints, both as a curative and as a preventive.

The medicinal virtues of the plant are probably largely due to its caffeine content, which is higher than in any other plant source and 2½ times that of coffee. The plant was introduced into France by a physician who had been working in Brazil. It

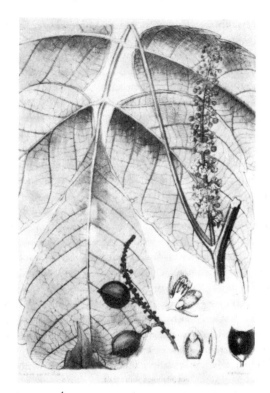

GUARANÁ: The most caffeine-rich plant, it has been successfully employed to alleviate the pain of migraine and to arrest diarrhea.

came to be employed in the treatment of migraine and nervous headaches, neuralgia, paralysis, urinary-tract irritation, and other ailments, as well as continuing to be administered for chronic diarrhea.

The caffeine explains the efficacy of Guaraná in alleviating the pain of migraine headaches, and the tannins undoubtedly act as an astringent to alleviate diarrhea.

Dose: The beverage, which is also used medicinally, is prepared from 1 teaspoon of Guaraná to a glass or cup of sweetened water.

HELLEBORE, AMERICAN
Veratrum viride

PARTS USED: Rhizome
OTHER COMMON NAMES: Green Hellebore, Indian Poke, Itch Weed, Veratrum, False Hellebore

Botanical Description: The American hellebore, known also by the names of Indian Poke, Poke Root, Swamp Hellebore, and others (see above) has a perennial, thick, fleshy root, the upper portion of which is tunicated, the lower solid and beset with numerous whitish fibers or radicles. The stem is annual, round, striated, pubescent, and solid, from 3 to 6 feet in height, furnished with bright green leaves, and terminating in a panicle of greenish-yellow flowers. The leaves gradually decrease in size as they ascend. The lower are from 6 inches to a foot long, oval, acuminate, plaited, nerved, and pubescent; and embrace the stem at their base, thus affording it a sheath for a considerable portion of its length. Those on the upper part of the stem, at the origin of the flowering branches, are oblong lanceolate. The panicle consists of numerous flowers distributed in racemes with downy peduncles. Each flower is accompanied with a downy pointed bract much longer than its pedicle. There is no calyx, and the corolla is divided into 6 oval acute segments, thickened on the inside at their base, with the three alternate segments longer than the others. The six stamens have recurved filaments, and roundish 2-lobed anthers. The germs are 3, with recurved styles as long as the stamens. Some of the flowers have only the rudiments of pistils. Those on the upper end of the branchlets are barren, those on the lower portion fruitful. The fruit consists of 3 cohering capsules, separating at top, opening on the inner side, and containing flat imbricated seeds.

This indigenous species of *Veratrum* is found from Canada to Carolina, inhabiting swamps, wet meadows, and the banks of mountain streamlets. Early in the spring, before the stem rises, it bears a slight resemblance to the *Ictodes foetidus*, with which it is very frequently associated; but the latter sends forth no stem. From May to July is the season for flowering. (U.S.D.)

Medicinal Uses: Like its European cousin, the Black Hellebore, this herb is highly toxic, producing distressing nausea and extreme depression of the circulation and the nervous system, and its use in generalized herbal practice as a home remedy is to be avoided.

As with many other toxic herbs, minute doses of Hellebore are an important remedy in the homeopathic discipline of medicine; the homeopathic preparations are used as nervines and more es-

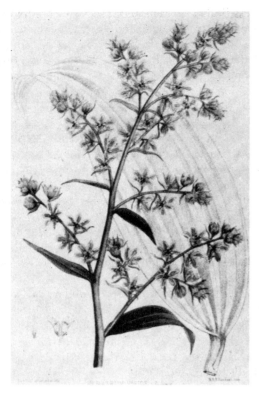

HELLEBORE, AMERICAN: Like its European cousin, the Black Hellebore, this herb is highly toxic, producing distressing nausea and extreme depression of the circulation and the nervous system. It is to be avoided as a home remedy.

pecially for their sedative action on the circulation. It is reported by homeopaths that "in suitable doses, it can be relied upon to bring the pulse down from 150 beats per minute to 40 bpm or even to 30 bpm." However, even the homeopathic tests warn of the dangers of overdosing and prescribe as an antidote in case of accidental poisoning "morphine or laudanum in a little brandy or ginger."

In regular medicine, Hellebore was used for its irritant and sedative action in a wide range of complaints, including pneumonia, gout, rheumatism, typhoid and rheumatic fevers, and local inflammations.

American Hellebore preparations are well known to contain a complex mixture of steroid alkaloids (including jervine, pseudojervine and veratroidine) that have been, and are still used by the medical profession to treat severe cases of high blood pressure and related cardiovascular conditions, including tachycardia. It must be pointed out, however, that this is one of our most potent drug plants. It is effective only in selected types of high blood pressure, and has many potential side effects if used over a long period of time.

A related species, *V. californicum,* or False Hellebore, is a famous contraceptive plant of Indian tribes of Nevada and surrounding regions. Shoshones and other Native Americans employ a root decoction daily for three weeks to insure sterility. The plant is called by its Shoshone name, *'div-oh-savva,* meaning "sterile."

Dose: EXTREME CAUTION. When prescribed as a tincture, 8 ounces of the dried root to 16 ounces of diluted .835 alcohol is macerated for 2 weeks, then expressed and filtered.

Tincture: Dose is 0.6–1.8 milliliters. Of the fluidextract, 0.065–0.13 grams.

HELLEBORE, BLACK
Helleborus niger

PARTS USED: Rhizome

OTHER COMMON NAMES: Indian Poke, Itchweed, Christmas Rose

Botanical Description: The root of the Black Hellebore is perennial, knotted, blackish on the outside, white within, and sends off numerous long, simple, depending fibers, which are brownish-yellow when fresh, but become dark brown upon drying. The leaves are pedate, of a deep green color, and stand on long footstalks which spring immediately from the root. Each leaf is composed of 5 leaflets, 1 terminal, and 2, 3, or 4 on each side supported on a single partial petiole. The leaflets are ovate lanceolate, smooth, shining, coriaceous, and serrated in their upper portion. The flower stem, which also rises from the root, is 6 to 8 inches high, round, tapering, reddish towards the base, and bears 1 or 2 large, pendent, roselike flowers, accompanied with floral leaves, which supply the place of the calyx. The petals, 5 in number, are large, roundish, concave, spreading, and of a white or pale rose color, with occasionally a greenish tinge. There are two varieties of the plant—the *Helleborus niger humilifolius,* and

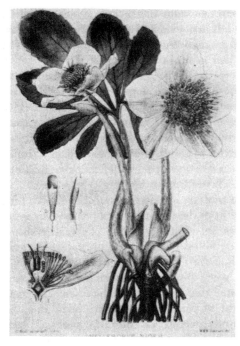

HELLEBORE, BLACK: This perennial herb is quite toxic, and its usage in herbal medicine was restricted by physicians who were fully aware of its poisonous properties.

Helleborus niger altifolius—in the former of which the leaves are shorter than the flower stem, in the latter longer.

This plant is a native of the mountainous regions of southern and temperate Europe. It is found in Greece, Austria, Italy, Switzerland, France, and Spain. It is cultivated in gardens for the beauty of its flowers, which expand in the middle of winter, and have, from this circumstance, given rise to the name of Christmas Rose, by which the Black Hellebore is sometimes called. (U.S.D.)

Medicinal Uses: This perennial plant is quite toxic, and its usage in herbal medicine was restricted by physicians, who were fully aware of its poisonous properties. Used properly by a knowledgeable herbalist or physician, Hellebore has been given as a purgative; to excite sneezing; to provoke menstrual evacuation; and, externally applied, to cause blistering and inflammation of the skin.

Perhaps it is most famous for its use in dropsy.

99

The plant contains the cardiac glycoside hellebrin, as well as many related chemical substances which would explain the claimed beneficial effects for this plant in dropsy.

There is a peculiar story regarding Black Hellebore. In 1806 a group of French prisoners were suffering from hemeralopia (blindness from sunset to sunrise). After attempting a variety of treatments, a powdered snuff of Black Hellebore was given to them; they recovered in a few days. At the same time they reported a welcome side-effect—relief from dyspeptic symptoms!

The root has also been used throughout history, dating from the ancients, as a remedy for insanity. Its reputed efficacy in such psychiatric disorders was attributed to its drastic purgative property of expelling the "black bile" from which such maladies were thought to originate. One can only presume that the doctors believed the patient, brought to the doors of death with this violent purgative, would be literally shocked back to reality, the fear of further treatment being more than sufficient incentive to quit irrational behavior. The brutal treatment of the mentally ill by continual application of violent drugs remains one of the most tragic chapters in medical history, a chapter not yet finished.

Dose: CAUTION. Toxic.

HEMLOCK
Conium maculatum

PARTS USED: Entire plant, except root
OTHER COMMON NAMES: Conium, Poison Hemlock, Spotted Hemlock

Botanical Description: This is an umbelliferous plant, having a biennial spindle-shaped whitish root, and an herbaceous branching stem, from 3 to 6 feet high, round, hollow, smooth, shining, slightly striated, and marked with brownish-purple spots. The lower leaves are tripinnate, more than a foot in length, shining, and attached to the joints of the stem by sheathing petioles; the upper are smaller, bipinnate, and inserted at the divisions of the branches; both have channelled footstalks, and incised leaflets which are deep green on their upper surface and paler beneath. The flowers are

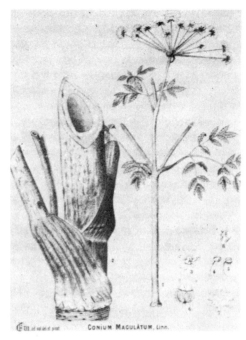

CONIUM MACULATUM, Linn.

HEMLOCK: Famed as the Athenian state poison administered as a mode of execution, the plant contains the poisonous alkaloid coniine. In small quantities sedative and antispasmodic effects have been experienced but its high toxicity presents a potentially fatal risk you should not run.

very small, white, and disposed in compound terminal umbels. The general involucre consists of from 5 to 7 lanceolate, reflected leaflets, whitish at their edges; the partial involucre, of 3 or 4, oval, pointed, spreading, and on one side only. The petals are cordate, with their points inflected, 5 in number, and nearly equal. The stamens are spreading, and about as long as the corolla; the styles diverging. The fruit is roundish ovate, striated, and composed of 2 planoconvex seeds, which have on their outer surface five crenated ribs.

The hemlock is a native of Europe, and has been introduced into the United States, where it is now naturalized. It grows usually in bunches along the roadsides or in waste grounds, and is found most abundantly in the neighborhood of old settlements. Its flowers appear in June and July. The whole plant, especially at this period, exhales a fetid odor, usually compared to that of the urine of cats; and narcotic effects are experienced by those who breathe for a long time air impregnated with the effluvia. The plant varies in narcotic power according to the climate and character of the weather, being most active in hot and dry seasons, and in warm countries. The hemlock of Greece, Italy, and Spain is said to be much more energetic than that of the north of Europe. As a general rule, those plants are most active which grow in a sunny exposure. The proper season for gathering the leaves is when the plant is in flower; they are most active about the time when the flowers begin to fade. The footstalks should be rejected, and the leaflets quickly dried, either in the hot sun, or on tin plates before a fire. They should be kept in boxes or tin cases excluded as much as possible from the air and light, by exposure to which they lose their fine green color, and become deteriorated in medical virtues. The same end is answered by pulverizing them, and preserving the powder in opaque and well stopped bottles. (U.S.D.).

Medicinal Uses: Sedative and antispasmodic when used medicinally, Hemlock is a deadly poison which in sufficient doses paralyzes the motor centers. It appears to be well established by scientists and historians that the poison administered as a mode of execution of state criminals at Athens was principally, if not wholly, composed of the juice of the leaves and the green seeds of this plant.

Conium was first mentioned as a medicinal by Dioscorides, who reported the use of an external plaster in the treatment of herpes and other skin eruptions. From that time on we find a veritable explosion of diseases this plant was reputed to cure, ranging from cancer of the breast to syphilis, epilepsy, ulcers, and jaundice, to mention only a few.

However, when we read the following account of the death of Socrates, we can only wonder at the herbalists who used Hemlock successfully, and without incurring charges of homicide:

No more fitting introduction to the action of this virulent spinal irritant could be written than the description, in Plato's *Phaedo,* of the death of Socrates: "And Crito, hearing this, gave the sign to the boy who stood near; and the boy departing, after some time returned, bringing with him the man who was to administer the poison, who brought it ready bruised in a cup. And Socrates, beholding the man, said: 'Good friend, come hither; you are experienced in these affairs—what is to be done?' 'Nothing,' replied the man, 'only when you have drank the poison you are to walk about until a heaviness takes place in your legs; then lie down—this is all you have to do.' At the same time he presented the cup. Socrates received it from him with great calmness, without fear or change of countenance, and regarding the man with his usual stern aspect he asked: 'What say you of this potion? Is it lawful to sprinkle any portion of it on the earth, as a libation, or not?' 'We only bruise,' said the man, 'as much as is barely sufficient for the purpose.' 'I understand you,' said Socrates; 'but it is certainly lawful and proper to pray the gods that my departure from hence may be prosperous and happy, which I indeed beseech them to grant.' So saying, he carried the cup to his mouth, and drank it with great promptness and facility.

Thus far most of us had been able to refrain from weeping. But when we saw that he was drinking, and actually had drank the poison, we could no longer restrain our tears. . . . But he observing us, exclaimed, 'What is it you do, my excellent friends? I have sent away the women that they might not betray such weakness. I have heard that it is our duty to die cheerfully, and with expressions of joy and praise. Be silent, therefore, and let your fortitude be seen.' At this address we blushed, and suppressed our tears. But Socrates, after walking about, now told us that his legs were beginning to grow heavy, and immediately lay down, for so he had been ordered. At the same time the man who had given him the poison examined his feet and legs, touching them at intervals. At length he pressed violently upon his foot, and asked if he felt it. To which Socrates replied that he did not. The man then pressed his legs and so on, showing us that he was becoming cold and stiff. And Socrates, feeling it himself, assured us that when the effects had ascended to his heart, he should be gone. And now the middle of his body growing cold, he threw aside his clothes, and spoke for

the last time: 'Crito, we owe the sacrifice of a cock to Aesculapius. Discharge this, and neglect it not.' 'It shall be done,' said Crito; 'have you anything else to say?' He made no reply, but a moment after moved, and his eyes became fixed. And Crito, seeing this, closed his eyelids and mouth."
—Charles F. Millspaugh, *American Medicinal Plants* (New York: Dover Publications), 1974, pp. 268–69.

Dose: DANGEROUS. Avoid.

Hemlock contains the poisonous alkaloid coniine in all parts of the plant. Very small amounts of Hemlock will produce effects that explain the medicinal uses of this plant. However, the high toxic risk of using even dilute extracts of Hemlock, for any human condition, cannot be discounted.

HENBANE
Hyoscyamus niger

PARTS USED: Seeds, leaves, and root
OTHER COMMON NAMES: Hyoscyamus, Black Henbane, Poison Tobacco

Botanical Description: Henbane is a biennial plant, with a long, tapering, whitish, fleshy, somewhat branching root, bearing considerable resemblance to that of Parsley, for which it has been eaten by mistake. The stem is erect, round, branching, from 1 to 3 feet in height, and thickly furnished with leaves. These are large, oblong ovate, deeply sinuated, with pointed segments, undulated, soft to the touch, and at their base embrace the stem. The upper leaves are generally entire. Both the stem and leaves are hairy, viscid, and of a sea-green color. The flowers form long, one-sided, leafy spikes, which terminate the branches, and hang downwards. They are composed of a calyx with 5 pointed divisions, a funnel-shaped corolla with 5 unequal, obtuse segments at the border, 5 stamens inserted into the tube of the corolla, and a pistil with a blunt round stigma. Their color is an obscure yellow, beautifully variegated with purple veins. The fruit is a globular 2-celled capsule, covered with a lid, invested with the persistent calyx, and containing numerous small, irregular, brown or ash-colored seeds, which are discharged by the horizontal separation of the lid. The whole plant has a rank offensive smell.

This species of *Hyoscyamus* is found in the northern and eastern sections of the United States, occupying waste grounds in the vicinity of the older settlements, particularly graveyards, old gardens, and the foundations of ruined houses. It is rare, however, in this country, of which it is not a native, having been introduced from Europe. In Great Britain, France, Germany, and other parts of the Continent, it grows abundantly along the roads, around villages, amidst rubbish, and in uncultivated places. It flowers in June and July.

H. albus, so named from the whiteness of its flowers, is used in France indiscriminately with the former species above, which it resembles exactly in medicinal properties.

All parts of the *Hyoscyamus niger* are possessed of activity. Much of the efficacy of Henbane depends upon the time at which it is gathered. The leaves should be collected soon after the plant has flowered. Those of the second year are asserted to be greatly preferable to those of the first. The latter are less clammy and fetid, yield less extractive matter, and are medicinally much less efficient. (U.S.D.)

Medicinal Uses: Related to Belladonna, Henbane is a poisonous plant, extremely dangerous in overdose. Its action is similar to that of Belladonna, but its effects on the cerebrum and motor centers are more pronounced, while its stimulant action on the sympathetic nervous system is less. Overdose can produce headache, nausea, vertigo, extreme thirst, dry burning skin, dilated pupils, loss of sight and voluntary ocular motion, and in extreme cases, mania, convulsions, and death. Use by the amateur herbalist is obviously quite risky, since the toxic effects can be swift and fatal. Administered properly, and in correct doses, Henbane is a valuable folk remedy, and has been employed in traditional medicine as a sedative, anodyne, calmative, and antispasmodic. It is similar to atropine in its ability to dilate the pupil of the eye. The dried leaves have been smoked for toothache.

Dose: CAUTION!

All parts of the Henbane plant are known to contain atropine and hyoscyamine (with trace amounts of scopolamine), and thus preparations containing any part of this plant would have anodyne properties when applied externally. They would also be effective preparations for the treatment of stomach ulcers, but in order to gain a sedative effect (primarily due to scopolamine), one would have to take a dangerously high dose.

See important side effects and precautions on the use of Henbane preparations, which are described in the article on Belladonna.

HENNA
Lawsonia alba

PARTS USED: Leaves and fruit
OTHER COMMON NAMES: Mignonette Tree, Reseda

Botanical Description: A tree or shrub 6 to 20 feet high, with or without spines, native of north Africa and southern Asia. Leaves are opposite, short-stemmed, oval or narrower, 0.5 to 1.5 inches long. Fragrant flowers—white (var. *alba*) to red (var. *rubra*)—develop in panicles at branch tips, each flower to 0.25 inch in diameter, with four sepals, four wrinkled, short-clawed petals, stamens usually eight, style long. The fruiting capsule is globose, brittle, less than 0.25 inch in diameter, and is partly enclosed by the calyx. (Neal)

Medicinal Uses: Henna has recently experienced a renewed popularity as a hair dye, having been in use for that purpose since antiquity. Henna leaves were used by people of ancient civilizations to dye the manes and tails of their horses; the Arabs have employed the leaves for centuries to dye their beards, nails, palms and soles. Henna imparts a reddish tint to the hair. Mixed with Indigo, it imparts a fine blue-black gloss to beard and hair.

Interestingly, the mummies of ancient Egypt were found wrapped in henna-dyed cloth. In Africa the flowers are used to give a fine scent to pomades and oils.

In India the leaves were made into an astringent gargle. The fruits have been thought to stimulate the menstrual function. The leaves, in powdered form, have been used both internally and exter- nally to treat various skin diseases, including leprosy. In Arabic medicine the powder was employed in the treatment of jaundice, most likely on the basis of coloration (as implied by the Doctrine of Signatures); it is unlikely that Henna benefited the patient at all, and perhaps it only turned him more yellow.

Extracts of Henna leaves have been shown to act in a manner similar to Ergot with respect to inducing uterine contractions. It is therefore quite possible that extracts of this plant could induce menstruation and be effective emmanagogues. In test tube experiments, extracts of the leaves of Henna have shown good antibacterial activity, although not specifically against the leprosy bacillus, which is not possible to test against since it does not grow in non-living tissues. The active principle for these effects most likely is the coloring principle, lawsone.

The topical application of two chemical components of this shrub, lawsone and dihydroxyacetone, has been reported useful as a protective filter against ultraviolet light for people with chlorpromazine-induced light sensitivity. Experimentally, a water extract of the leaves inhibited gram-positive and gram-negative bacteria. Antitumor activity in experiments with mice tends to support folkloric uses of Henna as an anticancer agent.

Dose: Approximately ½ ounce of leaves to 1 pint of water; leaves may be cut small or granulated into powder as required. Water boiled separately and poured over the plant material and steeped for 5 to 20 minutes, depending on the desired effect. Drunk hot or warm, 1 to 2 cupfuls per day.

HOLLY
Ilex aquifolium (European Holly), *I. opaca* (American Holly)

PARTS USED: Leaves and berries

Botanical Description: A small evergreen tree, 4 to 30 feet high, much branched, the young shoots very smooth, pliant, of a fine green color; bark ash-colored, very compact; wood hard, heavy, yellowish-white, darker toward the center. Leaves persistent, alternate,

103

petiolate, coriaceous, deep shining green, ovate, undu-lated, and furnished at the margins with strong sharp spines. Flowers small, numerous, on short peduncles, somewhat umbellate, springing from the axils of the leaves. Calyx small, slightly hairy, mostly 4-toothed. Corolla rotate, in 4 deep divisions, of a whitish color. Stamens 4 (sometimes 5, and then the other parts of the flower have a corresponding development), spreading, with subulate filaments, attached to the base of the corolla. Ovary sessile, 4-celled, and terminated by 4 sessile obtuse stigmas. (The pistile in some flowers is altogether wanting.) Fruit a shining, scarlet berry, nearly spherical, and includes 4 bony, channelled nuts, each containing a single seed.

Distribution: Europe from southern Norway to Tur-key, and the Caucasus, western Asia. In copses and woods in England, and is frequently planted as an ornamental shrub. Flowers May to August. (B.F.M.)

Medicinal Uses: The leaves of *Ilex aquifolium,* the European species of this evergreen, were used for their ability to increase perspiration. In infu-sion, they were also employed to treat inflamma-tions of the mucous membranes, pleurisy, gout, and smallpox. The leaves enjoyed a brief reputa-tion in France as a cure for intermittent fevers. The berries were said to have purgative, emetic and diuretic properties, and the juice of the berries has been used in the treatment of jaun-dice.

Holly leaves are known to contain theobromine, which explains the diaphoretic and febrifuge effects attributed to herbal teas prepared from them. No studies have been reported on the berries of this plant.

The American holly, *I. opaca,* was used for essentially the same purposes. Two species grow-ing in the southern United States, *I. vomitoria* and *I. dahoon,* were used by North Carolina Indians in ritual as well as in medicine. A decoc-tion made from the toasted leaves, known as Black Drink or Yaupon, had emetic properties.

Dose: To reduce the effects of intermittent fevers, an infusion of the powdered leaves was taken 2 hours *before* the paroxysm in the dose of 3.9 grams; 10 or 12 berries are the emetic dose.

HOLY THISTLE
Cnicus benedictus

PARTS USED: Leaves and flowering tops
OTHER COMMON NAMES: Blessed Thistle, Spotted Thistle, Cardin

Botanical Description: The Holy Thistle is an annual herbaceous plant, the stem of which is about 2 feet high, branching toward the top, and furnished with long, elliptical, rough leaves, irregularly toothed, barbed with sharp points at their edges, of a bright green color on their upper surface, and whitish on the under. The lower leaves are deeply sinuated, and stand on footstalks; the upper are sessile, and in some measure decurrent. The flowers are yellow, and surrounded by an involucre of 10 leaves, of which the 5 exterior are largest. The calyx is oval, wooly, and composed of several imbricated scales, terminated by rigid, pinnate, spinous points.

This plant is a native of the south of Europe, and is cultivated in gardens in other parts of the world. It has become naturalized in the United States. The period of flowering is June, when its medicinal virtues are in greatest perfection. It should be cut when in flower, quickly dried, and kept in a dry place.

It has a feeble unpleasant odor, and an intensely bitter taste, more disagreeable in the fresh than the dried plant. (U.S.D.)

Medicinal Uses: The Holy Thistle has been recorded as a medicinal since the first century A.D. Credited with the medical virtues of a diuretic, diaphoretic, febrifuge, and cholagogue, it has been used to treat a variety of ailments. It is a bitter tonic and a good appetite stimulant, and is still used today to treat indigestion. At one time this herb was ascribed the nearly supernatural qualities of a "cure all," but current knowledge yields no evidence to support such a belief.

While there is no direct experimental evidence that preparations of Holy Thistle leaves will give the emetic effect claimed by some writers, if given in large enough quantity most any plant would produce emesis due to the presence of low con-centrations of irritant principles. On the other hand, the use of leaf decoctions as a bitter tonic is well founded. The bitter principle in this plant is known to be cnicin, and human experiments have shown that extracts of Holy Thistle stimulate the production of gastic juices.

Although widely used as an herbal tea for the treatment of amenorrhea (absence of menses), there is no experimental evidence that Holy Thistle seeds have this effect.

Dose: Approximately ½ ounce of leaves and flowering tops to 1 pint of water. Water boiled separately and poured over the plant material and steeped for 5 to 20 minutes, depending on the desired effect. Drunk hot or warm, 1 to 2 cups per day.

HOP
Humulus lupulus

PARTS USED: Strobiles

Botanical Description: The root of the Hop is perennial, and sends up numerous annual, angular, rough, flexible stems, which twine around neighboring objects in a spiral direction, from left to right, and climb to a great height. The leaves are opposite, and stand upon long footstalks. The smaller are sometimes cordate; the larger have 3 or 5 lobes; all are serrate, of a deep green color on the upper surface, and, together with the petioles, extremely rough, with minute prickles. At the base of the footstalks are 2 or 4 smooth, ovate, reflexed stipules. The flowers are numerous, axillary, and furnished with bracts. The male flowers are yellowish-white, and arranged in panicles; the female, which grow on a separate plant, are pale green, and disposed in solitary, peduncled aments, composed of membranous scales, ovate, acute, and tubular at the base. Each scale bears near its base, on its inner surface, 2 flowers, consisting of a roundish compressed germ, and 2 styles, with long filiform stigmas. The aments are converted into ovate membranous cones or strobiles, the scales of which contain each at their base two small seeds surrounded by a yellow, granular, resinous powder.

The Hop is a native of North America and Europe. The part of the plant used, as well in the preparation of malt liquors as in medicine, is the fruit or strobiles. These when fully ripe are picked from the vine, dried

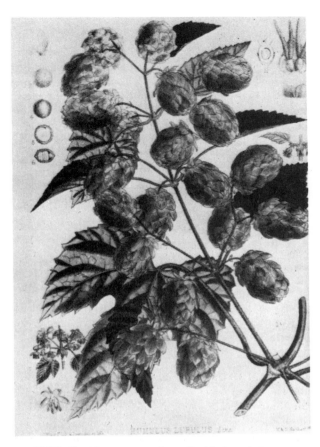

HOPS: Best known as an ingredient in beer brewing, the hops plant has also been used traditionally in the treatment of hysteria, restlessness, and insomnia.

by artificial heat, packed in bales, and sent into the market, under the name of Hops.

They consist of numerous thin, translucent, veined, leaflike scales, which are of a pale greenish-yellow color, and contain near their base two small, round, black seeds. Though brittle when quite dry, they are pulverized with great difficulty. Their odor is strong, peculiar, somewhat narcotic and fragrant; their taste very bitter, aromatic, and slightly astringent. Their aroma, bitterness, and astringency are imparted to water by decoction; but the first-mentioned property is dissipated by long boiling. The most active part of Hops is a substance secreted by the scales, and in the dried fruit existing upon their surface in the form of a fine powder. This substance is called lupulin. (U.S.D.)

Medicinal Uses: Best known as an ingredient in the brewing of beer, in which it is valued for its flavoring and perservative properties, the Hop plant has also been used traditionally in the treatment of hysteria, restlessness, and insomnia.

105

For this latter ailment, pillows stuffed with Hops have been used to produce sleep in nervous disorders; users of such pillows are advised to moisten them with water and glycerin or spirits before placing them under the head of the patient, to prevent rustling of the contents. External applications have been considered useful for arches, pains, and swellings.

The dried strobiles of Hops contain a complex mixture of substances known as "hop acids" (although not all of them are acids), which are all very bitter substances. Some of these hop acids are very effective sedatives, as determined from animal experiments. However, it is most likely that an essential oil in Hops also contributes to the sedative effects, although the active principle(s) in the oil has (have) not yet been identified.

Dose: An infusion prepared with ½ ounce of Hops and a pint of boiling water was given in the dose of 4 fluid ounces. As a fluidextract the usual dose was 2.0-5.8 grams. In making Hop pillows, the dried herb should be moistened with water diluted with a trace of glycerin to prevent rustling of the dried strobiles, which might upset the insomniac more than offering a calming influence.

HOREHOUND, WHITE
Marrubium vulgare

PARTS USED: Leaves and flowering tops
OTHER COMMON NAMES: Hoarhound

Botanical Description: The White Horehound has a perennial fibrous root, and numerous annual stems, which are quadrangular, erect, very downy, and from 12 to 18 inches high. The leaves are roundish ovate, dentate or deeply serrate, wrinkled, veined, hoary on the under surface, and supported in pairs upon strong footstalks. The flowers are white, and disposed in crowded axillary whorls. The calyx is tubular, and divided at the margin into 10 narrow segments, which are hooked at the end. The corolla is also tubular, with a labiate margin, of which the upper lip is bifid, the under reflected and 3-cleft, with the middle segment broad and slightly scalloped. The seeds are 4, and lie in the bottom of the calyx.

This plant is a native of Europe, but has been

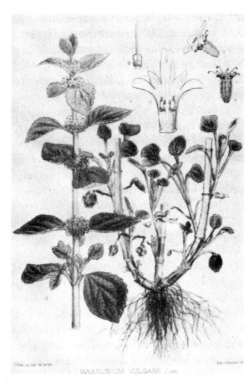

WHITE HOREHOUND: Containing a high concentration of mucilage, the leaves have been used to ease the irritation accompanying sore throats.

naturalized in this country, where it grows on the roadsides, and flowers in July and August. It is also cultivated in our gardens.

The herb has a strong, rather agreeable odor, which is diminished by drying, and is lost by keeping. Its taste is bitter and durable. The bitterness is extracted by water and alcohol. (U.S.D.)

Medicinal Uses: A very popular folk remedy, Horehound is mainly tonic and laxative in its action, but has also been considered valuable for removing obstructions in the system. It is also used to treat chronic hepatitis, and a wide range of ill health due to malignancies, advanced pulmonary tuberculosis, leukemia, malaria, and hysteria.

In domestic use, however, it is more often employed in respiratory complaints, for the treatment of sore throats, to promote the expectoration of phlegm in bronchitis, for asthma, pulmonary consumption, and for obstinate cough.

White Horehound has a high concentration of mucilage, which would be expected to ease the irritation accompanying sore throats.

Dose: 1 teaspoon of leaves and/or flowering tops per cup of boiling water. Drink when cold; 1 tablespoon at a time, 1 cup per day.

HORSECHESTNUT
Aesculus hippocastanum

PARTS USED: Nuts, Leaves, Bark

Botanical Description: Tree 40 or 50 feet high, sending off numerous spreading branches, covered with a rough brown bark. The wood is rapidly formed, is white and soft, but soon decays. Leaves digitate, composed of seven large, obovate, acuminate, serrate, light green leaflets, proceeding from the extremity of a common petiole. Flowers in terminal, somewhat panicled, racemes, or rather short peduncles. Calyx tubular, monophyllous, divided at the margin into 5 obtuse teeth. Corolla consists of 5 unequal spreading petals, ovate, somewhat undulated at the margin, white, and inserted by narrow claws into the calyx, with a rose-colored or yellowish mark at the base. Stamens 7, with awl-shaped, curved, tapering filaments, about the length of the petals, and oblong, somewhat incumbent anthers. Ovary roundish, 3-cornered, and 3-celled; style simple, short, filiform, acute, terminated by a pointed stigma. Fruit a coriaceous, 3-celled, 3-valved capsule, beset externally with short spines, and containing usually 2 large, roundish, shining seeds, destitute of albumen; embryo curved, inverted, with thick, very fleshy, cohering cotyledons; plumule very large, 2-leaved; radicle, conical, curved, and turned towards the hilum.

Distribution: This well known tree migrated originally from the north of Asia, by Constantinople, about the middle of the sixteenth century; it is not known in what year, but Matthiolus is the first botanist who mentions it. In the time of Clusius, it was so rare that when he left Vienna, to which city much of the fruit was brought from Constantinople in 1588, he saw only one tree, which was not more than twelve years old. That it was very little known in England in 1630–40 may be gathered from Parkinson, who states in his *Paradisus* that he cultivated it in his orchard as a fruit tree, esteeming the nuts superior to the ordinary sort. It is

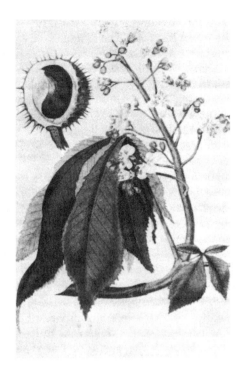

HORSECHESTNUT: The powdered kernel of the nut causes sneezing, and the oil (extracted with ether) has been used in France as a topical remedy for rheumatism. The active principle, escin, is widely used in Europe for vascular problems, including varicose veins.

now very common in the United States and England, and offers a magnificent spectacle during the month of May, when its flowers are in full perfection. (B.F.M.)

Medicinal Uses: The powdered kernel of the nut causes sneezing, and the oil extracted with ether from the kernels has been used in France as a topical remedy for rheumatism. A decoction of the leaves was formerly employed in the United States as a treatment for whooping cough, while the seed oil has been considered useful against sunburn and as a prophylactic against snow blindness. The nuts have been said to contain narcotic properties, and a tincture is very useful against hemorrhoids.

The active principle of Horsechestnut seeds is known to be the complex triterpene glycoside escin. Escin is widely used in Europe as an anti-inflammatory agent for a variety of conditions, in addition to being used for a number of vascular

107

problems, including varicose veins. It is most effective when injected, but is beneficial in some inflammatory conditions when taken by mouth.

The leaves of *A. glabra,* the Ohio Buckeye, were felt to be quite efficacious in the treatment of chest congestions. Buckeye seeds contain constituents similar to those in *A. hippocastanum* seeds, and thus would be expected to have a beneficial effect in the treatment of portal congestion.

Dose: A decoction of the bark, when used for fevers, was given in the dose of 16 grams (½ ounce) of the bark in 24 hours.

A leaf decoction was made from 1 teaspoon of the plant material, boiled in a covered container with 1 pint of water for about ½ hour, at a slow boil. Liquid allowed to cool slowly in the *closed* container. Drunk cold, 1 swallow or 1 tablespoon at a time, 1 to 2 cups per day.

A tincture of the seeds is dabbed on hemorrhoids as needed, while California Indians combined bear fat with the nut kernel as a paste for the same ailment.

INDIAN CORN
Zea mays

PARTS USED: Silk and oil from corn grains
OTHER COMMON NAMES: Maize

Botanical Description: The common food crop, known world wide.

Medicinal Uses: Employed as a mild stimulant diuretic, Corn silk, from this annual grass, was believed to aid acute and chronic cystitis and was also used to treat gonorrhea. In cases of dropsy associated with heart disease, it was considered particularly effective, being a fine diuretic.

The Chickasaw tribe of North America squeezed the oil from the Corn grains and rubbed it directly into the scalp as a dandruff remedy. Corn meal has also been used as an emollient poultice for skin problems.

Corn starch is an effective antidote for iodine poisoning, simply swallowed.

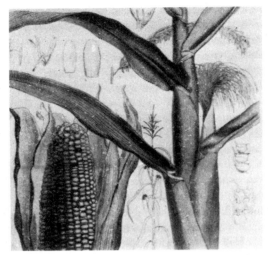

INDIAN CORN: Employed as a mildly stimulant diuretic, corn silk, from this annual grass, was believed to aid acute and chronic cystitis and to treat gonorrhea.

Dose: Steep a handful of the silk. Can be drunk or administered as an enema.

IPECAC
Cephaelis ipecacuanha (Euphorbia ipecacuanha)

PARTS USED: Root
OTHER COMMON NAMES: Ipecacuanha Root, Poaya

Botanical Description: This is a small shrubby plant, with a root from 4 to 6 inches long, about as thick as a goose-quill, marked with annular rugae, simple or somewhat branched, descending obliquely into the ground, and here and there sending forth slender fibrils. The stem is 2 or 3 feet long; but being partly under ground, and often procumbent at the base, usually rises less than a foot in height. It is slender; in the lower portion leafless, smooth, brown or ash-colored, and knotted, with radicles frequently proceeding from the knots; near the summit pubescent, green, and furnished with leaves seldom exceeding 6 in number. These are opposite, petiolate, oblong obovate, acute, entire, from 3 to 4 inches long, from 1 to 2 broad, obscurely green and somewhat rough on their upper

108

surface, pale, downy, and veined on the under. At the base of each pair of leaves are deciduous stipules, embracing the stem, membranous at their base, and separated above into numerous bristle-like divisions. The flowers are very small, white, and collected to the number of 8, 12, or more, each accompanied with a green bract, into a semiglobular head, supported upon a round, solitary, axillary footstalk, and embraced by a monophyllous involucre deeply divided into 4, sometimes 5 or 6 obovate pointed segments. The fruit is an ovate, obtuse berry, which is at first purple, but becomes almost black when ripe, and contains 2 small planoconvex seeds.

The plant is a native of Brazil, flourishing in moist, thick, and shady woods, and abounding most within the limits of latitudes 8° and 20° S. It flowers in January and February, and opens its fruit in May. (U.S.D.)

Medicinal Uses: The name *Ipecacuanha*, from the language of the Brazilian aborigines, has been applied to various emetic roots of South America. The Portuguese learned of this Indian remedy for bowel problems when they settled Brazil, and the root was introduced to Europe around 1672 as a remedy for dysentery. Originally sold in Paris as a secret remedy, the plant showed such value in bowel affections that no less a personage than Louis XIV eventually heaped a large sum of money and public honors on the physician who popularized its use, on the condition that he make it public.

Like many other similar drugs, ipecac is emetic only in large doses; in intermediate doses it is nauseant, diaphoretic, and expectorant; in small doses it is a mild stomach stimulant, increasing the appetite and aiding digestion. Very small doses have also been used to treat the vomiting of pregnancy. When used as a nauseant, ipecac was also observed to exert a sedative effect on the vascular system; hence it came to be employed for hemorrhages, particularly of the uterus.

After it was introduced in Europe, ipecac appeared to work extremely well in some cases of dysentery, while it did nothing in others. It was later shown that the drug has no value against bacteria; since there are two types of dysentery, one due to a specific amoeba and one due to a

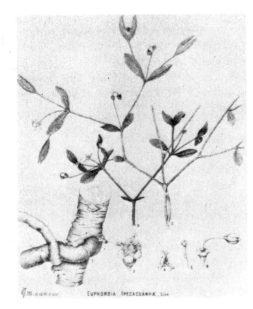

IPECAC: Originally sold in Paris as a secret remedy for bowel affections, ipecac is a potent emetic. The fluid extract is about 20 times more potent than the syrup and several deaths have been reported due to confusing the two forms.

bacillus, ipecac is useless against the latter, bacillary form, while its amebecidal properties account for its being considered probably the most efficacious remedy available against the amoebic type of dysentery.

The major active constituents of Ipecac root are the alkaloids emetine and cephaeline. These are potent drugs that can cause adverse effects on the heart, but in proper dosage, they are not appreciably absorbed from the stomach or intestinal tract, and thus the bad effects are rarely encountered.

Perhaps the major use for Ipecac is in the form of *syrup* of ipecac, which is widely publicized as a useful vomitive (emetic) to administer when people (especially children) have accidentally swallowed a poisonous substance, and it is desired to remove the poison by using an emetic agent. If the proper amount is administered, emesis will take place within 15–20 minutes, and no adverse effects are noted. Unfortunately, there have been a large number of cases in which *fluidextract* of ipecac has been *erroneously* used for this purpose, and several deaths have been recorded due to

109

such mistakes. *Fluidextract* of ipecac is about twenty times more potent than *syrup* of ipecac.

When used for its expectorant effect, very small doses of ipecac are required.

Dose: CAUTION. Do *not* use the fluidextract, unless advised by a physician. Syrup is far less dangerous.

IVY
Hedera helix

PARTS USED: Leaves, Berries, and Exudate
OTHER COMMON NAMES: True or English Ivy

Botanical Description: An evergreen climbing shrub, throwing out roots from the side by which it comes in contact with other substances; branches tortuous and flexible; wood soft, light, and porous. Leaves, when young, lanceolate and entire; at a more advanced period they become cordate, 3- or 5-lobed; and subsequently, when it has arrived at the top of any support, the branches shorten, and form into large bushy heads, and the leaves become ovate and undivided; all the leaves are petiolate, coriaceous, thick, shining, deep green, often veined with whitish lines. Flowers small, pale green, collected into spherical, simple umbels, at the summit of the branches; pedicels generally covered with stellate pubescence. Calyx very small, 5-toothed. Petals, oblong, acute, reflexes, light yellowish green. Stamens 5, alternate with the petals, erect, with subulate filaments inserted beneath a large disk, which crowns the ovary; anthers cleft at the base. Ovary inferior, turbinate, crowned by a very short style and simple stigma. Fruit smooth, globose, purplish black, rather succulent, about the size of a pea, crowned by the remains of the calyx, 1-celled, 3- to 5-seeded. Seeds large, oblong, angular, convex on the outer, angular on the inner side.

Distribution: Europe, Northern Africa, western Asia, to the Himalayas. In England it is very frequent in woods, on the trunks of trees, on the walls of ruined buildings, and on rocks. Flowers October to November, ripening its berries in March and April. (B.F.M.)

Medicinal Uses: The resinous substance which exudes through incisions in the bark has been used in medicine under the name Ivy gum as a stimulant and an emmenagogue (stimulating the menstrual function), and, when placed in cavities of teeth, to relieve toothache. Externally the resin has been used to heal sores, ulcers, etc.

Fresh Ivy leaves have been used as a dressing for wounds and sores that exude pus, and in decoction the leaves have been used to treat skin ulcers and various eruptions. The leaves were also employed as an insecticide.

The berries have been used as a purgative and emetic as well as to induce perspiration; in smaller doses they have been recommended as a cathartic.

The young twigs are a good source of a yellow and brown dye.

Dose: No recommended dosages for internal use.

For external application, an infusion may be prepared using approximately 1 ounce of resin to 1 pint of water. Water boiled separately and poured over the resin and steeped for 5 to 20 minutes, depending on the desired strength.

The leaves, for external use, are applied fresh, after being bruised and/or macerated.

JALAP
Ipomoea purga (Exogonium jalapa)

PARTS USED: Root
OTHER COMMON NAMES: Jalapa, Vera Cruz Jalap, High John Root, High John the Conqueror

Botanical Description: The root of this plant is a roundish somewhat pearshaped tuber, externally blackish, internally white, with long fibers proceeding from its lower part, as well as from the upper root-stalks. The stem is round, smooth, much disposed to twist, and rises to a considerable height upon neighboring objects, about which it twines. The leaves are heart-shaped, entire, smooth, pointed, deeply sinuated at the base, prominently veined on their under surface, and supported upon long footstalks. The lower leaves are nearly hastate, or with diverging angular points. The flowers, which are large and of a lilac-purple color, stand upon peduncles about as long as the petioles. Each peduncle supports 2, or more rarely, 3 flowers. The calyx is without bracts, 5-leaved, obtuse, with 2 of the divisions

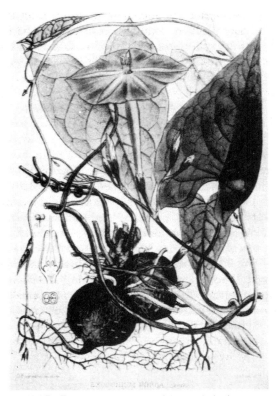

JALAP: The cathartic action of this resin is due to a complex chemical structure which contains long-chain fatty acids linked to glycerin.

external. The corolla is funnel-form. The stamens are 5 in number, with oblong, white, somewhat exserted anthers. The stigma is simple and capitate.

The Jalap plant is a native of Mexico, and derived its name from the city of Xalappa, in the state of Vera Cruz. (U.S.D.)

Medicinal Uses: Jalap is a powerful cathartic, and was used widely during the seventeenth century in Europe as a purgative and to reduce fluid retention of tissues and organs in dropsical complaints. At one time in the United States, Jalap root was administered in cases of complaints due to liver congestion, including constipation, headache, loss of appetite, and fever accompanied with vomiting of bile.

Jalap root resin is well known to act as a powerful hydragogue cathartic, resulting in profuse watery stools when preparations of this plant are taken orally by humans. The action is due to a complex resin mixture which contains long chain fatty acids linked to glycerin.

The cathartic action of Jalap is so harsh, powerful, and unpleasant that it is doubtful whether it should be used for any purpose.

We have been unable to verify any diuretic effect for this plant as reported in the scientific literature, nor any useful property that would allay the symptoms of dropsy.

Dose: CAUTION. Do not use.

JASMINE, YELLOW
Gelsemium sempervirens

PARTS USED: Root

OTHER COMMON NAMES: Gelsemium Root, Yellow Jessamine, Carolina Jessamine

Botanical Description: The Yellow or Carolina Jessamine is one of the most beautiful climbing plants of our southern states, ascending lofty trees, and forming festoons from one tree to another, and during its flowering season, in the early spring, scenting the atmosphere with its delicious odor. The stem is twining, smooth, and shining; the leaves perennial, opposite, nearly persistent, short, petiolate, lanceolate, entire, dark green above, and paler beneath; the flowers in axillary clusters, large, of a deep-yellow color, and fragrant, with a very small, 5-leaved calyx, and a funnel-shaped corolla, having a spreading, 5-lobed, nearly equal border. The fruit is a flat, compressed capsule, divisible into 2 parts, 2-locular, and furnished with flat seeds, which adhere to the margins of the valves. The plant grows in rich, moist soils along the seacoast from Virginia to the south of Florida and Texas. The flowers are said to be poisonous. *Gelsemium elegans*, of upper Burma, is an extremely poisonous creeper which contains gelsemine or an allied alkaloid.

This official plant must not be confounded with the true yellow jasmine of Madeira, often planted in the southern states; this is the *Jasminum odoratissimum*, which also has very fragrant yellow flowers. (U.S.D.)

Medicinal Uses: Yellow Jasmine was formerly employed as an arterial sedative and as an agent to reduce very high fevers. During the latter half of the nineteenth century it was given to treat

111

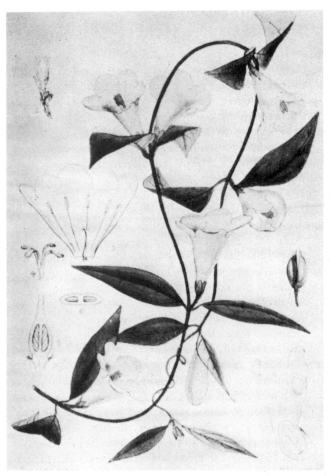

JASMINE, YELLOW: Gelsemine has very potent analgesic effects of a specific type that have led to its valuable use in the relief of pain due to *tic douloureux* (trigeminal neuralgia), which is a condition relating to nerve pain in the cheek.

spasmodic diseases such as asthma and whooping cough.

The rhizomes and roots contain a complex mixture of alkaloids, the major and most important one being gelsemine. Gelsemine has very potent analgesic effects of a specific type that has led to its valuable use in the relief of pain due to *tic douloureux* (trigeminal neuralgia), which is a condition relating to nerve pain in the cheek. The use of Yellow Jasmine to treat this condition is not without risk, however, since gelsemine does have a high order of toxicity.

Resembling Hemlock in its action, Yellow Jasmine may lead to death by asphyxia.

Due to recognized dangers of *Gelsemium* poisoning, use of the plant declined by World War I.

Dose: CAUTION. Not recommended for amateur use. A very potent drug. Overdose can cause death: 35 drops of a bark tincture have caused

death in 1½ hours; while 0.7 milliliter proved fatal to a 3-year-old boy! When *prescribed*, the dose is usually 0.6 milliliter of the tincture or 0.12 milliliter of the fluidextract.

JIMSON WEED
Datura stramonium

PARTS USED: Leaves
OTHER COMMON NAMES: Datura, Thornapple, Jamestown Weed, Nightshade

Botanical Description: Jimson Weed is an annual plant, of rank and vigorous growth, usually about 3 feet high, but in a very rich soil sometimes rising 6 feet or more. The root is large, whitish, and furnished with numerous fibers. The stem is erect, round, smooth, somewhat shining, simple below, dichotomous above, with numerous spreading branches. The leaves, which stand on short round footstalks in the forks of the stem, are 5 or 6

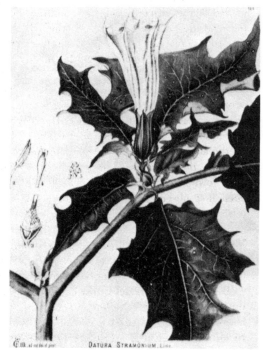

DATURA STRAMONIUM. Linn.

JIMSON WEED: All parts of the plant contain Belladonna-like alkaloids which render it both medicinal and toxic. The violent mania and other mental symptoms produced led to its use in treating insanity and epilepsy, with some reported success.

112

inches long, of an ovate triangular form, irregularly sinuated and toothed at the edges, unequal at the base, of a dark-green color on the upper surface, and pale beneath. The flowers are large, axillary, solitary, and peduncled; having a tubular, pentangular, 5-toothed calyx, and a funnel-shaped corolla with a long tube, and a waved plaited border, terminating in 5 acuminate teeth. The upper portion of the calyx falls with the deciduous parts of the flower, leaving its base, which becomes reflexed, and remains attached to the fruit. This is a large, fleshy, roundish-ovate, 4-valved, 4-celled capsule, thickly covered with sharp spines, and containing numerous seeds attached to a longitudinal receptacle in the center of each cell. It opens at the summit.

Two varieties of this species of *Datura* have been described: one with green stems and white flowers; the other with a dark reddish stem, minutely dotted with green, and purplish flowers striped with deep purple on the inside. The latter variety, however, is considered by most botanists as a distinct species, being the *D. tatula* of Linnaeus. The properties of both are the same.

It is doubtful to what country this plant originally belonged. In the United States it is found everywhere in the vicinity of cultivation, frequenting dung-heaps, the roadsides and commons, and other places where a rank soil is created by the deposited refuse of towns and villages. Its flowers appear from May to July or August, according to the latitude. Where the plant grows abundantly, its vicinity may be detected by the rank odor which it diffuses to some distance around. All parts of it possess medicinal properties. The leaves may be gathered at any time from the appearance of the flowers till the autumnal frost. In the common language of this country, the plant is most known by the name of Jamestown Weed, derived probably from its having been first observed in the neighborhood of that old settlement in Virginia. (U.S.D.)

Medicinal Uses: All parts of the plant contain Belladonna-like alkaloids which render it both medicinal and toxic. Jimson Weed is very similar to Belladonna in its action in both large and small doses, both in its toxicity and in its therapeutic action. The two plants were used interchangeably to check secretions, stimulate circulation, stimulate respiration, overcome spasm of the involuntary muscles, and externally as a local anodyne.

Atropine poisoning may follow external as well as internal application. Interestingly, the violent mania and other mental symptoms produced by the plant led to its use in treating insanity and epilepsy, with some reported success.

Homeopathic doses were administered to treat skin eruptions, hemorrhoids, hysteria, and neuralgias. In spasmodic asthma, the leaves, smoked in cigarettes, or their steam, inhaled from an infusion, reportedly provided great temporary relief and facilitated expectoration, but extreme caution was advised in any such use of the plant.

While Jimson Weed is used for about the same purposes as described for Belladonna, and contains the same active constituents, Jimson Weed usually contains higher concentrations of scopolamine than does Belladonna. Because of this, *Datura stramonium* has been used to some extent by the drug culture as an hallucinogen, either by taking extracts orally, or by smoking the plant parts. There are a large number of published medical reports that confirm this effect in humans.

Jimson Weed is also very effective in relieving the symptoms of asthma by either burning the leaves and inhaling the smoke, or by inhaling the smoke from *stramonium* cigarettes. The active alkaloids are volatile and pass with the smoke into the lungs. They then exert their effect by relaxing the smooth muscle of that organ, which is constricted during an asthmatic attack, thereby allowing the person to breathe more freely.

As with Belladonna, similar precautions in use must be observed because of the powerful action of this plant.

Dose: CAUTION. Very potent drug.

JUNIPER
Juniperus communis

PARTS USED: Berries
OTHER COMMON NAMES: Viscum, Juniper Mistletoe, Mistletoe

Botanical Description: This is an erect evergreen shrub, usually small, but sometimes attaining a height of 12 or 15 feet, with numerous very close branches. The leaves are narrow, longer than the fruit, entire, sharply

113

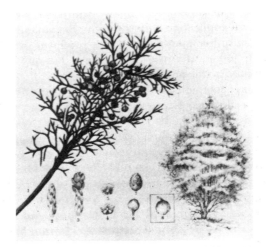

JUNIPER BERRY: The primary source of flavoring for gin, the aromatic berries show experimental value in treating arthritis. The principal use, however, has been as a diuretic, and this effect has been demonstrated in animals.

pointed, channelled, of a deep green color, somewhat glaucous on their upper surface, spreading, and attached to the stem or branches in threes, in a verticillate manner. The flowers are dioecious and disposed in small, ovate, axillary, sessile, solitary aments. The fruit is a globular berry, formed of the fleshy coalescing scales of the ament, and containing 3 angular seeds.

The common Juniper is a native of Europe; but has been introduced in this country, in some parts of which it has become naturalized. The common Juniper flowers in May, but does not ripen its fruit till late in the following year. All parts of the plant contain a volatile oil, which imparts to them a peculiar flavor. The wood has a slight aromatic odor, and was formerly used for fumigation. A terebinthinate juice exudes from the tree and hardens on the bark. The fruit and tops of Juniper are the only officinal parts.

The berries are sometimes collected in this country. But, though equal to the European in appearance, they are inferior in strength, and are not much used. The best come from the south of Europe, particularly from Trieste and the Italian ports. They are globular; more or less shrivelled; about as large as a pea; marked with three furrows at the summit, and with tubercles from the persistent calyx at the base; covered with a glaucous bloom, beneath which they are of a shining blackish-purple color; and containing a brownish-yellow pulp and three angular seeds. They have an agreeable somewhat

aromatic odor, and a sweetish, warm, bitterish, slightly terebinthinate taste. These properties, as well as their medicinal virtues, they owe chiefly to an essential oil which may be separated by distillation. (U.S.D.)

Medicinal Uses: Juniper berries have a gently stimulant and diuretic action, and impart an odor of violets to the urine. Taken in large quantities, they occasionally produce irritation of the urinary passages. Their principal use is as an adjuvant to more powerful diuretics in problems of fluid retention. The berries are also used medicinally as carminatives, stomachics, antiseptics, and stimulants. The volatile oil distilled from the berries was used as a carminative to aid the expulsion of intestinal flatulence, and also as a diuretic.

While the USFDA considers this plant an "unsafe herb," there are no known data to substantiate this opinion.

Juniper berries, the primary source of flavoring for gin, have been used as an herbal remedy for a number of conditions. The aromatic berries have been employed in folk medicine to lower serum cholesterol and as an anticancer remedy. Experimentally, antitumor activity has been shown in animals.

The primary use, however, has been as a diuretic, and this effect has been shown in animals. The active diuretic principle has been shown to be a simple terpene, terpinen-4-ol.

Although there is no direct experimental evidence that Juniper berries would be effective in the treatment of gout, studies have been conducted in humans that indicate a value in treating arthritis. Both gout and arthritis are acute inflammatory conditions, and drugs effective for one of these conditions are usually found useful in the other.

The mildly stimulant effect attributed to Juniper berries is due to the action of constituents in the essential oil.

Dose: 3 ounces of the berries to 1 pint of boiling water, poured over the berries and steeped for 5 to 20 minutes, depending on the desired effect. Drunk hot or warm, 1 cup every 4 or 5 hours, to which may be added extract of Dandelion, or cream of tartar.

KAVA-KAVA
Piper methysticum

PARTS USED: Root
OTHER COMMON NAMES: Ava

Botanical Description: The genus *Piper* includes a large number of subtropical plants, which are mostly shrubs, and rarely herbs or trees. A number of the species are of great economic importance. *Piper methysticum* is a shrub, several feet high, indigenous to many of the South Sea islands. It has green, jointed stems, swollen at the joints, and with alternate, heart-shaped leaves about 5 to 8 inches long and nearly as wide, the petioles about 1 inch long, the blades with 11 to 13 prominent veins originating at the base. Flowers are borne in narrow spikes, the 2 sexes, it is said, on separate plants. Kava is a native of Pacific islands, and in early times it was distributed eastward through tropical islands by migrating people, who valued the root as the source of a drink and of medicine. In Hawaii more than 15 varieties were known. In many islands of the Pacific, Kava has long played an important part in the life of the people, being used in ceremonies, festivals, and as a sign of good will. (U.S.D. & Neal)

Medicinal Uses: The root is used to prepare a beverage, the ceremonial drink of many inhabitants of Melanesia and Polynesia, which is reputedly sedative, aphrodisiac, tonic, stimulant, diuretic, and diaphoretic. While both men and women drink Kava nowadays, in former times tribal custom forbade women to partake; furthermore, the beverage was prepared through mastication of the root by young virgins, for the men's ceremonial purposes. The root has a faint but characteristic odor, an aromatic, bitter, pungent taste, with a slight local anesthesia resulting.

Animal studies clearly point out a marked ability of extracts of Kava to calm experimentally enraged animals. The principle responsible for this effect has not been discovered.

A number of compounds referred to as "Kava pyrones," for example, kawain, dihydrokawain, methysticin, and dihydromethysticin, are claimed to have mild sedative and tranquilizing effects. Kawain is marketed in Europe as a mild sedative for the elderly. Extracts of Kava, and most of the Kava pyrones, have been shown to have antiseptic properties in test tube experiments.

Regular and prolonged use of Kava extracts results in the production of a skin rash, which is pigmented yellow. This condition, among Kava users in the South Pacific, is known as "Kawaism." The condition subsides following restriction of the Kava beverage, with no ill effects. It is important to remember that this plant has been utilized for its calming effects in Oceania since antiquity. While the introduction of alcohol has created many social problems, those groups still using this plant in its traditional way enjoy a mild insulation from life's vicissitudes.

Dose: The Fiji Islanders take one large handful of the dried, powdered root and wrap it in a cheesecloth. In one quart of *cold* water they knead the Kava-Kava until the liquid is a *dark* chalky gray. They stir and drink at once, several cupfuls, unsweetened. They then add water, reknead the root, and drink as desired until sedation is felt.

KINO
Pterocarpus marsupium, P. indicus, P. echinatus

PARTS USED: Exudate (juice from incisions in trunk of tree)
OTHER COMMON NAMES: Gummi, Narra, Bibla, Prickly Narra, Padauk

Botanical Description: Large, handsome trees, sometimes developing buttresses, with a large crown of foliage and, in season, masses of flowers, *Pterocarpus* species are from southeastern Asia, Malaysia, India, and the Philippines. *P. marsupium* has 5 to 7 oval, leathery leaflets, notched at the tip, petals yellow or white, the calyx bearing dark brown hairs. Next to Teak and Rosewood, it is the most widely cultivated tree in India. Kino, an oily gum, is extracted from the bark.

The Prickly Narra (*P. echinatus*) from the Philippines is similar, differing mainly in having each pod with slender spines over the central area where the single seed lies. (Neal)

Medicinal Uses: Kino is the name given to the juice that exudes from incisions in the trunk of the

115

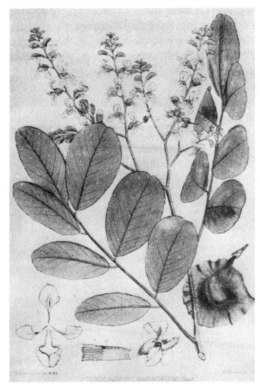

KINO: The juice from this tree is a powerful astringent and has seen much folkloric use to check discharges from wounds, scrapes, and skin ulcers.

tree *Pterocarpus marsupium*. It was deemed a powerful astringent and as such was used externally to check discharges from wounds, scrapes, and skin ulcers. In combination with Opium or chalk mixtures, it was administered to treat non-inflammatory diarrheas; it was never given in the presence of fever. Its action is primarily due to the presence of a tannin-like substance, kinotannic acid, which also gives it application in the treatment of leucorrhea by injection. It has also been used to treat passive hemorrhages of the intestines and uterus, diabetes, and as a gargle to relax the throat. Aromatic substances were often added to the Kino to make it more palatable.

A related species, from Africa, *P. angloensis* (Bloodwood), used as a substitute for Indian teak, is famed as an aphrodisiac. The roots are used for this activity in the Congo, Angola, Tanganyika, Mozambique, and the Transvaal.

Dose: For internal use—.05–2.0 grams of powdered exudate, dissolved in 1 cup of boiling water, taken 1 cup per day, 1 tablespoon at a time.

For external use, powdered exudate is applied directly to the affected area.

LAVENDER
Lavandula officinalis (L. vera and *L. spica)*

PARTS USED: Flowers (and oil)

Botanical Description: The common Lavender is a small shrub, usually rising not more than 2 or 3 feet, but sometimes attaining an elevation of 6 feet. The stem is woody below, and covered with a brown bark; above, is divided into numerous slender, straight, herbaceous, pubescent, quadrangular branches, furnished with opposite, sessile, narrow, nearly linear, entire, and green or glaucous leaves. The flowers are small, blue, and disposed in interrupted whorls around the young shoots, forming terminal cylindrical spikes. Each whorl is accompanied with two bracts. The corolla is tubular and labiate, with the lower lip divided into three segments, the upper larger and bifid. The filaments are within the tube.

The plant is a native of southern Europe, and covers vast tracts of dry and barren land in Spain, Italy, and the south of France. It is cultivated abundantly in our gardens, and in this country flowers in August. All parts of it are endowed with properties similar to those for which the flowers are used; but these only are officinal. The spikes should be cut when they begin to bloom.

Lavender flowers have a strong fragrant odor, and an aromatic, warm, bitterish taste. They retain their fragrance a long time after drying. Alcohol extracts their virtues; and a volatile oil upon which their odor depends rises with that liquid in distillation. The oil may be procured separately by distilling the flowers with water. (U.S.D.)

Medicinal Uses: Oil distilled from Lavender flowers is used medicinally as an aromatic stimulant, mild carminative, and tonic, to treat nervous languor and headache. The flowers, as well as the oil, are employed chiefly in perfumery, but their fragrance also led to their use to disguise nasty-smelling herbal and other pharmaceutical preparations.

116

Chemically, the plant contains l-linalyl acetate, geraniol, and linalol. Lavender flowers contain large amounts of a highly aromatic oil, and have definite spasmolytic, antiseptic, and carminative activity. These activities are all attributed to the essential oil, and its aromatic principles.

Bunches of the dried flowers are used to make sachets and for imparting a gentle scent to linen.

Interestingly, the oil (known as "oil of aspic") is also utilized in varnishes to dilute delicate colors in china paintings.

Dose: 1 teaspoon of the flowers, cut small or granulated, to 1 cup of boiling water. Water boiled separately and poured over the plant material and steeped for 5–20 minutes, depending on the desired effect. Drunk cold, a large mouthful at a time, 1 cup during the day.

LETTUCE, WILD
Lactuca elongata

PARTS USED: Latex

Botanical Description: This indigenous species of Lettuce is biennial, with a stem from 3 to 6 feet in height, and leaves of which the lower are runcinate, entire, and clasping, the lowest toothed, and the highest lanceolate. They are all smooth on their under surface. The flowers are in corymbose panicles, small, and of a pale yellow color. The stem and leaves yield, when wounded, a milky juice in which the virtues of the plant reside.

The Wild Lettuce grows in all latitudes of the United States, from Canada to the Carolinas. It is found in woods, along roads, and in fertile soils, and flowers in June and July. (U.S.D.)

Medicinal Uses: The medicinal effects of Lettuce (there are about 100 wild species) depend upon the milky juice which exudes on laceration of the stem or the flower stalks. This juice later becomes brownish, resembling opium. The medicinal preparation, which consists of the juice in hardened, evaporated form, is known as lactucarium. The juice possesses narcotic and sudorific qualities. It has very mild pain-allaying and calmative effects, somewhat like a weak dose of opium. It may best be employed as a mild

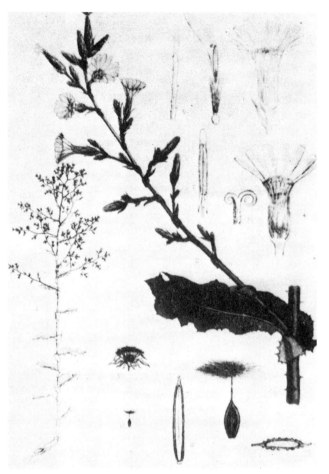

LETTUCE, WILD: The white latex which exudes on laceration possesses narcotic qualities somewhat like those of a weak dose of opium.

sedative. It was also used as a draught in constipation, intestinal disorders such as engorgements, and for other gastric upsets. Mentioned by the Greeks Dioscorides, Galen, and Theophrastus, among others, Lettuce has been in use as a painkiller and relaxant since ancient times. More recently, it has been revived to some extent among the drug culture in the form of a commercial preparation known as "Lettuce Opium."

Lactucarium, found in this and other species of Lettuce, is obtained by wounding the plants in the flowering season when their vessels are filled with juice and so irritable that they often spontaneously burst or are ruptured by very slight accidental injuries. In color, taste, and odor, lactucarium strongly resembles opium.

The fresh milky latex from Wild Lettuce plants contains a sedative principle known as lactupicrin. The best way to collect this juice is by placing

117

successive small pieces of cotton on the cut stem and throwing them into a little water. After a quantity has accumulated, the water holding in solution the contents of the pieces of cotton is evaporated, and an extract thus procured. An easier way to collect the latex is by macerating in water the stems and leaves, just after the seeds have matured and before the plant decays. The maceration is to be continued for 24 hours, then the liquid is boiled for 2 hours, and finally evaporated in shallow basins.

Dose: When used for its sedative effects, the latex of Wild Lettuce was taken in a dose of 3.0 to 12 grams every 24 hours.

LICORICE
Glycyrrhiza glabra

PARTS USED: Dried root and subterranean stem
OTHER COMMON NAMES: Sweet Wood

Botanical Description: The Licorice plant has a perennial root, which is round, succulent, tough, and pliable, furnished with sparse fibers, rapid in its growth, and in a sandy soil penetrates deeply into the ground. The stems are herbaceous, erect, and usually 4 or 5 feet in height; have few branches; and are garnished with alternate, pinnate leaves, consisting of several pairs of ovate, blunt, petiolate leaflets, with a single leaflet at the end, of a pale green color, and clammy on their under surface. The flowers are violet or purple, formed like those of the pea, and arranged in axillary spikes supported on long peduncles. The calyx is tubular and persistent. The fruit is a compressed, smooth, acute, one-celled legume, containing from one to four small kidney-shaped seeds.

The plant is a native of the south of Europe, Barbary, Syria, and Persia; and is cultivated in England, the north of France, and Germany. This species is also abundantly produced in the south of Russia. (U.S.D.)

Medicinal Uses: Among the ancient Greeks Licorice root had a reputation for quenching thirst, and was used in this connection in the treatment of dropsy. It is an excellent demulcent, and hence has been given to treat irritated urinary, bowel, and respiratory passages. It was often given in combination with Senega and Mezereon (see articles on these plants), when these drugs were used on persons with irritated or inflamed eliminatory organs. The root also reportedly had expectorant and laxative properties. Children suck on Licorice sticks both as candies and also as a remedy for coughs. Licorice is a valuable flavoring adjunct to medicines with unpleasant tastes; and the powdered root was used in the preparation of pills, both to give them more substance and to coat the surfaces to prevent their sticking together.

The multitude of pharmacological effects of Licorice rhizomes and roots are practically all attributed to the presence of a triterpene saponin called glycyrrhizin.

Glycyrrhizin is about fifty times sweeter than sugar, and has a powerful cortisone-like effect. In fact, several cases have been reported in the medical literature in which humans ingesting 6–8 ounces of licorice candy daily for a period of several weeks are "poisoned" due to the cortisone-like effects of the licorice extract in the candy. Proper treatment restores patients to normal.

In addition, Licorice rhizomes and roots have a high mucilage content. When mixed with water, the resulting preparation has a very pleasant odor and taste, and acts as an effective demulcent on irritated mucous membranes, such as accompany a sore throat.

Dose: 1 teaspoon of the root or subterranean stem, boiled in a covered container with 1½ pints of water for about ½ hour, at a slow boil. Liquid allowed to cool slowly in the *closed* container. Drunk cold, 1 swallow or 1 tablespoon at a time, 1 to 2 cups per day.

LILY-OF-THE-VALLEY
Convallaria majalis

PARTS USED: Root, fruit, flowers
OTHER COMMON NAMES: Convallaria, May Lily, May-Blossom

Botanical Description: The fragrant, little, white, bell-shaped flowers, which hang on slender stems along one side of the main, erect, 4- to 10-inch stem, are popular for wedding bouquets. The flowers, only 0.25 inch long, have 6 tiny blunt lobes curving back from the mouth of the bell. The 2 or 3 oblong or oval leaves which rise from near the ground measure 5 to 12 by 1 to 2.5 inches. They are borne on short petioles. Though the plants grow wild over a wide area, from Europe to eastern Asia and from Virginia to South Carolina, all are the same species, and no other species is known from other regions. They grow best in shade. (Neal)

Medicinal Uses: Convallaria has long been used to expel worms from the intestinal tract, and as a popular remedy for dropsy.

The flowers were believed to stimulate the secretions of the mucous membranes of the nose, and were employed in the treatment of apoplexy, epilepsy, coma, and vertigo. Spirits distilled from the flowers were applied externally on sprains and to treat rheumatism.

The root has the same recorded properties as the flowers, and in extract was additionally used for its gentle stimulant and laxative properties.

The major traditional use for Lily-of-the-Valley seems to be as a cardiotonic. Its action is then explained fully on the basis of the presence of cardiac glycosides similar in structure and effect to the *Digitalis* glycosides. The major cardiac glycoside in Lily-of-the-Valley is convallatoxin.

Since there are no advantages of *Convallaria* as a cardiotonic over the effects of *Digitalis purpurea* (Foxglove), it has not been used extensively in the United States. It is used, however, rather extensively in Europe at the present time.

Dose: Of either the flowers or the root, as a cardiotonic, 0.32–0.65 gram. CAUTION. This plant has a powerful digitalis-like effect.

LOBELIA
Lobelia inflata

PARTS USED: Leaves and seeds
OTHER COMMON NAMES: Indian Tobacco, Wild Tobacco, Asthma Weed

Botanical Description: The Indian Tobacco is an annual or biennial indigenous plant, usually a foot or more in height, with a fibrous root, and a solitary, erect,

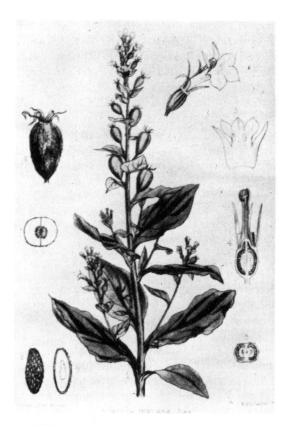

LOBELIA: The leaves and flowering tops of this annual contain lobeline, which is used to stimulate respiration in newborn infants and as a smoking deterrent when used in small doses.

angular, very hairy stem, much branched about midway, but rising considerably above the summits of the highest branches. The leaves are scattered, sessile, oval, acute, serrate, and hairy. The flowers are numerous, disposed in leafy terminal racemes, and supported on short axillary footstalks. The segments of the calyx are linear and pointed. The corolla, which is of a delicate blue color, has a labiate border, with the upper lip divided into 2, the lower into 3 acute segments. The united anthers are curved, and enclose the stigma. The fruit is an oval, striated, inflated capsule, crowned with the persistent calyx, and containing, in 2 cells, numerous very small, brown seeds.

This species of Lobelia is a very common weed, growing on the roadsides, and in neglected fields, throughout the United States. Its flowers begin to appear toward the end of July and continue to expand in succession till the occurrence of frost. The plant when

119

wounded or broken exudes a milky juice. All parts of it are possessed of medicinal activity; but the root and inflated capsules are most powerful. The plant should be collected in August or September, when the capsules are numerous, and should be carefully dried. It may be kept whole, or in the state of powder.

Dried Lobelia has a slight, irritating odor, and when chewed, though at first without much taste, soon produces a burning acrid impression upon the posterior parts of the tongue and palate, very closely resembling that produced by tobacco, and attended, in like manner, with a flow of saliva and a nauseating effect upon the stomach. The powder is of greenish color. The plant yields its active properties readily to water and alcohol; and water distilled from it retains its acrid taste. (U.S.D.)

Medicinal Uses: This controversial herb was the mainstay of the system of herbal medicine introduced by Samuel Thomson, who wrote in the third edition of his *Botanic Family Physician* (Boston, 1831): "In consequence of their [accredited doctors] thus forming an erroneous opinion of this herb, which they had no knowledge of, they undertook to represent it as a deadly poison; and in order to destroy my practice, they raised a hue and cry about my killing my patients by administering it to them." Thomson's book is largely given over to passionate protestations toward the medical establishment, which he felt was persecuting him.

Lobelia was reported useful in treating bronchitis, laryngitis, asthma, and convulsive and inflammatory disorders such as epilepsy, tetanus, diptheria, and tonsillitis. As a muscle relaxant, Lobelia was employed in midwifery to alleviate rigidity of the pelvic musculature during childbirth, according to the recommendations of one of Thomson's followers. Used externally in a poultice with Slippery Elm and a little soap, Lobelia was helpful in bringing abscesses and boils to a head.

The precautions about the poisonous potential of the plant are always mentioned by herbalists other than those practicing the Thomsonian system. Lobelia, along with twenty-six other plants, has been declared an "unsafe herb" by the U.S. Food and Drug Administration, which describes it as "a poisonous plant which contains the alkaloid

lobeline, plus a number of other pyridine alkaloids. Overdoses of the plant or extracts of the leaves or fruits produce vomiting, sweating, pain, paralysis, depressed temperatures, rapid but feeble pulse, collapse, coma and death in the human being." The effects of excessive doses, classified by herbalists as "acro-narcotic," are similar to those of tobacco; hence its popular name, Indian Tobacco.

Lobelia leaves and flowering tops do contain the alkaloid lobeline, which is known to relax smooth muscle, and thus would give rise to an antispasmodic effect. Extracts of the leaves have been shown experimentally to have expectorant properties, most likely due to the lobeline content.

Lobeline is used to stimulate respiration in newborn infants. It is a popular smoking deterrent when used orally in small doses. Human experimental evidence attests to its value in aiding smokers to drop the habit, contradicting the possibly excessive cautions of the USFDA.

Dose: The tincture, used in asthma, was given in doses of 0.9 millimeter every hour(!). The fluidextract, used as an antispasmodic, was given in doses of 0.13–0.5 gram.

MADDER
Rubia tinctorum

PARTS USED: Root
OTHER COMMON NAMES: Dyers' Madder

Botanical Description: The root of the Dyers' Madder is perennial, and consists of numerous long, succulent fibers, varying in thickness from the size of a quill to that of the little finger, and uniting at top in a common head, from which also proceed side-roots that run near the surface of the ground, and send up many annual stems. These are slender, quadrangular, jointed, procumbent, and furnished with short prickles by which they adhere to the neighboring plants upon which they climb. The leaves are elliptical, pointed, rough, firm, about 3 inches long and nearly 1 inch broad, having rough points on their edges and midrib, and standing at the joints of the stem in whorls of 4, 5, or 6 together. The branches rise in pairs from the same joints, and bear small yellow flowers at the summit of each of their subdivisions. The fruit is a round, shining, black berry.

The plant is a native of the south of Europe, and is cultivated in France and Holland. (U.S.D.)

Medicinal Uses: The principal use of the Madder root has been as the source of a red dye for fabrics. Madder seemingly became popular as a medicinal only because of its very unusual ability to impart a red color to the urine and bones when taken internally, especially in young animals. It does not dye the surrounding tissues and seems to concentrate on the bones nearest the heart. It enjoyed a striking reputation among the ancient Greek physicians for its reported ability to promote the flow of urine and menstruation, cure dysentery and jaundice, and aid in childbirth. Its use to promote menstruation and its inclusion in remedies for dropsical complaints, as well as its employment to treat internal wounds and bruises, may have been traceable to the early physicians' belief that a plant that could dye urine and bones as well as the beaks and feet of birds which fed upon it must be good for the blood and bones. More recently Madder roots and rhizomes have been used for their tonic and astringent properties.

Dyers' Madder has become virtually obsolete in medicine in more recent times. However, Madder roots are known to cause contractions of uterine muscle in certain types of laboratory experiments. In some cases, contraction of uterine muscle can result in the induction of menstruation, and thus would have beneficial effects in women suffering from amenorrhea. We have been unable to locate experimental evidence that would substantiate the use of Madder in treating dropsy. Nevertheless, the bruised roots and leaves have attained some reputation as a facial for the removal of freckles!

Dose: 1 teaspoon of the root, boiled in a covered container of 1½ pints of water for about ½ hour, at a slow boil. Liquid allowed to cool slowly in the *closed* container. Drunk cold, 1 swallow or 1 tablespoon at a time, 1 to 2 cups per day.

MAGNOLIA
Magnolia glauca, and other *Magnolia* species

PARTS USED: Bark and root bark
OTHER COMMON NAMES: White Bay, Beaver Tree, Sweet Magnolia

Botanical Description: The medicinal properties which have rendered the bark of the Magnolia official are common to most if not all of the species composing this splendid genus. Among the numerous trees which adorn the American landscape, these are most conspicuous for the beautiful richness of their foliage, and the delicious odor of their flowers; and the *M. grandiflora* of the southern states rivals in magnitude the largest inhabitants of our forests.

Magnolia glauca. This species of Magnolia, which in the northern states is often nothing more than a shrub, sometimes attains in the South the height of 40 feet. The leaves are scattered, petiolate, oval, obtuse, entire, glabrous, thick, opaque, yellowish-green on their upper surface, and of a beautiful pale glaucous color beneath. The flowers are large, terminal solitary, cream-colored, strongly odorous, often scenting the air to a considerable distance. The calyx is composed of 3 leaves; the petals, from 8 to 14 in number, are obovate, obtuse,

MAGNOLIA: Owing to their ability to produce sweating, the barks of various Magnolias have long been used to treat fevers. Used in place of Cinchona, Magnolia has been administered for longer periods of time without side effects.

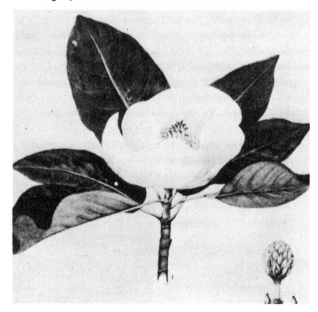

concave, and contracted at the base; the stamens are very numerous, and inserted on a conical receptacle; the germs are collected into a cone, and each is surmounted by a linear recurved style. The fruit is conical, about an inch in length, consisting of numerous imbricated cells, each containing a single scarlet seed. This escapes through a longitudinal opening in the cell, but remains for some time suspended from the cone by a slender thread to which it is attached.

M. glauca extends along the eastern seaboard of the United States, from Cape Ann in Massachusetts to the shores of the Gulf of Mexico. It is abundant in the Midwest and South, usually growing in swamps and morasses; and is seldom met with in the interior of the country west of the Rocky Mountains. It begins to flower in May, June, or July, according to the latitude. (U.S.D.)

Medicinal Uses: Owing to their diaphoretic properties, the barks of various Magnolias were taken to mitigate the ravages of malarial as well as other intermittent fevers. Used in place of Cinchona, Magnolia could be administered for longer periods of time with no side effects. It was also employed as a remedy for rheumatism at one time, and is a gently stimulant aromatic tonic. There is some record of the Magnolia bark's usefulness as a substitute for tobacco and as an aid for breaking the habit of chewing tobacco.

M. officinalis is prized in Chinese herbalism as a tonic, and is considered aphrodisiac. In Mexico, *M. Schiedeana* is used to treat scorpion stings, in a flower decoction applied topically. Perhaps most interesting of all medicinal properties of Magnolias is reported of a species found in Brazil *(M. pubescens)*. The stems, leaves, and seeds contain saponins capable of stupefying fish and are used for this purpose by fishermen wanting an easier catch.

Dose: For medicinal applications, 1 teaspoon of the bark, cut small or granulated, is boiled in a covered container with 1½ pints of water for about ½ hour, at a slow boil. Liquid allowed to cool slowly in the *closed* container. Drunk cold, 1 swallow or 1 tablespoon at a time, 1 cup per day.

MAIDENHAIR FERN
Adiantum pedatum, A. capillus-veneris

PARTS USED: Herb
OTHER COMMON NAMES: Venus' Hair

Botanical Description: Many forms of these popular ornamental pot plants are known. Most species originated in warm parts of America. They can be recognized by the large or small, 4-sided, oblong, or wedge-shaped subdivisions of the fronds, the margins of which are more or less notched, and by the slender, wiry stems, which may be dark and shiny. Spores are borne at the tips or in notches of the last subdivisions, the edge being rolled back to cover them, thus making an indusium. (*Adiantum* is Greek for "unwetted," referring to the smooth, waterproof fronds.) (Neal)

Medicinal Uses: Most commonly employed to relieve coughs of colds and nasal congestion, Maidenhair Fern was felt to relieve thirst and fever, as well as stimulate secretions of the bronchopulmonary mucous membranes and facilitate their removal. In this latter function as an expectorant, it was used for asthma and other pulmonary congestive disorders.

A dandruff remedy reported by some herbalists consisted of the ashes of this fern, combined with vinegar and olive oil, and applied to the scalp.

Extracts of a related fern, *Adiantum caudatum*, have been studied in animals. These experiments indicate that extracts of the fern are capable of relaxing smooth muscle, a finding that is in support of the use of *A. pedatum* and *A. capillus-veneris* for asthma. Further work is obviously necessary before one can validate the effectiveness of these herbal remedies.

Dose: For medicinal use, one teaspoonful of the herb is added to 1 cup of boiling water. Drunk cold, 1 tablespoon at a time, up to a total of 1 to 2 cups per day.

MALE FERN
Dryopteris filix-mas (Aspidium filix-mas)

PARTS USED: Rhizome

OTHER COMMON NAMES: Aspidium

Botanical Description: The Male Fern has a perennial, horizontal root, from which numerous annual fronds or leaves arise, forming tufts from a foot to 4 feet in height. The stipe or footstalk, and midrib, are thickly beset with brown, tough, transparent scales; the frond itself is oval lanceolate, acute, pinnate, and of a bright green color. The pinnae or leaflets are remote below, approach more nearly as they ascend, and run together at the summit of the leaf. They are deeply divided into lobes, which are of an oval shape, crenate at the edges, and gradually diminish from the base of the pinna to the apex. The fructification is in small dots in the back of each lobe, placed in 2 rows near the base, and distant from the edges.

The Male Fern is indigenous, growing in shady pine forests from New Jersey to Virginia. It is a native also of Europe, Asia, and North Africa. In the American plant, the leaflets are said to be more obtuse, and oftener doubly serrated than in the European.

The proper period for collecting the root is during the summer, when it abounds more in the active principle than at any other season. It deteriorates rapidly when kept, and in about two years becomes entirely inert. The roots of other species of fern are frequently substituted for the officinal; and in the dried state it is difficult to distinguish them. (U.S.D.)

Medicinal Uses: The ancient Greeks Theophrastus, Dioscorides, and Pliny all recommended Male Fern for use in expelling tapeworms and other parasitic worms from the intestines; they advised combining the fern with wine and barley meal. The Male Fern was widely used for these purposes during the nineteenth century, after a certain Madame Nouffer sold her secret remedy to Louis XVI for 18,000 francs. It was often taken on an empty stomach, followed in two hours by a dose of castor oil or other mild purgative. Excessive doses can be poisonous, so this fern was always used very carefully.

Dose: The oleoresin from the rhizomes of Male Fern is a well-known anthelmintic, owing its activity to a complex mixture of substances known collectively as "filicin." Male Fern oleoresin is almost exclusively used to remove tapeworms from the intestinal tract. When used properly it is quite safe, but if used improperly it can be more toxic to the person taking it than to the tapeworm.

Thus, before using Aspidium oleoresin, a person should maintain a fat-free diet for 24 hours. A saline cathartic such as citrate of magnesia should then be taken, but not oily cathartics. The reason for this is that the filicin is very poisonous if it is absorbed into the body from the intestine. It will only do this if there is fat or oil present. The cathartic will not remove the tapeworm since it has "hooks" on its head (scolex) that attach to the intestine wall. When a single dose of Aspidium oleoresin is taken, the filicin numbs and/or para-

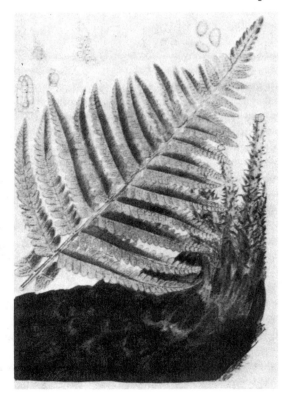

MALE FERN: The oleoresin from these rhizomes is a well-known treatment for tapeworms. If used improperly, it can be more toxic to the person taking it than it is to the tapeworm.

123

lyzes the tapeworm and it releases its hold on the intestinal wall. After a short period of time another dose of the *saline* (not oily) cathartic is taken and the tapeworm is flushed out of the body.

It is important that the feces be examined to see if the head (scolex) of the tapeworm has been removed. Tapeworms can be up to 15 or more feet in length, and practically all of the worm could be flushed out of the body, but if the scolex remains, it will continue to reproduce and form another full-size parasite.

MANDRAKE
Podophyllum peltatum (American Mandrake),
Mandragora officinarum (European Mandrake)

PARTS USED: Root

OTHER COMMON NAMES: Podophyllum, May-Apple, Devil's Apple

Botanical Description: *Podophyllum peltatum.* The May-Apple, known also by the name of Mandrake, is an indigenous herbaceous plant, and the only species belonging to this genus. The root is perennial, creeping, usually several feet in length, about ¼ inch thick, of a brown color externally, smooth, jointed, and furnished with radicles at the joints. The stem is about 1 foot high, erect, round, smooth, divided at top into 2 petioles, and supporting at the fork a solitary 1 flowered peduncle. Each petiole bears a large peltate, palmate leaf, with six or seven wedge-shaped lobes, irregularly incised at the extremity, yellowish-green on the upper surface, paler and slightly pubescent beneath. The flower is nodding. The calyx is composed of three oval, obtuse, concave, deciduous leaves. The corolla has from 6 to 9 white, fragrant petals, which are obovate, obtuse, concave, with delicate transparent veins. The stamens are from 13 to 20, shorter than the petals, with oblong yellow anthers of twice the length of the filaments. The stigma is sessile, and rendered irregular on its surface by numerous folds or convolutions. The fruit is a large oval berry, crowned with the persistent stigma, and containing a sweetish fleshy pulp, in which about 15 ovate seeds are embedded. It is, when ripe, of a lemon-yellow color, interrupted by round brownish spots.

The plant is extensively diffused throughout the United States, growing luxuriantly in moist shady

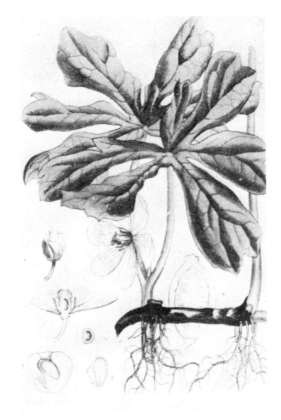

MANDRAKE (AMERICAN): The fantastic myths and legends surrounding the Mandrakes result from the uncanny likeness to a human form that the root configuration often develops.

woods, and in low marshy grounds. It is propagated by its creeping root, and is often found in large patches. The flowers appear about the end of May and beginning of June; and the fruit ripens in the latter part of September. The leaves are said to be poisonous. The fruit has a subacid, sweetish, peculiar taste, agreeable to some palates, and may be eaten freely with impunity. From its color and shape it is sometimes called Wild Lemon. The root is the officinal portion; and is said to be most efficient when collected after the falling of the leaves. It shrinks considerably in drying. (U.S.D.)

Medicinal Uses: *American Mandrake:* The fantastic myths and legends surrounding the Mandrakes result from the uncanny likeness to a human form that the root configuration often develops. The more closely it resembles the human figure, the more highly is the root valued in folkloric medicine. It was such a prized commodity at one time that collectors invented dire horror stories surrounding inappropriate methods of collection, predicting horrible consequences, to discourage entrepreneurs from trading.

The plant is a poisonous narcotic (USFDA unsafe herb list, March 1977). It was widely used by the ancients for its narcotic value and as an anesthetic prior to surgery. "Morion," or "Death Wine," said to have been administered previous to the torture, was made from it.

The rhizomes and roots of American Mandrake contain the toxic and irritant principles podophyllotoxin, alpha-peltatin, and beta-peltatin. They are responsible for the well established purgative effect of this plant. However, there is no scientific evidence that this plant has sedative, anodyne or aphrodisiac effects as has been claimed by some folkloric practitioners.

American Mandrake has been employed in cases of chronic constipation for its cathartic effect, as well as in problems arising from liver congestion, and also as a remedy for ridding people of worms. The resin derived from the root was considered a safe and reliable substitute in all cases where mercury was indicated, earning this plant its nicknames, "Vegetable Mercury" and "Vegetable Calomel."

European Mandrake: In appearance, European Mandrake is similar to Ginseng, in that the root often takes on the appearance of a human body with its appendages. It has therefore gained a reputation as an aphrodisiac, which is probably based on the "doctrine of signatures," with no real scientific rationale existing for this type of effect.

Mandrake is, however, related to *Atropa* species and contains tropane alkaloids similar in structure and biological effects to those in *A. belladonna*. Hence, the anodyne, sedative, and poisonous effects attributed to the use of this plant have a sound basis in fact. It was formerly given prior to surgical operations for its effects.

For side effects and contraindications to the use of European Mandrake, the reader should refer to the article on Belladonna; these would apply also to the European Mandrake.

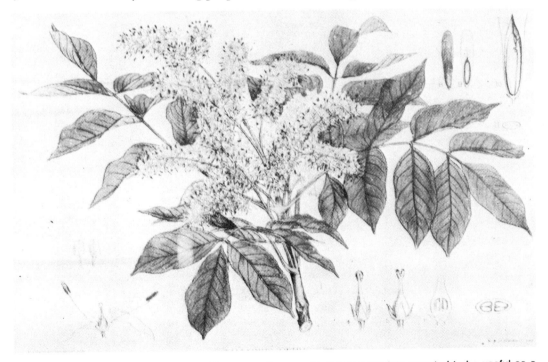

MANNA: Not the Manna of the Bible, this tree produces a dried sugar exudate reported to be useful as a gentle laxative.

European Mandrake should not be confused with American Mandrake, which is treated above.

Dose: American Mandrake: CAUTION. Safer purgatives than the American Mandrake exist.

MANNA
Fraxinus ornus

PARTS USED: Dried exudate from bark
OTHER COMMON NAMES: Flowering Ash

Botanical Description: Manna is not the product of one plant exclusively. Besides the *Fraxinus ornus* indicated by the pharmacopoeias, it is afforded by several other species of the same genus, among which *F. rotundifolia*, *F. excelsior*, and *F. parviflora* are particularly mentioned. Substances known as Manna are collected from plants of other genera in North Africa and in India, but are considered much inferior to that obtained from the different species of ash.

The Flowering Ash is a tree of moderate height, usually from 20 to 25 feet, very branching, with opposite, petiolate, pinnate leaves, composed of 3 or 4 pairs of leaflets, and an odd one at the extremity. The leaflets are oval, acuminate, obtusely serrate, about 1½ inches in length, smooth, of a bright green color, and stand on short footstalks. The flowers are white, and usually expand at the same time with the leaves. They grow in close panicles at the extremity of the young branches, and have a very short calyx with four teeth, and a corolla composed of four linear lanceolate petals.

Both this species of *Fraxinus* and *F. rotundifolia* are natives of Sicily, Calabria, and Apulia; and both contribute to supply the Manna of commerce. During the hot months, the juice exudes spontaneously from the bark, and concretes upon its surface; but as the exudation is slow, it is customary to facilitate the process by making deep longitudinal incisions on one side of the trunk. In the following season these are repeated on the other side, and thus alternately for 30 or 40 years, during which the trees are said to yield Manna. Straws or clean chips are frequently placed so as to receive the juice, which concretes upon them. The Manna varies much in its character, according to the mode of collection and nature of the season, and the period of the year in which the exudation takes place. That procured in Sicily is said to be the best. (U.S.D.)

Medicinal Uses: This is not the manna of the Bible. Most botanists agree the Scriptural manna was probably the lichen *Lecanora esculenta*, from which bread may be produced; others say it was from the shrub *Tamarix mannifera*.

Manna is the name given to the dried saccharine exudate of the "Manna-Ash" tree. The Manna exudes spontaneously from the bark, but for commercial purposes, when it is cultivated as a crop, incisions are made in the trunk to produce a larger yield.

In combination with Senna or Rhubarb, whose taste is concealed by the aromatic Manna, the effect is purgative. Taken alone, Manna is a gentle laxative which may occasionally produce the side effects of stomach gas and some cramping pains. Generally, however, it is considered safe for children. The principal constituent is mannite, or Manna sugar, which possesses similar laxative properties to the exudate, and is often employed in Italy for that purpose.

Manna contains a high concentration of sugar alcohols, primarily mannitol. These sugar alcohols, when taken orally, cause fluids surrounding the intestinal tract to be drawn inside of the intestine. This results in an increased volume of fluid within the lower bowel, which causes a laxative effect.

Dose: Approximately ½ ounce of the dried exudate, powdered, to 1 pint of water. Water boiled separately and poured over the plant material and steeped for 5 to 20 minutes, depending on the desired effect. Drunk hot or warm, 1 to 2 cups per day.

MARIGOLD
Calendula officinalis

PARTS USED: Flowers
OTHER COMMON NAMES: Calendula, Pot Marigold, Marybud, Holigold

Botanical Description: Grown for its showy flowers, this hairy, branching, variable annual, 1 to 2 feet high, is a native of southern Europe. The leaves are both basal and alternate on the stems, narrow, 2 inches long or more, entire or fine-toothed, thick, stemless. The flower heads, solitary on long stalks, are 1.5 to 4 inches in diameter, open only during the day, the ray florets cream to orange, the central florets yellow to brownish and in globose, double heads concealed by the numerous rays. The flower heads, which resemble those of other marigolds, are sometimes used to flavor stews. The fruits are without pappus and all but the central ones are curved. (Neal)

Medicinal Uses: Calendula, applied locally as a tincture, oil, or lotion, is considered a "natural antiseptic" by homeopaths. The crushed petals may be combined with olive oil to form an ointment for external application to cuts, bruises, sores, and burns.

The infusion was used to soothe watery, irritated eyes, and for relief in bronchial complaints. The Marigold, frequently used as a home remedy in liver disorders, was also thought to induce perspiration in fever.

The flowers contain an essential oil, an amorphous bitter compound, and calendulin. Ex-

perimentally, Marigold flower extracts have been shown to lower blood pressure and to have sedative effects in several animal species, and it thus seems that the use of Marigold tea would have a beneficial effect in these conditions as well.

An Austrian patent was issued in 1955 for the use of extracts of Marigold flowers as an emollient in the treatment of burns in humans.

Marigold is a common adulterant of Saffron.

Dose: The medicinal dose is 1 to 4 grams of granulated flowers per cup of boiling water, 1 cup per day.

MARIJUANA
Cannabis sativa

PARTS USED: Flowering tops
OTHER COMMON NAMES: Cannabis, Indian
  Hemp, Grass, Pot, Bhang, Dagga

Botanical Description: *Cannabis sativa,* the hemp

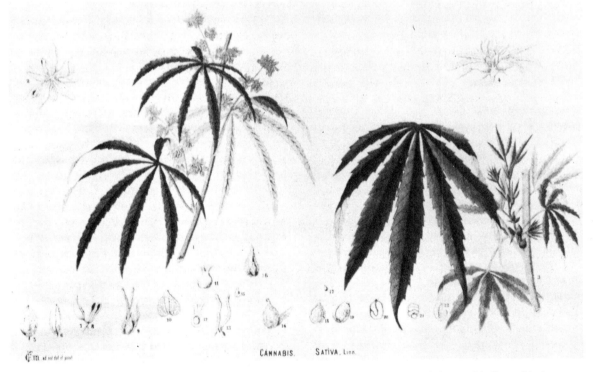

CANNABIS. SATIVA, Linn.

MARIJUANA (Cannabis): Currently an illegal drug in almost every country of the world, Cannabis has nevertheless enjoyed a long and respectable history as a medicinal agent.

127

plant, is an annual, from 4 to 8 feet or more in height, with an erect, branching, angular stem. The leaves are alternate or opposite, and digitate, with 5 to 7 linear-lanceolate, coarsely serrated segments. The stipules are subulate. The flowers are axillary; the staminate in long, branched, drooping racemes; the pistillate in erect, simple spikes. The stamens are 5, with long pendulous anthers; the pistils 2, with long, filiform, glandular stigmas. The fruit is ovate and 1-seeded. The whole plant is covered with a fine pubescence, scarcely visible to the naked eye, and somewhat viscid to the touch.

C. sativa is a native of the Caucasus, Persia, and the hilly regions of northern India. It has been cultivated in many parts of Europe and Asia, and largely in our western states. It is from the Indian variety exclusively that the medicine was formerly obtained, the heat of the climate apparently favoring the development of its active principle. (U.S.D.)

Medicinal Uses: Currently an illegal drug in almost every country of the world, Cannabis has enjoyed a long and respectable history as a medicinal agent. As early as 2737 B.C., the plant was included in the pharmacopoeia of the Chinese Emperor Shen Nung. The ancient Scythians used it in their funeral rites, and seeds have been found in funerary urns dating back to the fifth century B.C.

Cannabis was formerly used in medicine to treat insomnia, allay pain, and soothe restlessness. Held to be narcotic and antispasmodic, it was recognized in the 1918 *U.S. Dispensatory* as a general nerve sedative, used in hysteria, mental depression, and neurasthenia.

Its anodyne and soporific action resembles that of Opium, but without the undesirable aftereffects of constipation and appetite loss. As an antispasmodic and anodyne, Cannabis has been given in the treatment of neuralgias, spasmodic coughs as in pertussis and asthma, in tetanus and hydrophobia and other painful spasmodic diseases. The herbalist Culpepper recommended Cannabis in the treatment of colic, bloody noses, and jaundice.

Inhalation of Cannabis smoke produces great exhilaration and can cause muscle fatigue to temporarily disappear. These psychic effects of the drug have made it useful as a nervine and stimulant for raising the spirits.

Besides its medicinal applications, Hemp is an important fiber crop; it has been observed that plants grown in colder climates yield better fiber while those from warmer climates have more pronounced intoxicant and medicinal properties, owing to a higher content of the resin which contains the active principles.

The fruits, known as Hemp seeds, are a popular ingredient in bird seed. At one time they were employed medicinally in the treatment of mucous membrane inflammations.

Currently, it is estimated that one in seven Americans twelve years of age or older has used Marijuana, and this number seems to have stabilized over the past two or three years. Although many refer to Marijuana as a "narcotic" or "hallucinogen," in a strict scientific sense neither term is applicable. Marijuana is not "addicting," nor does it produce true hallucinations, except in extremely high doses. Pharmacologists have been unable really to place Marijuana into a neat "category" for purposes of explaining its effects; it is a drug in a class by itself. However, it is safe to say that currently the most popular use for Marijuana is as a recreational euphoriant.

The major active euphoric principle in Marijuana is a substance known as Δ-9-tetrahydrocannabinol (Δ9-THC). It is an extremely unstable substance in the pure form, but in the living or dead plant it is quite stable. Although some botanists, with reasonable arguments, claim that three major species of Marijuana exist, i.e., *Cannabis sativa* (most common), *Cannabis indica,* and *Cannabis ruderalis,* most chemical and pharmacological evidence seems to support the existence of only one species, i.e., *Cannabis sativa.*

It is amazing to learn that there is only one plant—*Cannabis sativa*—known to contain Δ-9-THC, or compounds related to this principle.

Recent clinical experience demonstrates that Cannabis has a wide range of useful applications in medicine. Certain types of glaucoma that are resistant to conventional types of treatment can be controlled by smoking Marijuana. Administration of THC to cancer patients who experience nausea and vomiting as a common side effect of chemotherapy produces relief of these symptoms. Marijuana or its constituents do not, however, have useful anticancer properties.

Other remarkable effects of THC, based on results of human studies, are to relieve pain, control seizures of epilepsy, relieve symptoms of asthma, and to act as a sedative. Indeed, if it were not for the adverse publicity over the past several decades, most of which has not been based on fact, Marijuana and THC would probably be widely used in the practice of medicine.

It is now well established that the use of Marijuana in the treatment of pain, to induce sleep, and for other maladies, has been fully justified on the basis of solid scientific evidence.

Dose: As required.

MARSHMALLOW
Althaea officinalis

PARTS USED: Root and leaves
OTHER COMMON NAMES: Wymote, White Mallow, Mortification Root

Botanical Description: The Marshmallow is an herbaceous perennial, with a perpendicular branching root, and erect wooly stems, 2 to 4 feet or more in height, branched and leafy toward the summit. The leaves are alternate, petiolate, nearly cordate on the lower part of the stem, oblong-ovate and obscurely 3-lobed above, somewhat angular, irregularly serrate, pointed, and covered on both sides with a soft down. The flowers are terminal and axillary, with short peduncles, each bearing 1, 2, or 3 flowers. The corolla has 5 spreading, obcordate petals, of a pale-purplish color. The fruit consists of numerous capsules united in a compact circular form, each containing a single seed. The plant grows throughout Europe, inhabiting salt marshes, the banks of rivers, and other moist places. It is found also in this country on the borders of salt marshes. In some parts of the Continent, it is largely cultivated for medical use. The whole plant abounds in mucilage. Both the leaves and root are officinal, but the latter only is employed to any extent in this country. The flowers

are sometimes to be found in the shops, but are scarcely used.

The roots should be collected in autumn from plants at least two years old. They are cylindrical, branched, as thick as the finger or thicker, from 1 foot to 1½ feet long, externally of a yellowish color which becomes grayish by drying, within white and fleshy. They are usually prepared for the market by removing the epidermis. (U.S.D.)

Medicinal Uses: Marshmallow root is an excellent demulcent and emollient. The decoction is taken internally to relieve irritation and inflammation of the mucous membranes. The crushed leaves and flowers are boiled and applied externally in poultice form as a soothing dressing for scrapes, chafing, and other irritated skin conditions.

The ancient Greeks praised the virtues of Marshmallow and seemed to consider it a medicinal that would help cure any ailment. Hippocrates especially felt it was an immense aid in the treatment of wounds. During the Renaissance, Marshmallow was used by herbalists to aid sore throats, stomach problems, gonorrhea, leucorrhea, and toothache, and as a gargle to treat mouth infections.

Marshmallow root is well known to have a very high mucilage content. When the mucilage comes into contact with water it swells and forms a very soft, soothing, and protective gel. Thus, the external application of water extracts of this plant will have a demulcent and emollient effect on mucous membranes, or on the skin, or will have a lubricant effect. We can find no experimental data that would suggest a true "analgesic" effect for Marshmallow. However, if a water extract of Marshmallow was applied to a burn or skin abrasion, its emollient effect would reduce the amount of pain from the burn or abrasions, and in this context, it would have pain-relieving properties.

Dose: ½ teaspoon of the crushed root, boiled for ½ hour, strained, and mixed well with honey. Drunk cold, 1 to 2 tablespoonfuls at a time, 1 to 2 cups per day.

129

MEADOW SAFFRON
Colchicum autumnale

PARTS USED: Corn (bulb); seeds
OTHER COMMON NAMES: Colchicum

Botanical Description: The Meadow Saffron is a perennial bulbous plant, the leaves of which appear in spring, and the flowers in autumn. Its manner of growth is peculiar, and deserves notice, as connected in some measure with its medicinal efficacy. In the latter part of summer a new bulb begins to form at the lateral inferior portion of the old one, which receives the young offshoot in its bosom, and embraces it half round. The new plant sends out fibers from its base, and is furnished with a radical spathe, which is cylindrical, tubular, cloven at top on one side, and half under ground. In September from 2 to 6 flowers, of a purplish rosy color, emerge from the spathe, unaccompanied with leaves. The corolla consists of a tube 5 inches long concealed for two-thirds of its length in the ground, and of a limb divided into 6 segments. The flowers perish by the end of October, and the rudiments of the fruit remain under ground till the following spring, when they rise upon a stem above the surface in the form of a 3-lobed, 3-celled capsule. The leaves of the new plant appear at the same time, so that in fact they follow the flower instead of preceding it, as might be inferred from the order of the seasons in which they respectively show themselves. The leaves are radical, spear-shaped, erect, numerous, about 5 inches long, and 1 inch broad at the base. In the mean time, the new bulb has been increasing at the expense of the old, which having performed its appointed office perishes, while the former, after attaining its full growth, sends forth new shoots from itself, and in turn decays. Each parent bulb has two offsets.

The *C. autumnale* is a native of the temperate parts of Europe, where it grows wild in moist meadows. Various attempts have been made to introduce its culture into this country, but with no very encouraging success; though small quantities of the bulb of apparently good quality have been brought into the market. The officinal portions are the bulb and seed. The root, botanically speaking, consists of the fibers which are attached to the base of the bulb. (U.S.D.)

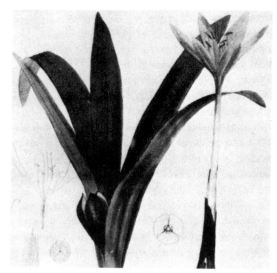

MEADOW SAFFRON: All parts of the plant contain the alkaloid colchicine, which has a specific action in relieving the pain and inflammation associated with gout.

Medicinal Uses: This beautiful plant has long been known for its potent medicinal properties. The generic name is derived from Colchis, a town in Natolia (near the Black Sea), which abounded in this and other medicinal plants, and "perhaps gave rise to some of the poetical fictions respecting the enchantress Medea, who was not infrequently called Colchis, from the place of her birth." (Country people in nineteenth-century England called the flowers "Naked Ladies" "because they come up naked, without any leaves or cover.")

Colchicum has been used in home remedies to treat gout, rheumatism, and dropsy, but owing to varying times of collection of the corms, with varying degrees of success. Climate and soil influence the potency, but the season of collection is most important. In spring, when the corms are most potent they are often eaten by animals, with fatal results. The old French name, *Tue-chien*, intimates that dogs are especially vulnerable to the poison.

All parts of the Meadow Saffron plant contain the alkaloid colchicine, which has a specific action in relieving the pain and inflammation associated with gout. However, only a very small amount of colchicine will produce this effect, and if larger than necessary quantities are taken, severe toxic effects will occur.

Instances are recorded where death ensued within a day after about 4 grams of the wine of Colchicum had been taken for dropsy. (The seeds possess the same properties as the bulbs and are used for the same purposes.)

The toxic alkaloid colchicine is so potent as to be used in experimental genetics to induce "new permanent characteristics in plants and animals."

Dose: CAUTION. Not for home use. When used in medicine, the alcohol extract was given in a dose of 0.016–0.065 gram. The fluidextract was given in a dose of 0.12–0.5 milliliter; the tincture was given in a dose of 0.3–0.9 milliliter; while Colchicum wine was given in a dose of 0.6–2.5 milliliters.

"Wine of Colchicum seed is made by mixing together 10 milliliters of fluidextract of Colchicum seed, 15 milliliters of alcohol, and 75 milliliters of sherry wine. In gout this wine is frequently given in connection with magnesium sulphate." (U.S.D.) As little as 9.3 milliliters of the wine have caused death!

MEZEREON
Daphne mezereum

PARTS USED: Bark, Berries

Botanical Description: *Daphne mezereum* is a very hardy shrub, 3 or 4 feet high, with a branching stem, and a smooth dark-gray bark, which is very easily separable from the wood. The leaves spring from the ends of the branches, are deciduous, sessile, obovate lanceolate, entire, smooth, of a pale-green color, somewhat glaucous beneath, and about 2 inches long. They are preceded by the flowers, which appear very early in spring, and sometimes bloom even amidst the snow. These are of a pale-rose color, highly fragrant, and disposed in clusters, each consisting of 2 or 3 flowers, forming together a kind of spike at the upper part of the stem and branches. At the base of each cluster are deciduous floral leaves. The fruit is oval, shining, fleshy, of a bright-red color, and contains a single round seed.

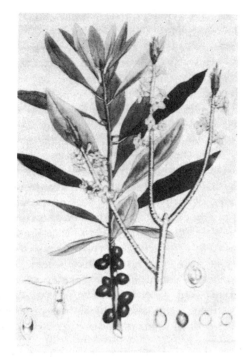

MEZEREON: In animal experiments, the active principle of this plant inhibits experimental tumors. However, this component itself may be a co-carcinogen and for this reason the plant is not recommended for home use.

Another variety produces white flowers and yellow fruit.

This species of *Daphne* is a native of Great Britain and the neighboring continent, in the northern parts of which it is particularly abundant. It is cultivated in Europe both for medicinal purposes and as an ornamental plant, and is occasionally found in our own gardens. It flowers in February, March, or April, according to the greater or lesser mildness of the climate. (U.S.D.)

Medicinal Uses: While the berries and bark of Mezereon have reportedly been useful in European folk medicine (to cure paralysis of the mouth), the plant is a strong *internal* poison. However, an ointment made of the berries gained a folkloric reputation in northern Europe as a treatment for cancer, canker sores, and ulcerous lesions.

Earlier, Linnaeus stated that the Swedes applied the bark to parts bitten by poisonous reptiles and rabid animals.

Mezereon contains an extremely irritant substance, known as mezerein, that is toxic to cells. In animal experiments, mezerein, as well as extracts of Mezereon, inhibit experimental tumors. These properties explain most of the effects claimed for this plant.

It must be pointed out that mezerein is a chemical substance closely related to other substances classified as co-carcinogens. This means that, by itself, the substance cannot cause cancer. However, it will increase the cancer-causing effects of other chemical substances when they are put together. Thus, it is possible that the use of Mezereon by a tobacco user will increase the risk of cancer, due to this additive effect. Other environmental cancer-causing agents, which we are all exposed to continuously, could possibly react with mezerein and enhance the production of cancer cells in humans who are exposed to both types of agents.

For these reasons, one must understand the risk potential in using Mezereon for any purpose.

Dose: Not for home use.

MISTLETOE
Viscum album (European Mistletoe);
Phoradendron flavescens (American Mistletoe)

PARTS USED: Berries, leaves, and wood

Botanical Description: Mistletoe, or in Anglo-Saxon, Mistiltan, is thought to be derived from *mistl*, different, and *tan*, twig, being so unlike the tree it grows upon.

A parasitical plant, with a root firmly attached to the wood of the tree on which it grows. Stem firm, succulent, bright yellowish green, 1 to 2 feet high, divided into numerous dichotomous branches. Leaves opposite, persistent, obovate-lanceolate, obtuse, coriaceous, thick, with parallel ribs, quite entire, light green. Flowers dioecious, in sessile axillary heads, of about 5 flowers. Male flowers have an obsolete calyx, a corolla of 4 ovate petals united at the base, each bearing a single compressed sessile anther with many cells opening by pores; female flowers very small; calyx forming an obscure margin; corolla of 4 ovate equal decidous petals united at the base; ovary inferior, crowned by the border of the calyx; stigma sessile, obtuse. Fruit a smooth, whitish, succulent, globose berry, containing a solitary, cordate, compressed seed. Seed has sometimes 2, occasionally 3 embryos.

Distribution: Europe, northern Asia, America. Parasitic chiefly on apple trees, it is also found upon the Hawthorn, Service, Pear tree, Lime tree, Walnut, and Willow, and rarely upon the Oak. Flowers March to May, and berries ripen in October. (B.F.M.)

Medicinal Uses: This parasitic plant was sacred to the Druids, and was supposedly used therapeutically by that mysterious ancient people as a cure for sterility and epilepsy, and as an antidote to poisons. Its medicinal use is recorded over centuries. Hippocrates, Dioscorides, and Galen highly extol the virtues of the glutinous extract of Mistletoe as an external remedy; but only Hippocrates, among these greats, recommends it internally, in disorders of the spleen.

Mistletoe is considered briskly purgative and emetic. Through the early part of this century it was thought to have beneficial effects on nervous conditions, but by 1917 it was already out of vogue as a nervine.

The glutinous substance viscin is obtained by boiling the bark in alcohol; this material was felt to be beneficial as an external application for irritated and chafed skin. American Mistletoe was used to arrest postpartum and other uterine hemorrhage. The leaves and branches are diuretic and the drug obtained from them was thought to aid asthma and whooping cough.

Accounts on the use and safety of "Mistletoe" preparations in the scientific literature are at best confusing. In most cases, the conclusions drawn are erroneous. The reason for this is that most people consider "Mistletoe" to be a single plant. The situation is not so simple. A large number of Mistletoes grow naturally in the United States and Canada, but *Viscum album* does not. All of the North American Mistletoes are classified in the related group of plants, *Phoradendron*. The European Mistletoe is correctly referred to as *Viscum album*; the American Mistletoe can be any one of a number of species, but most commonly *Phoradendron flavescens*.

Several reports can be found that suggest ingestion of "Mistletoe" or "Mistletoe berries" results in adverse effects and even death (in animals and small children). In carefully checking into each of these reports, there is good reason to believe that they are incorrect. It was found that either there was no evidence by a qualified person that the plant material ingested was really a "Mistletoe," or there was no evidence that the plant material was even ingested. When one considers that up until about 1968, "Mistletoe" (*Viscum album*) preparations were official in the pharmacopoeias of several European countries as a means of treating high blood pressure, it is difficult to believe that such a plant could result in the toxic effects described by some.

On the other hand, there is both animal and human test evidence available that *Viscum album* preparations do have sedative (nervine) properties, but we have not been able to find good evidence that an emetic effect will result from use of such preparations.

A point of caution relative to the use of *Viscum album* preparations is that one should make absolutely sure that he or she is not taking at the same time any prescription medicine that contains a monoamineoxidase inhibitor, since the mixture will cause very serious side effects. A constituent of *Viscum album* is well established to be tyramine. Tyramine will not have any appreciable effects in humans when taken by mouth, unless a monoamineoxidase inhibitor is taken at the same time. In this case, a serious drop in blood pressure will result. This should not be a cause for alarm, since many foods, as well as Chianti wine, contain large amounts of tyramine, and the same caution holds true for them as with *Viscum album* preparations.

American Mistletoe, *Phoradendron flavescens*, is a plant that is parasitic on a number of different woody species. Extracts have been used by the medical profession to prevent postpartum hemorrhage and to aid in the induction of labor at term in pregnancy. It was used most frequently in the mid-1800s in the United States, and was claimed at that time to be superior over Ergot preparations (see article on Ergot for additional details).

There is no evidence that American Mistletoe, if taken before sexual relations, will prevent conception. However, it is quite possible that taken shortly after fertilization has occurred, menstruation might be induced. In that case it would be acting as an early abortifacient.

Previous remarks under *Viscum album* (European Mistletoe), which has similar effects to those of *Phoradendron flavescens*, are worth recalling. Note especially that American Mistletoe also contains tyramine, and the same precautions for this plant should be observed as for the European Mistletoe.

Dose: Because of the confusion surrounding this herb, there is no recommended dose of Mistletoe for domestic use. However, when used in medicine the leaves and wood were given in the dose of 3.9 grams. To lower blood pressure, a water extract of 0.2 gram daily was prescribed.

MORNING GLORY
Ipomoea purpurea and other *Ipomoea* species

PARTS USED: Seeds

Botanical Description: The genus *Ipomoea* consists of annual or perennial herbs or woody vines, shrubs, or trees; stems erect to trailing, creeping or twining and climbing; leaves sessile to long-petioled, simple or palmately compound (in one species pinnately cut almost to midrib, appearing compound), entire or toothed or shallowly to deeply lobed; flowers axillary or terminal, solitary to numerous; peduncles and pedicels various; sepals 5, commonly laterally overlapping; corolla 5-angled or shallowly 5-lobed, salverform to funnelform or campanulate, usually large, variously colored, usually open for less than 24 hours (morning, daytime, or night); stamens included or exserted; ovary 1- to 3-celled; style simple; stigma globose or with 2 or 3 globose lobes; capsule 1- to several-seeded, variously dehiscent or (a few species) indehiscent.

Over 600 species (often referred to 6 to 10 unsatisfactorily distinguishable genera), warm-temperate and tropical regions of both hemispheres.

Ipomoea tricolor. Glabrous annual high-climbing vine; leaf blades cordate, acuminate, 5–15 centimeters long, 4–12 centimeters wide; peduncles several- to many-flowered; sepals ovate-lanceolate, acute; corolla blue or purple to red or white or multicolored, 5–9 centimeters long. Commonly cultivated, July–October; native of Mexico. (Texas)

Medicinal Uses: A great deal of confusion revolves around the use of Morning Glory as an herbal remedy. This is due to more than one plant species being used widely. A great deal of difference in effect occurs, depending on whether the seeds or the roots are used.

The most common cultivated garden ornamental Morning Glory is *Ipomoea purpurea*. No part of this species is capable of producing hallucinogenic effects. However, the roots contain a complex mixture of fatty acid–like substances that produce a rather harsh purgative effect.

In recent years, the seeds of *Ipomoea violacea* (*Ipomoea tricolor*) have been widely employed as a hallucinogen in North America. Ironically, this use was known in Mexico for centuries for a plant known as Badoh Negra, and it was only about two decades ago that Badoh Negra was botanically authenticated as *Ipomoea violacea*.

The hallucinogenic effect of this plant is due to chemical substances very closely related to lysergic acid diethylamide (LSD). The active compounds are found in trace amounts in all parts of the plant, highest concentrations being found in the seeds.

More than 175 horticultural variants of *Ipomoea violacea* are known, but the lysergic acid–like substances have only been found in seven of these.

Early controversy arose as to whether or not Morning Glory seeds were, in fact, hallucinogenic, since some persons taking the seeds claimed this effect; others failed to experience the effect. This variance in experience is explained by the fact that the seeds are very hard and if boiled in water, the active constituents will probably not be extracted. Similarly, when the whole seeds have been taken by mouth, most people who've used them have found that the seeds were not digested and thus that little or no effect was experienced.

It has been estimated that about 350 seeds are required to produce hallucinations in most humans.

Dose: CAUTION. See above.

MOTHERWORT
Leonurus cardiaca

PARTS USED: Tops and leaves
OTHER COMMON NAMES: Lion's Tail, Throw-Wort, Roman Motherwort

Botanical Description: Perennial. Stems stout, erect, up to 1.5 meters tall, finely pubescent on the angles and nodes. Leaves long-petioled, the larger broadly ovate to suborbicular, palmately lobed and sharply toothed, the upper progressively smaller and proportionately narrower, those subtending verticils commonly oblong and merely 3-toothed. Bracts subulate, rarely half as long as the calyx. Calyx-tube 5-angled, 5-ribbed, nearly glabrous, 3–4 millimeters long; calyx-lobes nearly as long as the tube, the lower two somewhat the larger and strongly deflexed. Corolla pale pink, the upper lip white-villous.

Native of central Asia; formerly cultivated as a home remedy and now established in waste places, roadsides, and gardens, Nova Scotia to Montana, south to North Carolina, Tennessee, and Texas. Flowers June to August. (B&B)

Medicinal Uses: While most uses of this aromatic, perennial herb, as evidenced by the common name, have been directed toward the female anatomy, recent evidence has confirmed its utility in heart problems. Employed in douche form, it has been recommended as a treatment for vaginitis. The plant has been employed to provoke menstruation and to aid the continuation of the flow of the lochia following childbirth. Reportedly it was used to calm epileptics during the seventeenth century, and more recently it has been employed as a nerve tonic and sedative, especially for administration after childbirth.

After flowering the herb is richest in its drug component, consisting of various glycosides, resins, tannins, saponins, and organic acids. Experimentally, Motherwort extracts have been reported to have cardiotonic effects based on experiments involving application of extracts of the plant on isolated animal hearts. The action was confirmed in whole animals. Hot-water extracts also show sedative and anti-epileptic effects in animals. These experiments tend to confirm the accuracy of the species epithet (*cardiaca*).

Dose: 1 teaspoon of leaves and tops to 1 cup of boiling water. Taken cold, 1 mouthful at a time, to 1 or 2 cups per day.

MUGWORT
Artemisia vulgaris

PARTS USED: Leaves and flowering tops
OTHER COMMON NAMES: St. John's Plant

Botanical Description: Root about the thickness of the finger, perennial, creeping, ligneous, furnished with numerous strong fibers. Stem nearly herbaceous, erect, cylindrical, channelled, branched, reddish, sometimes covered with whitish pubescence, 3 or more feet high. Leaves alternate, pinnatifid, incised; deep green above, white and cottony beneath; upper much less divided with nearly linear segments. Flowers in axillary racemose spikes; each flower ovate, sessile, composed of several small pale purplish florets seated on a naked receptacle. Involucre of a few narrow, imbricated, wooly scales. Florets of the circumference female, subulate, bifid at the limb, about 5 in number; those of the center, or disk, hermaphorodite, with a filiform tube and 5-cleft limb; segments acute and revolute. Stamens 5; filaments setaceous; anthers cylindrical, united into a tube. Ovary ovate, obtuse, glabrous, surmounted with a setaceous style passing through the tube of the anthers (in the perfect florets), tipped with a bifid revolute stigma. Fruit an obovate pericarp, or achene, destitute of pappus.

Distribution: Europe (Arctic), Northern Africa, Siberia, western Asia to the Himalayas. Common in waste places, hedgerows, etc., in Britain. Flowers July to September. (B.F.M.)

Medicinal Uses: The leaves of the common Mugwort were used to make "moxas." The term *moxa* designates a small mass of combustible matter, which, by being burnt slowly in contact with the skin, produces an eschar (a slough or scab produced from cauterization). Cauterization by fire, as a treatment for disease, has been commonly practiced from the earliest periods of history by primitive tribes as well as by the highest civilizations. The ancient Egyptians and Greeks were acquainted with the use of moxa; as were the ancients in China, Japan, and other Asian countries. The early Portuguese navigators brought the practice from Asia to Europe. In the 1830s moxas were a popular remedy in France for amaurosis, loss of taste, deafness, paralytic affections of the muscles, asthma, chronic catarrh and pleurisy, phthisis, chronic engorgement of the liver and spleen, rachitis, diseased spine, coxalgia, and other forms of scrofulous and rheumatic inflammation of the joints. The *British Flora Medica* has this to say:

> The dried leaves, bruised in a mortar, and rubbed between the hands until the downy part is separated from the woody fibre, and rolled into little cones, is a good substitute for Chinese moxa. The part is first moistened and then a cone of the moxa is applied, which is set on fire at the apex and gradually burns down to the skin, producing a dark-coloured spot; by repeating this painful process an eschar is formed, and this on separation leaves an ulcer which may be kept open or healed as circumstances may require.

Hippocrates recommended Mugwort taken internally to aid in the delivery of the placenta; Dioscorides used it to expedite labor and delivery. It has also been used as a tonic and as a cure for intermittent fevers.

Mugwort is one of the most commonly employed herbal preparations for the treatment of amenorrhea, i.e., use as an emmenagogue. We have records showing that it is used in the Philippines, Vietnam, India, Korea, China, Portugal, Europe, and in the United States for this purpose. There is evidence that water extracts of Mugwort will cause a stimulation of uterine muscle in the test tube; thus, on a theoretical basis, it could act as an emmenagogue in humans. There is no really effective means to establish whether or not a substance has an emmenagogue effect in animals or in humans, and thus it is difficult to use evidence such as this in support of this effect. However, when a plant is used for the same purpose in as many geographically separated areas as is Mugwort, this adds credibility to the alleged effect.

Certain of its extracts injected into laboratory

animals give rise to a sedative effect. Thus, it is possible that this sedative effect could be beneficial in a person with epilepsy, an illness in which Mugwort has been employed.

Dose: Approximately ½ ounce of leaves or flowering tops to 1 pint of water. Water boiled separately and poured over the plant material and steeped for 5–20 minutes, depending on the desired effect. Drunk hot or warm, 1 to 2 cups per day, at bedtime and upon awakening.

MULBERRY, BLACK
Morus nigra

PARTS USED: Fruit

Botanical Description: This species of Mulberry is

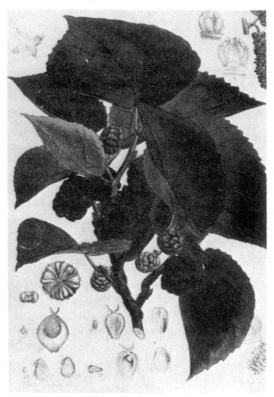

BLACK MULBERRY: Mulberries are very rich in grape sugar, which gives rise to a laxative effect. The juice has long been used as a remedy for children and aged persons suffering from mild constipation.

distinguished by its cordate ovate, or lobed, unequally toothed, and scabrous leaves. It is a tree of middle size, supposed to have been brought originally from Persia into Italy, and thence spread over Europe and America. Its leaves afford food for the silkworm; and the bark of the root, which is bitter and slightly acrid, has been employed as a vermifuge, especially in cases of the tapeworm. But the fruit is the only portion that has been officially recognized as medicinal.

This is oblong oval, of a dark reddish-purple, almost black color; and consists of numerous minute berries united together and attached to a common receptacle, each containing a single seed, the succulent envelope of which is formed by the calyx. It is inodorous, has a sweet, mucilaginous, acidulous taste, and abounds in a deep red juice. The sourish taste is due to the presence of tartaric acid.

Our native mulberry, the fruit of *M. rubra,* is quite equal to that of the imported species. *M. alba,* originally from China, and now extensively cultivated as a source of food for the silkworm, bears a white fruit, which is sweeter than the others. (U.S.D.)

Medicinal Uses: The leaves of this useful tree furnish food for silkworms; it is cultivated extensively for this purpose. Mulberries are very rich in grape sugar, surpassed only by cherries and grapes. The sweet mucilaginous acidulous taste makes the juice quite refreshing for feverish patients, with the added property of being mildly laxative. The juice is a good remedy for children and aged persons suffering from mild constipation. The syrup has also been used as a detergent, applied to thrush of the mouth, and given as a gargle for sore throat.

The fruits of this plant contain large concentrations of certain sugars that can give rise to a laxative effect if taken in large enough quantities.

Dose: ½ ounce of fresh juice per pint of hot water. Drink 1 to 2 cups per day, 1 tablespoon at a time.

MULLEIN
Verbascum thapsus

PARTS USED: Leaves and flowers
OTHER COMMON NAMES: Velvet Dock, Velvet Plant, Flannel Leaf

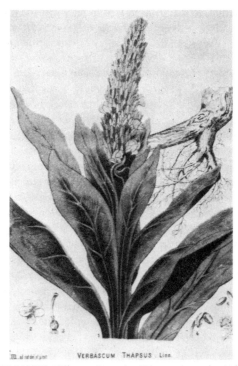

MULLEIN: Taken internally, this common herb is often used to soothe the throat and lungs, to allay pain, and for its antispasmodic effect. The leaves contain high concentrations of mucilage, which accounts for these effects.

Botanical Description: This is a biennial plant, with an erect, round, rigid, hairy stem, which rises from 3 to 6 feet in height, and is irregularly beset with large sessile, oblong or oval, somewhat pointed leaves, indented at the margin, wooly on both sides, and decurrent at the base. The flowers are yellow, and disposed in a long, close, cylindrical, terminal spike.

The Mullein is common throughout the United States, growing along the roadsides and in neglected fields, and springing up abundantly in newly cleared places, at the most remote distance from cultivation. It is nevertheless considered by many botanists as a naturalized plant, introduced originally from Europe, where it is also abundant. It flowers from June to August. The leaves and flowers have been employed in medicine. Both have a slight, somewhat narcotic smell, which in the dried flowers becomes agreeable. Their taste is mucilaginous, herbaceous, and bitterish, but very feeble. They impart their virtues to water by infusion. (U.S.D.)

Medicinal Uses: Mullein is a formidable medicinal with many recommended uses. It has been given to cattle to treat coughs from pulmonary ailments. Various species of Mullein were recommended by early herbalists for colic, coughs, all chest ailments, hemorrhoids, gout, and warts.

Internally demulcent, Mullein soothes the throat and lungs. It is also diuretic, allays pain, and is antispasmodic. It does not have a very pleasant taste, so the addition of aromatics, together with boiling the herb in milk, have been advised.

Mullein leaves have high concentrations of mucilage, which is responsible for the emollient and demulcent effects of water extracts of this plant. In its application as an external emollient, a fomentation of Mullein leaves in hot vinegar and water makes an agreeable application to piles and itching complaints. Boiled with lard, it makes an ointment for dressing wounds. Fomentations or poultices of the leaves or flowers beaten up with Linseed meal have been applied to burns, scalds, and boils. The steam was often inhaled to relieve cold symptoms such as nasal congestion and throat irritation.

Dose: The medicinal preparation consists of 1 teaspoon of leaves, steeped in 1 cup of boiling water. Drunk cold, 1 to 2 cups per day, 1 tablespoon at a time.

MUSTARD
Sinapis alba, S. nigra

PARTS USED: Seeds
OTHER COMMON NAMES: White Mustard, Black Mustard

Botanical Description: *Sinapis nigra.* The Common or Black, Mustard is an annual plant, with a stem 3 or 4 feet in height, divided and subdivided into numerous spreading branches. The leaves are petiolate, and variously shaped. Those near the root are large, rough, lyrate-pinnate, and unequally toothed; those higher on the stem are smooth and less lobed; and the uppermost are entire, narrow, smooth, and dependent. The flowers are small, yellow, with a colored calyx, and stand closely together upon peduncles at the upper part of the

137

branches. The pods are smooth, erect, nearly parallel with the branches, quadrangular, furnished with a short beak, and occupied by numerous seeds.

Sinapis alba. The White Mustard is also an annual plant. It is rather smaller than the preceding species. The lower leaves are deeply pinnatifid, the upper sublyrate, and all irregularly toothed, rugged with stiff hairs on both sides, and of a pale green color. The flowers are in racemes, with yellow petals, and linear, green, calycine leaflets. The pods are spreading, bristly, rugged, roundish, swelling in the position of the seeds, ribbed, and provided with a very long ensiform beak.

Both plants are natives of Europe and cultivated in our culinary gardens; and *S. nigra* has become naturalized in some parts of this country. Their flowers appear in June. The seeds are kept in the shops both whole and in the state of very fine powder, as prepared by the manufacturers for the table. (U.S.D.)

Medicinal Uses: Powdered Mustard seeds are a common condiment; they promote the appetite and stimulate the gastric mucous membrane, with some effect on pancreatic secretions, thereby aiding digestion. By virtue of these effects they can sometime relieve obstinate hiccough.

Mustard is also a valuable emetic, when it is desired to empty the stomach without accompanying depression of the system, as in cases of narcotic poisoning. Taken whole, the seeds are laxative and can aid in upset stomach due to acid indigestion.

An important use of mustard is externally, as a rubefacient (reddening the skin, producing local congestion, the vessels becoming dilated and the supply of blood increased); with longer applications vesication, or blister formation, occurs, drawing deeper fluids to the surface. Mustard poultices may be mixed with alcohol, almond oil, or olive oil. The poultice should be carefully attended, as too long an application can result in pain and tissue damage.

Black and White Mustard seeds both contain highly irritating so-called "mustard-oil" glycosides, typified by "mustard oil," or allyl isothiocyanate. The irritant effect is mild in water extracts, but in concentrated extracts, the irritation can actually induce blistering. A combination of mild irritation due to the mustard-oil

glycosides, in addition to a high fat content, causes the laxative effect of Mustard seeds. In larger doses, the irritant action of the mustard-oil glycosides causes emesis.

Mustard plasters are still widely used, and their effective utility requires special handling. The mustard plaster is simply a thin layer of defatted Mustard seeds, applied to a piece of paper with a suitable glue. Prior to use, the mustard plaster is dipped into lukewarm (never hot) water. This contact with water sets off a chemical reaction in which the end-product is "mustard oil." The plaster is then applied for a short period of time. While the plaster is in contact with the skin, the mustard oil causes a mild irritation, which causes blood to rush to the area of application. The additional blood supply serves to produce an anti-inflammatory response, relax muscles, and in general provide relief from muscle strains and similar ailments. It must be pointed out that the mustard plaster should not be allowed to remain in contact with the skin for any prolonged period of time, or it will result in the formation of blisters. The blisters are very painful and there is always a possibility that infection will result. However, mustard plasters, applied externally for periods up to 15 minutes, will usually not result in blistering, and are quite safe and effective for those whose skin is of normal sensitivity.

Mustard oil itself is used in many proprietary ointments intended for external application for the relief of minor aches and pains, much the same as mustard plaster.

Dose: CAUTION. Mustard plasters can rarely be taken for more than 10 or 15 minutes. As an emetic (especially used in narcotic poisoning), mustard powder was given in the quantity of 3.9–7.7 grams.

MYRRH
Commiphora myrrha

PARTS USED: Oleo-gum resin from stem

Botanical Description: *Commiphora myrrha* is a small tree, with a stunted trunk, covered with a whitish-gray bark, and furnished with rough abortive branches terminating in spines. The leaves are ternate, consisting of obovate, blunt, smooth, obtusely denticulate leaflets, of which the 2 latter are much smaller than that at the end. The fruit is oval-lanceolate, pointed, longitudinally furrowed, of a brown color, and surrounded at its base by the persistent calyx. The tree grows in Arabia, in dwarfish thickets, interspersed among Acacias and Euphorbiaceae. The juice concretes spontaneously upon the bark.

Formerly the best myrrh was brought from the shores of the Red Sea by way of Egypt and the Levant, and hence received the name of Turkey myrrh, while the inferior qualities, imported from the East Indies, were commonly called India myrrh.

It appears to be established that *C. myrrha* produces myrrh, but it is probable that it is also yielded by other trees belonging to the genus *Commiphora*, a genus which includes more than 60 species, natives of Arabia and Africa. (U.S.D.)

Medicinal Uses: Myrrh has been used for thousands of years as an ingredient in incense and perfumes. As a medicinal, it is a stimulant tonic, and expectorant, and was most commonly administered to patients suffering from chest problems in order to stimulate mucous secretions and promote their drainage.

A second major area of usage concerned the female reproductive organs. Myrrh was taken to stimulate the menstrual flow or to bring it on, even when the patient had never menstruated. In this connection it was often combined with aloes for the laxative properties contributed by the latter. Myrrh was also applied to spongy gums and mouth ulcers.

The gum-resin was used by the ancients for embalming. A gentle rubefacient in external application, myrrh was employed to make a plaster where it was desirable to produce blisters slowly and with a minimum of pain (see "Dose," below, for instructions on how to make this plaster).

The use of myrrh to allay the pain and hasten healing of mouth ulcers and spongy gums in children is based on the known presence of astringent tannins in this resinous exudate. Direct experimental evidence is lacking in support of the use of myrrh as a stimulating tonic and expec-

torant, but constituents are present in myrrh that are known to stimulate gastric secretions and to relax smooth muscle in the lungs. Should the myrrh itself produce these effects, there is a rational basis for these actions.

Dose: For internal complaints, an infusion is prepared with approximately ½ ounce of myrrh to 1 pint of water. Water boiled separately and poured over the plant material and steeped for 5 to 20 minutes, depending on the desired effect. Drunk hot or warm, 1 to 2 cups per day.

An *external* plaster of Myrrh was made by rubbing together powdered Myrrh, Camphor, and Balsam of Peru, 1½ oz. each, adding to 32 oz. of lead plaster previously melted, and stirring well until the plaster thickens on cooling.

A formula for incense, prepared by the ancient Hebrews, appears in the Chasidic prayer book (*Siddur Tehillat Hashem*, Rabbi Nissen Mangel, 1978):

The Lord said to Moses: Take fragrant spices . . . and you shall make it into incense, a compound expertly blended, well-mingled, pure and holy. . . . Aaron shall burn upon the altar the incense of fragrant spices; every morning when he cleans the cup [of the *Menorah*], he shall burn it. And toward evening, when Aaron lights the Menorah, he shall burn it; this is a continual incense-offering before the Lord throughout your generations.

The Rabbis have taught: How was the incense prepared? The incense contained the following eleven kinds of spices: (1) balm, (2) onycha, (3) galbanum, (4) frankincense—each one weighing seventy *maneh;* (5) myrrh, (6) cassia, (7) spikenard, (8) saffron—each weighing sixteen *maneh;* (9) costus, twelve *maneh;* (10) aromatic bark, three [*maneh*]; (11) cinnamon, nine [*maneh*] . . . While the *Kohen* was grinding the incense, the overseer would say, "Grind it thin, grind it thin," because the [*rhythmic*] sound is good for the compounding of the spices.

139

NETTLE
Urtica dioica

PARTS USED: Roots, leaves, and seeds
OTHER COMMON NAMES: Great Stinging Nettle, Bigsting Nettle

Botanical Description: Root perennial, creeping, ligneous, fibrous. Stems erect, somewhat branched, quadrangular, hispid with rigid articulated pungent hairs, 2 to 4 feet high. Leaves opposite, petiolate, ovate-acuminate, cordate at the base, deeply serrated, rugose, dull dark green above, paler beneath, hispid on both sides, with 2 small, opposite, concave, reflected stipules at the base of the petiole. Flowers in long, pendent, somewhat branched clusters, frequently 2 from the axil of each leaf, male and female on separate plants (dioecious), seldom monoecious. Male flowers have a perianth of 4 ovate, obtuse, concave, spreading segments, and 4 setaceous filaments tipped with ovate-gibbous, 2-celled anthers. Female flowers consist of a perianth of 2 ovate, obtuse, pilose leaves, and a superior, ovate, glabrous ovary, terminated by a sessile, downy, spreading stigma. Fruit an ovate, compressed, polished nut, containing a single seed, and enveloped by the persistent perianth.

Distribution: Northern temperate regions (Arctic), South Africa, Andes, Australia. In England the Nettle is well known as one of the most common plants in waste places, and under walls and hedge-banks. Flowers June to September (B.F.M.)

Medicinal Uses: The Nettle has been used medicinally either to excite the skin locally, or to affect the nervous system generally. Used to heal burns and wounds, Nettle juice at one time formed the main component (93 percent) of a preparation known as Brandol, which was commercially marketed. The poisonous stinging hairs of the fresh Nettle will produce intense itching and stinging; however, both Pliny and homeopathic physicians used the juice to cure its own sting! The leaves will stimulate, irritate, and cause blisters, so they are used where a rubefacient is desired.

Nettle seeds are sometimes used in home remedies for hair troubles, coughs, and shortness of breath.

In the second and third centuries B.C., several practitioners made reference to the medicinal properties of Nettles. It was used as an antidote for Hemlock, a counterpoison for Henbane, and as a cure for snakebite and scorpion sting. It was reputedly an aid for gout, asthma, and tuberculosis. Other recorded applications of the plant are as a diuretic and to arrest uterine hemorrhages. The tops of the plants, boiled, are eaten as greens by many people as a pot herb and in soups. It is recommended as an emergency food plant and has been suggested as a possible source of chlorophyll, for commercial purposes.

Extracts of Nettle have been tested in animals and show anti-inflammatory effects, and also lower the amount of sugar in the blood.

Dose: For medicinal use one teaspoon of the granulated leaves or root is used per 1 cup of boiling water. Drunk cold, one tablespoon at a time, 1 cup per day.

NIGHTSHADE, BLACK
Solanum nigrum

PARTS USED: Leaves
OTHER COMMON NAMES: Garden Nightshade, Common Nightshade, Duscle, Hound's Berry, Morelle

Botanical Description: *Solanum nigrum*, the Common, Garden, or Black Nightshade, is an annual plant from 1 to 2 feet high, with an unarmed herbaceous stem, ovate, angular-dentate leaves, and white or pale violet flowers, arranged in peduncled nodding umbel-like racemes, and followed by clusters of spherical black berries, about the size of peas. There are numerous varieties of this species, one of which is a native of the United States. The leaves are the part employed as a medicine. (U.S.D.)

Medicinal Uses: Used to produce sweating, vomiting, and purging, Black Nightshade was felt to purify the blood of toxins. The North American Indians employed the plant internally as a treatment for tuberculosis and to expel worms. Both they and many other cultures used the plant to induce sleep.

OAK, WHITE
Quercus alba

PARTS USED: Bark and acorns
OTHER COMMON NAMES: Stone Oak

Botanical Description: A large tree reaching 80 feet in height, with many long, wide-spreading branches; bark pale or white, often marked with large black spots, young twigs glabrous. Leaves stalked, the petiole varying from ¼–¾ inch in length, 3–6 inches long, oval- or obovate-obling, tapering at the base, more or less deeply pinnatifid, with a few (4–6) ascending, obtuse, rounded, entire lobes, smooth on both surfaces when mature, thickly downy when young, bright light green above, glaucous and with the veins prominent beneath; stipulates linear, pubescent, caducous. Male catkins 1–3 inches long, slender, the rachis nearly glabrous; the parianth irregularly cut into 4–6 lobes; stamens 8. Fruit solitary or 2 together at the extremity of a stout peduncle, which varies in length from nearly an inch to scarcely a line, cup broadly hemispherical, rather shallow, gray, the scales ovate, acute, hard, becoming tubercular, strongly imbricate, pubescent; nut about an inch long, twice or thrice as long as the cup, ovoid.

This fine tree is found over a very large extent of North America, extending from the Red River, Lake Winnipeg, and Maine, in the north, to Texas and Florida in the south. It is especially abundant in Pennsylvania and Virginia, and grows by preference in rather moist ground. In England it is occasionally planted, having been first grown there in 1724.

It is of all the American oaks the kind most like the British species. (Bentley)

OAK, WHITE: Acorns are employed for their tonic and astringent properties. When applied locally, they tend to shrink hemorrhoids and often accelerate the healing of flabby ulcers.

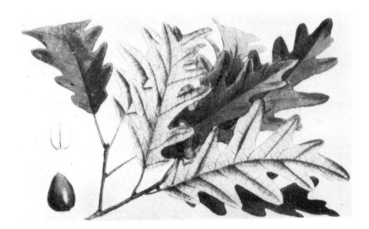

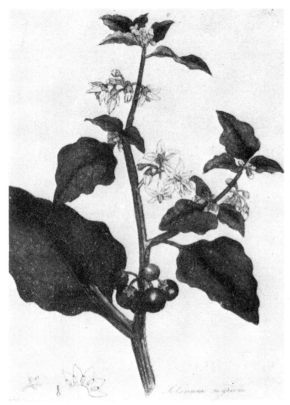

NIGHTSHADE, BLACK: Although the leaves have been applied externally in skin problems since the time of Dioscorides, these leaves and berries are poisonous, especially in the unripe state. As the fruit ripens, the toxic solanine-content level decreases.

The external application of the leaves in skin problems has been recorded since the ancient Greek Dioscorides; the Arabic physicians used the bruised leaves as an application for burns. A poultice of freshly crushed leaves or a compress soaked in a concentrated decoction was applied as an analgesic in cases of itching, hemorrhoids, and arthritis.

The leaves and berries are poisonous, especially in the unripe state. The berries are often involved in poisoning of children who find them attractive to eat. As the fruit ripens, the solanine (active principle) content gradually decreases to nontoxic levels. The ripe berries have sometimes been used to make preserves and pies. Boiling apparently also destroys the toxic principles.

Dose: For external use only, as a leaf poultice.

Medicinal Uses: The acorns are employed for their tonic and astringent properties. A decoction of these roasted nuts is an old German remedy for scrofula.

The bark is high in tannin content, which accounts for its astringent properties. It has not been used internally to a great extent, but a decoction of the bark has been found useful in treating chronic diarrhea, advanced dysentery, and other conditions. The principal use of the bark has been for external application, as an astringent wash, especially for flabby ulcers, as a gargle, and internally via injection for leucorrhea and hemorrhoids.

The chief use of Oak bark has always been not medicinal, but for tanning leather.

The inner bark of White Oak is known to contain about 10 percent of a tannin complex, often referred to as quercitannic acid. As with all tannins, it predictably exerts an astringent and mild antiseptic action, the latter effect being due primarily to the phenolic nature of the tannin complex. Thus, as reported in folklore accounts, decoctions or infusions of *Quercus alba* bark, when applied locally, would have an astringent effect, which would tend to shrink hemorrhoids and accelerate the healing of flabby ulcers.

Dose: Of the acorns—½ to 1 ounce decocted in 1½ pints of boiling water, allowed to simmer, at breakfast.

ONION, GARLIC

Allium cepa, Allium sativum and other *Allium* species

PARTS USED: Bulb

Botanical Description: *Allium* genus: Flowers perfect, in umbels. Perianth segments 6, uniform in color, but the inner circle often somewhat different in shape or size, withering and persistent below the capsule. Stamens 6, often adnate to the base of the perianth; filamenta of the epipetalous series often wider, or greatly flattened, or variously toothed; anthers short, intorse. Ovary 3-celled; ovules 1 or 2 in each cell. Capsule short, ovoid, globose, or obovoid; 3-lobed, loculicidal; seeds black, 1 or 2 in each cell. Biennial or

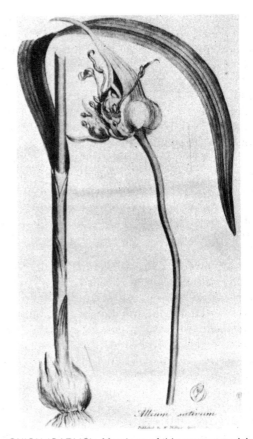

Allium sativum

ONION (GARLIC): Members of this genus are rich sources of sulphur which acts as a strong disinfectant. The plants also exert antibacterial effects, giving them a wide reputation as powerful home remedies.

perennial herbs from a coated bulb, with a strong odor of onion or garlic, the leaves usually narrow, basal or in the lower part of the stem, the scaperlike stem erect, terminated by an umbel subtended by 1–3 bracts, the flowers white to pink or purple, in some species wholly or partly replaced by sessile bulblets.

Allium cepa. Bulb globose to depressed. Stem inflated below the middle. Leaves basal, 5–15 millimeters in diameter. Umbel 5–10 centimeters in diameter, the pedicels greatly exceeding the greenish white flowers.

Native probably of southwest Asia; commonly cultivated and rarely adventive on waste ground. Blooms in summer. (B&B)

Medicinal Uses: Onions are a marvelous aid in the maintenance of good health through proper diet, eaten raw, boiled, or baked. There is sulphur in the onion, which acts as a strong disinfectant; so it seems there was more than simple superstitious belief connected with the hanging of a bunch outside the door to absorb the plague during the Middle Ages.

Onions are diuretic, stimulant and expectorant, and so were administered for colds and bronchial complaints. A syrup made from the juice is used as a cough medicine. The Onion was put to many of the same folkloric uses as Garlic (*A. sativum*), but to a lesser degree. Externally, poultices of boiled bulbs were applied to inflammatory tumors, boils and the like, to promote the formation and discharge of pus and to reduce painful tension. Onion juice was a recommended cure for deafness, dropped directly into the ear, or applied with a cotton pack. The juice was also applied topically for burns, chilblains, and insect bites and stings. In the sixteenth century, the crushed bulbs were often used to treat gunpowder burns as well as gunshot wounds. The juice was also mixed with vinegar as an application for the removal of freckles and old age spots!

Experimentally, Onion juice has been shown to produce a myriad of biological effects, including antibacterial and diuretic activities. The active compounds are very unstable after being formed, which is why fresh Onion must be used. Garlic, popular in many countries as a flavoring and for its healthful properties, contains selenicem, an important nutritional component.

Dose: At the sign of a cold or sore throat chew fresh Onions, holding the material in the back of the mouth for a few minutes, consciously inhaling the vapors.

As an application to the skin, for various problems, macerate fresh onions and apply directly.

OPIUM
Papaver somniferum

PARTS USED: Seed capsules
OTHER COMMON NAMES: Poppy

Botanical Description: An annual, with a thick, tapering, much-branched, yellow root. Stem reaching (in the

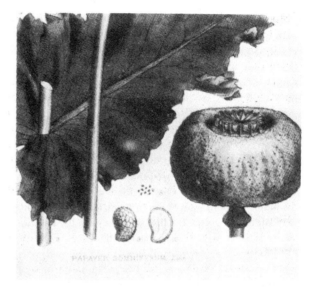

OPIUM: The mother of medicinal plants provides us with our most valuable pain-relieving agents.

cultivated plant) over 3 feet in height, and a diameter of ½ inch at the base, erect, cylindrical, solid, quite smooth or with a few scattered, bristly, horizontal hairs, pale green covered with a white bloom, more or less branched. Leaves rather numerous and closely placed, alternate, sessile, spreading horizontally, the lower ones never more than 6 inches long, oval-oblong, tapering at the base, deeply pinnatisect with acute segments, and deeply and irregularly dentate, the upper ones reaching as much as 10 inches in length, gradually becoming wider and with a more cordate base, the uppermost ones very broadly ovate, with a deeply cordate amplexicaul base, not pinnatisect but more strongly and deeply toothed, the teeth tipped with callous white points, all quite smooth and shining (or the root-leaves with a few bristly hairs beneath), rather thick, dull green, covered with a glaucous-white bloom, which is readily removed, slightly paler beneath, and with prominent veins, midrib very wide, nearly white. Flowers few, solitary, very large, 3–7 inches across, terminating the stem and branches, erect, buds ovate-ovoid, drooping. Sepals 2, broad, blunt, quite smooth, of the same color as the leaves, disarticulating and pushed away as the flowers expand. Petals 4, very large, decussate, the 2 outer wider than long and much overlapping the narrower inner ones, concave, undulated, with numerous closely placed veins, radiating from the stiff, thick, wedge-shaped base, satiny and shining, variable in size and

143

color, in the (English) cultivated plant pure snow-white with a pale greenish-yellow base, in the wild one pale violet, with a large wedge-shaped dark purple or nearly black spot at the base, crumpled in the bud, soon falling. Stamens very numerous, hypogynous, inserted in 5 or 6 rows on the under surface of the dilated gynophore, erect, filaments more than 1 inch long, narrow linear, flat and ribbon-shaped, slightly dilated at the top, white, anthers linear, about ¼ inch long, attached by a very narrow base to the filaments, cream-colored, becoming pale-brown and twisted after dehiscence. Ovary large, depressed globular, about 1 inch in diameter, the top scarcely on a level with the anthers, very suddenly contracted below into a neck (gynophore) about ¼ inch wide, which again dilates to form the receptacle which narrows off below into the peduncle, more or less faintly channelled vertically, quite smooth, pale green, 1-celled, with large spongy parietal placentae, equal in number to and beneath the stigmatic rays, passing nearly to the center, and bearing numerous ovules scattered over all parts of their surface; stigma sessile, peltate, narrower than the ovary, spreading or curved over its top, with 8–20 short, obtuse, oblong rays. Fruit usually more or less globular, often somewhat depressed, or ovoid, 1½–3 inches in diameter, supported on a neck (as in the ovary) and crowned by the persistent stigma, pericarp dry, hard, brittle, smooth, brownish-yellow usually speckled with black, indehiscent or dehiscing by small apertures beneath the stigmatic crown, 1-celled, with the dry papery placentae reaching about half-way to the center. Seeds very numerous, very small, reniform, white, gray, violet, or black, testa with a raised reticulated network, embryo slightly curved, in the axis of the oily endosperm. (Bentley)

Medicinal Uses: Although we consider this the mother of medicinal plants, the Latin name *Papaver* is thought to be derived from the Celtic *papa* (whence "pap," the soft food given to children), a food in which the Opium seeds were formerly boiled to induce sleep.

The use of Opium as a medicine can be traced back to the time of Hippocrates. It has been called the most important and valuable medicine of the whole materia medica, and "the source, by its judicious employment, of more happiness, and by its abuse, of more misery, than any other drug employed by mankind." (Pereira)

Laudanum (tincture of Opium) was regularly given to infants and small children during the nineteenth century to treat colic.

The gummy latex of this annual herb contains many alkaloids, including morphine, codeine, narcotine, laudenine, and papaverine. The highly addicting *synthetic* heroin is made by modifying morphine.

Various medicines made from Opium alkaloids are used for their sedative, hypnotic, narcotic, antispasmodic, and analgesic effects.

Poppy seeds used in baking will yield the plant simply by scattering them in a vacant lot!

There is no substitute for the narcotic abilities of Opium. Many terminally ill cancer patients in this country whose major concern is dying with dignity, drug addiction not being a problem of any concern whatever, are denied this most efficacious painkiller, to suffer out their last weeks and months in needless agony for themselves—and for their families, who must stand by helplessly.

It is the authors' fervent hope that Opium and its derivatives will once again be made available in this country to ease the suffering of the terminally ill, and, with proper controls, for use in place of the synthetic tranquilizers. Ultimately, we would like to see this plant regain its status as the valued natural drug it is.

The following formula for camphorated tincture of Opium (paregoric) was once a standard in medical practice.

4 grams powdered opium
4 grams benzoic acid
4 grams camphor
4 milliliters oil of anise

Macerate mixed drugs in stoppered container, with 40 milliliters of glycerin and 950 milliliters of diluted alcohol. Continue maceration with frequent agitation during 3 days, transfer mixture to a filter and, when the liquid has drained off completely, gradually wash the residue on the filter with enough alcohol to make one thousand milliliters of finished tincture.

144

ORCHID, WILD
Orchis spp.

PARTS USED: Tubers
OTHER COMMON NAMES: Salep

Botanical Description: Though never considered medicinal by any of the British colleges, nor by our national *Pharmacopoeia*, this substance deserves a slight notice, as it was frequently mentioned by writers on materia medica. The name is given to the prepared bulbs of the *Orchis mascula* and other species of the same genus. The Wild Orchid is a native of Europe, the Levant, and Northern Africa. Its bulbs, which are 2 in number, oval or roundish, internally white and spongy, are prepared by removing their epidermis, plunging them into boiling water, then stringing them together and drying them in the sun or by the fire. By this process they acquire the appearance and consistence which distinguish them as found in the shops. They were formerly procured exclusively from Asia Minor and Persia, but more recently have been prepared in France and perhaps other parts of Europe.

Salep is in small, oval, irregular masses, hard, horny, semitransparent, of a yellowish color, a feeble odor, and a mild mucilaginous taste. It is sometimes kept in the state of a powder. (U.S.D.)

Medicinal Uses: Orchids have enjoyed a widespread reputation as restoratives, rejuvenants, and aphrodisiacs, seemingly more because of the splendid and opulent flowers than from any specific excitant or stimulant properties. A product known as salep is prepared from the tubers of various *Orchis* species. The tubers are strung on strings, scalded to destroy their vitality, then dried to a hard consistency; after maceration in water they regain their original form and volume. These strings of dried tubers, or salep, are highly prized in India, Persia, and Turkey for restoring the strength of debilitated or aged persons, and especially as an aphrodisiac. One writer has speculated that it is the odor and appearance of the salep, and the tubers from which it is derived, that suggested its application as an aphrodisiac, on the basis of the "doctrine of signatures."

Fundamentally, the tubers are nutritive and compare favorably with tapioca and sago in the convalescent's diet. Salep has also been used to treat diarrhea, dysentery, and nervous fevers.

Dose: First macerate the tubers in cold water until they soften and then rapidly dry them. Take 1 to 2 ounces per day.

OREGON GRAPE
Berberis aquifolium

PARTS USED: Root
OTHER COMMON NAMES: Wild Oregon Grape, Rocky Mountain Grape, California Barberry, Berberis, Holly-Leaf Marberry, Trailing Mahonia

Botanical Description: The genus *Berberis* is a large one, comprising shrubs or trees widely distributed throughout temperate regions and in the mountains of the tropics. There are three well-defined medicinal groups: (1) The Rocky Mountain group, including *Berberis aquifolium*, which yields the Oregon Grape root. (2) The Asiatic group, which includes *B. aristata*, a shrub indigenous to India and to Ceylon, and is recognized by the British *Pharmacopoeia*. (3) The European group, which includes the common Barberry (*B. vulgaris*), naturalized in New England. Reportedly about 40 different species of *Berberis* have been used in medicine.

The Oregon Grape is a tall shrub, about 6 to 7 feet high, with evergreen, coriaceous, bright and shining leaves, and having numerous small, yellowish-green flowers in the early Spring, and later clusters of purple berries containing an acid pulp. It is a native in woods from Colorado to the Pacific Ocean, especially abundant in Oregon and northern California. The root, which was formerly official, occurs in pieces about a foot long, ¼ inch thick, of a brownish color, but yellowish within, yielding a bright lemon-colored powder. (U.S.D.)

Medicinal Uses: Oregon Grape has been used to treat jaundice, chronic hepatitis, syphilis, and scrofula. It was believed to have specific action on the spleen and was administered in cases of malaria where the spleen was dangerously enlarged; this was a risky procedure, however, since

145

the ability to produce contraction was so strong that there was a possibility of rupture and fatal hemorrhage if the herb was taken by a person whose spleen was dangerously softened.

The plant has also been considered diuretic, mildly tonic, and gently laxative. It has been applied topically for various minor skin irritations.

All *Berberis* species are quite similar in chemical composition, and hence would give rise to similar pharmacological effects. See remarks in article on Barberry *(Berberis vulgaris)* for further details.

Dose: The traditional medicinal preparation consists of 1 teaspoon of granulated root per 1½ pints of boiling water; steeped for ½ hour and strained. Take 1 tablespoon 3 to 6 times per day.

ORRIS
Iris germanica and other *Iris* species

PARTS USED: Rhizome
OTHER COMMON NAMES: German Iris, Flag Iris

Botanical Description: The Iris family includes about 60 genera and 1,000 species, most abundant in South Africa and South America. They are perennial herbs rising from a short and thick or long underground stem or a bulb. Members of the Iris and Amaryllis families are somewhat alike, and each family is supposed to have evolved along separate lines from the Lily family. The Iris family is known best for its ornamentals, especially for the many forms of Iris and Gladiolus. In their homelands, some species of *Crocus, Iris, Tigridia, Tritonia,* and other genera are used as food. Saffron Crocus has long been known as a dye, flavoring, and medicine. The underground rhizome of some Iris (Orris Root) is useful for medicine, dentifrice, perfume, and toilet powder.

Leaves more or less crowded at the base of the stem, long and narrow, mostly folded together lengthwise and overlapping at base in a fan shape, veins longitudinally parallel. Flowers single or clustered but not in raylike heads, with 2 or more bracts, perfect, radially symmetrical or not, tubular or not, having 6 nearly equal segments, or 3 more or less distinctly larger than the other 3; stamens 3; ovary inferior, 3- or 1-celled, many-

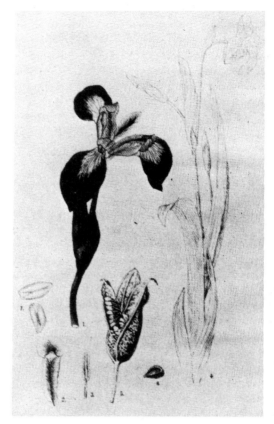

ORRIS ROOT (IRIS): Blue Flag (illustrated) is used for its emetic, diuretic, and cathartic effects. The rhizome contains an acrid resin and essential oil.

ovuled; style 3-parted, the branches either parted again or petal-like. Fruit a capsule. (Neal)

Medicinal Uses: Orris root is prepared by stripping away the outer layer of the rhizome and the roots. The remaining part is distilled to yield a solid oil. This oil (one part diluted with 3–4 parts alcohol) has a scent resembling that of violets; it is consequently of value in the perfume and cosmetics businesses.

Medicinally it is reputedly cathartic and diuretic, and in stronger doses it has been reported to be emetic. It was felt to be useful in treating dropsical conditions (water retention of tissues and/or organs). The root was also chewed as a coverup for bad breath.

Blue Flag *(Iris versicolor)*, another herbaceous perennial, found in the eastern states, is used for its emetic, diuretic, and cathartic effects. This rhizome contains an acrid resin and essential oil.

Dose: 1 teaspoon of rhizome, boiled in a covered container with 1½ pints of water for about ½ hour, at a slow boil. Liquid allowed to cool slowly in the *closed* container. Drunk cold, 1 swallow or 1 tablespoon at a time, 1 to 2 cups per day.

PANSY, WILD
Viola tricolor

PARTS USED: Herb, Flowers and Root
OTHER COMMON NAMES: Pansy, Johnny Jump-Up, Heart's Ease, Violet

Botanical Description: To give an accurate botanical description of *Viola tricolor* it is necessary first to describe the other Violets, *Viola odorata* and *Viola serpens*, although they are not medically active.

Viola odorata (Violet), a perennial herb, one of about 400 species of *Viola*, is a native of Eurasia and Africa. Many plants are grown on the French Riviera for their flowers, as a source of a favorite perfume, though a synthetic product now usually replaces the natural one. The plants with their tufts of dark green leaves are good for garden borders and for ground cover in partly shaded corners. They have horizontal underground stems, none above ground, and they have runners and tufted, heart-shaped to kidney-shaped, blunt-toothed leaves, 2 inches more or less long, on long stems. Flower stems with leafy bracts near the middle rise from leaf axils and bear 1 or 2 fragrant, violet, white-centered or white-lined, nodding flowers about 0.66 inch long, the lowest petal short-spurred, the side and upper petals paired, the sepals shorter, green, more or less pointed. Forms vary in size and color of flowers, some being white or pink, some double. Later in the year, after the showy flowers no longer appear, inconspicuous flowers, without petals, develop near the ground and produce many seeds. Fruiting capsules have 3 valves, which contract suddenly when dry and shoot out the seeds.

Viola serpens (Violet), a small, inconspicuous herb, wide-spreading or not, native from southeast Asia to Malaysia, is extremely variable. The ovate heart-shaped leaves, 1 to 2+ inches long, may be hairy or smooth,

blunt or pointed. Flowers are pale violet, odorless, 0.3 inch across.

Viola tricolor (Pansy), a European herb, living a year or longer, has long, branching stems bearing near the ground round heart-shaped leaves, and along the stems, wide to narrow-oblong, toothed leaves. The plant is grown for its large, attractive flowers, which are about 2 inches in diameter, have large, round petals, and are commonly colored blue, white, and yellow, the lowest petal short-spurred. (Neal)

Medicinal Uses: The herb, which contains mucilaginous material, functions as an external soothing lotion for boils, swellings, and skin diseases of various kinds. It is also a good and gentle laxative, also because of the mucilage. This part of the Pansy has been utilized to treat pectoral and nephritic diseases.

The flowers also have demulcent properties, again because of the mucilage, and are made into syrup and administered as a laxative for infants.

The root is both emetic and cathartic.

Sweet Violet (*V. odorata*) is much used as a flavoring and in candy making, while a leaf tea is a good cough remedy.

The Wonder Violet (*V. mirabilis*) is used in decoction in Ukrainian folk medicine to treat heart ailments, palpitation, and shortness of breath.

Dose: Flowers and herb—Approximately ½ ounce of flowers or herb to 1 pint of water. Water boiled separately and poured over plant material and steeped for 5 to 20 minutes, depending on the desired effect. Drunk hot or warm, 1 to 2 cups per day, at bedtime and upon awakening.

Root—1 teaspoon of the root, boiled in a covered container with 1½ pints of water for about ½ hour, at a slow boil. Liquid allowed to cool slowly in the *closed* container. Drunk cold, 1 swallow or 1 tablespoon at a time, 1 to 2 cups per day.

PAPAYA
Carica papaya

PARTS USED: Leaf and latex
OTHER COMMON NAMES: Melon-Tree, Pawpaw

Botanical Description: The Papaya, a native of tropical

147

America, is a favorite fruit in Hawaii, where the tree grows easily and quickly from seeds, from near sea level to an altitude of about 1,200 feet. Although the date of its introduction is not known, the Papaya may have arrived in Hawaii indirectly by way of Asia and the South Sea islands, before the white man came. At the latest, it arrived with him or soon afterward.

The trees are small, about 5 to 25 feet high, and though ordinarily unbranched, many develop several erect branches. The trunks are gradually tapering, are hollow within, and have light-colored bark, which contains a very caustic milky juice and is nearly smooth except for regular, heart-shaped scars. Ropes can be manufactured from the bark fiber. The smooth, broad leaves, 2 feet or more across, with milky juice, are deeply 7-lobed and again divided. They are clustered at the top of the trunk on hollow stems 2 feet or more long, and directly at their base, 5-petaled, cream-white, fragrant flowers and the fruit are borne. A tree should begin to bear a year after being set out, and though the best crops are produced during 3 or 4 years, trees have been known to bear for 15 years. During winter, fruit ripens slowly, hence the supply is then smallest. The fruit is globose to ovoid, with 5 shallow grooves, 6 to 12 inches long, more or less, yellow or green and yellow, thin-skinned, pulp white to orange or red, sweet, juicy, the central space ordinarily lined with small, hard, knobby, black seeds, covered with a gelatinous coat and a smooth, glistening skin.

In nature of flowers the trees vary considerably, about a dozen different kinds having been noted. One kind produces only fruit-bearing flowers; a second, only pollen-bearing; a third, both fruit and pollen-bearing; a fourth, all three kinds. Except the fruit-bearing, these forms are not constant, some pollen-bearing trees changing to fruit-bearing after being cut off at the top. Fruit develops from some pollen-bearing flowers, and it is of excellent quality. The fruit varies in shape and size, large Papayas weighing about 8 pounds, "solo" Papayas much less. Some pollinated and unpollinated fruits develop without containing seeds. (Neal)

Medicinal Uses: Although the Papaya is best known for its delicious fruit, fresh Papaya leaves were used medicinally as a dressing for wounds by the Indians indigenous to the tropical areas where the plant grows. They also wrapped meat in these leaves to make the flesh more tender.

In the Fiji Islands a filtrate of the inner bark is used to treat toothache, while the fresh milky white sap (latex) is applied directly on large boils and also utilized to treat wounds.

The dried latex of the Papaya is marketed under the names papayotin, papain or papoid, and is given to treat dyspepsia and gastric catarrh. In powder form it is applied to treat skin diseases, including warts and tubercule swellings. Much of this medicinal product is supplied from Ceylon and the West Indies. It is still employed as a meat tenderizer and is contained as an additive in one brand of beer to dissolve excess proteins, thereby making the beer more clear.

The enzyme chymopapain, a derivative of the latex of the Papaya, has been used on an experimental basis by neurosurgeons to dissolve herniated ("slipped") intervertebral discs in patients complaining of back pain.

Dose: Leaves wrapped directly on wounds. Latex used as needed; avoid internal use due to presence of protein-digesting properties.

PASSIONFLOWER
Passiflora incarnata

PARTS USED: Plant and flower

Botanical Description: All but about 40 species of the nearly 400 known species of *Passiflora* are natives of America; the 40 are natives of Asia, South Pacific islands, and Madagascar. They are commonly vines with tendrils at leaf axils. Most bear highly ornamental flowers, which develop at leaf axils and are accompanied by bracts. The calyx consists of a short to long tube bearing 5 sepals, 5 petals (rarely none), and a corona, or crown, between the base of the tube and the petals, consisting of a series of rings bearing threadlike or other processes or none. The 5 stamens are usually borne on the stalk of the ovary, which has 3 styles. The fruit is berrylike, and is often called granadilla or water lemon. Early European travelers in tropical America gave this strange flower the name Passionflower, as it suggested to them the passion or suffering of Christ: the 10 equal sepals and petals represented the crown of thorns, or halo; the 5 stamens, the five wounds; the 3 styles, the three nails; the tendrils, the cords or scourges; the

148

leaves, the hands of the persecutors. The white color symbolizes purity; the blue, heaven. (Neal)

Medicinal Uses: As a sedative, Passionflower has qualities unlike those of any other herb. It is very effective, with a pleasant taste, and yet surprisingly gentle. It is helpful in a variety of ailments, from insomnia, dysmenorrhea, nervous tension, and fatigue, to muscle spasms. It can be used with safety even for small children.

Passiflora incarnata may be our best tranquilizer yet. The dried leaves and stems both induce a natural sleep and calm hyperactive people.

This plant drug is used in Italy to treat hyperactive children; and in the Yucatan it is an old remedy for insomnia, hysteria, and convulsions in children. Interestingly, the early Algonquin Indians brewed this woody vine to soothe their nerves. The state flower of Tennessee appears to be a useful bridge between traditional medicine and modern ills, especially anxiety states. Physicians could well recommend this plant to patients who want to wean themselves from synthetic sleeping pills and tranquilizers.

Surprisingly, one kind of Passionflower (*P. quadrangularis,* or Giant Granadilla) was recently found to contain serotonin. Low levels of this compound in the cerebrospinal fluid of patients with chronic depression have led some researchers to speculate that adding it to circulating blood would relieve states of depression. This may be confirmed by the fact that LSD-like compounds which are used to induce clinical psychoses are known to have potent *anti*-serotonin activity; perhaps Passionflower therefore acts as a natural calming agent by promoting the transmission of subtle nerve impulses. It appears to aid concentration, alter perception, and gently shift mood.

Utilized since its "discovery" by early Jesuit missionaries in South America, Passionflower has no known toxicity in small doses.

Dose: For medicinal use, ½ to 1 teaspoon of the dried herb is used to 1 cup of boiling water. The resultant infusion may be taken every 3 to 4 hours.

As a fluidextract, 3–4 drops every 4 hours.

PATCHOULI LEAF
Pogostemon patchouli (P. cablin)

PARTS USED: Herb

Botanical Description: This is an odoriferous shrubby green leafed plant of the mint family, native to Silhat, Penang, and the Malay peninsula.

Medicinal Uses: The oil of the Patchouli was believed by the Arabs, Chinese and Japanese to prevent venereal disease, when applied prior to and during sexual intercourse.

It has a valuable property of fixing odors, giving it broad application in the perfumery business as an odor and scent preservative added to other fragrances.

Almost all essential oils from plants have inhibitory activity against some type of microorganism. However, they rarely are tested against the organisms responsible for venereal disease, and thus it is difficult to project whether or not the use of Patchouli oil as a prophylaxis for venereal diseases is valid.

Although the authors have not personally used Patchouli oil as an application to the genitalia to prevent venereal disease, we nevertheless pass on a word of caution. Virtually any essential oil, when applied undiluted to any mucous tissue, including the genitalia, produces a rush of heat to the area due to rapid evaporation and dilation of blood vessels in the area. This could produce a very uncomfortable condition if Patchouli oil was applied to the sensitive tissue of the penis and/or vagina!

Dose: No recommended dose. Not medically active for above folkloric usage. Ill effects, such as loss of appetite and sleep, and nervous attacks have been ascribed to the excessive employment of patchouli as a perfume.

PENNYROYAL
Hedeoma pulegioides (American Pennyroyal), *Mentha pulegium* (European Pennyroyal)

PARTS USED: Whole plant
OTHER COMMON NAMES: Tickweed, Squawmint, Hedeoma

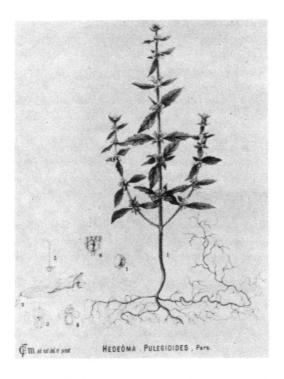

HEDEÔMA PULEGIOIDES, Pers.

PENNYROYAL: In laboratory studies, extracts of this aromatic plant are shown to stimulate the uterus. This could account for the menses-inducing effect.

Botanical Description: *Hedeoma pulegioides.* This is an indigenous annual plant, from 9 to 15 inches high, with a small, branching, fibrous, yellowish root, and a pubescent stem, which sends off numerous slender erect branches. The leaves are opposite, oblong lanceolate or oval, nearly acute, attenuated at the base, remotely serrate, rough or pubescent, and prominently veined on the under surface. The flowers are very small, of a pale-blue color, supported on short peduncles, and arranged in axillary whorls, along the whole length of the branches.

The plant is common in all parts of the United States, preferring dry grounds and pastures, and, where it is abundant, scenting the air for a considerable distance with its grateful odor.

Both in the recent and dried state it has a pleasant aromatic smell, and a warm, pungent, mintlike taste. It readily imparts its virtues to boiling water. The volatile oil upon which they depend may be separated by distillation, and employed instead of the herb itself.

This herb has been very erroneously confounded by some with the *Mentha pulegium,* or European Pennyroyal.

Mentha pulegium. This species of Mint is distinguished by its roundish prostrate stems, its ovate obtuse, somewhat crenate leaves, and its verticillate flowers. It is a native of Europe, and neither cultivated nor employed in this country. Our native Pennyroyal belongs to a different genus, *Hedeoma pulegioides,* described above. *M. pulegium* possesses similar properties, and is employed for the same purposes with the other Mints. (U.S.D.)

Medicinal Uses: Pennyroyal was employed in the Thomsonian system of medicine to check nosebleed; the patient sat with feet immersed in a tub of quite warm water while drinking a tea made from the plant. This was thought to equalize circulation and alleviate pressure to the head.

It is a gentle stimulant, and as an aid in relieving the common cold, a draught was often drunk at bedtime to promote perspiration, again with the feet soaking in hot water. It was also used the same way to bring on suppressed menstruation.

It is a very soothing tea, and produces a nice sense of comforting warmth.

The two species both have the medicinal properties of the official Mints, being stimulant, aromatic, carminative, and stomachic. The volatile oil has similar properties to the herb and is frequently used in domestic practice to promote the menstrual flow. Pennyroyal is considered inferior in its medicinal qualities to Peppermint, which largely superseded it in regular medicine, but Pennyroyal has continued to be popular in domestic practice.

Experimentally, extracts of Pennyroyal are known to stimulate the uterus in test tube studies, which could account for the menses-inducing effect. The active principle is known as pulegone. *Large doses* of this plant are known to produce nausea, vomiting, and *possible toxic effects.* A recent death was found to be the result of the ingestion of pennyroyal *essential oil, not* an infusion of the herb.

The alcoholic infusion has been used to treat

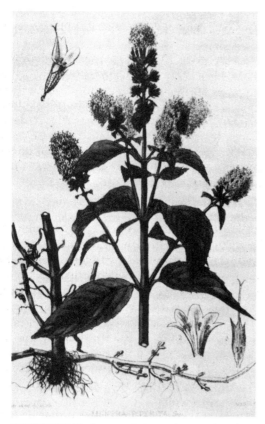

PEPPERMINT: A tea of these leaves is taken primarily for its soothing effects. Animal experiments confirm folkloric claims.

fainting, asphyxia and paralysis, asthma, hysteria, atonic gout, and flatulence.

Dose: 1 teaspoon per cup of boiling water. Water boiled separately and poured over the plant material and steeped for 5–20 minutes, depending on the desired effect. Drunk hot or warm, 1 to 2 cups. CAUTION, the essential oil has caused death.

PEPPERMINT
Mentha piperita

PARTS USED: Leaves and flowering tops

Botanical Description: Peppermint is a perennial herbaceous plant, with a creeping root, and erect, quadrangular, channeled, purplish, somewhat hairy stems, which are branched toward the top, and about 2 feet in height. The leaves are opposite, petiolate, ovate, serrate, pointed, smoother on the upper than the under surface, and of a dark-green color which is paler beneath. The flowers are small, purple, and disposed in terminal obtuse spikes, which are interrupted below. The calyx is tubular, furrowed, and 5-toothed; the corolla is also tubular, with its border divided into 4 segments, of which the uppermost is broadest, and notched at its apex. The anthers are concealed within the tube of the corolla; the style projects beyond it, and terminates in a bifid stigma. The 4-cleft germ is converted into 4 seeds, which are lodged in the calyx.

This species of mint is a native of Great Britain, whence it has been conveyed to the continent of Europe and to this country. In some parts of the United States it is largely cultivated for the sake of its volatile oil. We occasionally find it growing wild along the fences of our villages. The cultivators of this herb have observed that, in order to maintain its flavor in perfection, it is necessary to transplant the roots every 3 years. It should be cut for medical use in dry weather, about the period of the expansion of the flowers. These appear in August.

The herb, both in the recent and dried state, has a penetrating, grateful odor, somewhat resembling that of camphor. The taste is aromatic, warm, pungent, glowing, camphorous, bitterish, and attended with a sensation of coolness when air is admitted into the mouth. These properties depend on a volatile oil which abounds in the herb, and may be separated by distillation with water. Peppermint also contains camphor, which rises with the oil. The virtues of the herb are imparted to water, and more readily to alcohol. (U.S.D.)

Medicinal Uses: It is recorded that Peppermint was cultivated by the ancient Egyptians, and its usage is documented in the Icelandic pharmacopoeia of the thirteenth century. The most agreeable and powerful of the mints, it possesses aromatic, carminative, stimulant, antispasmodic and stomachic properties. It is frequently used to allay nausea, relieve stomach and bowel spasms and griping, and to promote the expulsion of flatus. It is often drunk after mealtimes as an aid to digestion. The volatile oil, which has been similarly used in medicine, is also employed as a flavoring agent in cordials and candies, and has also been added to less palatable medicines to mask disagreeable odors and/or tastes.

151

Peppermint tea is one of the most common herbal remedies, used primarily as a carminative and intestinal antispasmodic. These effects are all explained on the basis of animal experiments using the essential oil from Peppermint, or purified essential oil constituents, the results of which mimic the effects claimed in humans.

Dose: Approximately ½ ounce of leaves to 1 pint of water. Water boiled separately and poured over the plant material and steeped for 5 to 20 minutes, depending on the desired effect. Drunk hot or warm, 1 to 2 cups or more per day.

PERIWINKLE, TROPICAL
Catharanthus roseus, Vinca rosea

PARTS USED: Herb

OTHER COMMON NAMES: Madagascar Periwinkle, Cape Periwinkle

Botanical Description: An everblooming perennial herb or small shrub 1 to 2 feet high, from tropical America, it's popular in gardens for ground cover and edges. The short-stemmed, paired leaves are oblong, 1 to 3 inches long, tipped with a short point. The flowers are showy, 5-parted, rose-purple or white (var. *albus*) with or without a red throat, 1 to 1.5 inches in diameter, the 5 broad, spreading lobes terminating a narrow, inch-long tube. The calyx is small and has awl-shaped lobes. Each fruit consists of 2 erect, podlike, inch-long cylinders containing several cylindrical seeds. (Neal)

Medicinal Uses: The Tropical Periwinkle is an extremely important example of a traditional folk medicine whose use was investigated by a major pharmaceutical company, resulting in the discovery of two alkaloids with practical application in the treatment of cancer.

In 1953 Dr. Faustino Garcia reported at the Pacific Science Congress that the plant, taken orally, is a folkloric remedy in the Philippines for the treatment of hyperglycemia. Researchers at the Lilly Company, conducting a general survey of many folk remedy plants through preliminary testing in a cancer-screening program, found that the Periwinkle showed striking anticancer activity in test animals.

While the Tropical Periwinkle is a pantropical plant that is often cultivated in temperate climates as an ornamental, the leaves have been used most extensively as an oral insulin substitute; proprietary products have been sold in Africa and the Philippines for this purpose.

At least seven or eight scientific publications are available in which investigators have reported no effect on blood sugar levels in normal, as well as diabetic, animals, when aqueous extracts of Periwinkle leaves were administered orally. Other studies have been published in which hot-water extracts of the leaves of this plant were given to diabetic patients, but in every instance there was no significant benefit to the patients.

In the early 1960s it was discovered that extracts of the leaves of *C. roseus* would significantly prolong the life of mice in which leukemia had been clinically induced. This finding eventually led to the discovery of two potent anticancer drugs, vincaleukoblastine (vinblastine, VLB) and leurocristine (vincristine, VCR), both of which are now available on a worldwide basis for the treatment of human cancer.

Vincristine is one of our most important anticancer drugs, being most useful for the treatment of childhood leukemias. Vinblastine is of lesser importance, but is effective in treating certain types of Hodgkin's disease.

Since vincristine does have neurotoxic side effects, and vinblastine can cause a marked decrease in the number of white blood cells, these must be considered as very potent drugs. Thus, it cannot be recommended that the Tropical Periwinkle be used as a herbal remedy, since the danger of potential life-threatening complications is very real.

Vinca major and *Vinca minor:* Both of these "Periwinkles" are often confused with the Tropical Periwinkle *(Catharanthus roseus)*, and although *Vinca* and *Catharanthus* are related in being members of the Dogbane (Apocynaceae) family, they are chemically and pharmacologically quite different.

Although *Vinca major* (Greater Periwinkle) and *Vinca minor* (Lesser Periwinkle) are somewhat different in chemical makeup, they have both been used externally to stop hemorrhages; such effect most likely being due to astringent tannins present in both plants. Any effect of preventing menstrual hemorrhaging (menorrhagia) could be due to vincamine, an indole alkaloid present in both species, which has been shown to contract uterine muscle in test tube experiments. Neither of these effects has been confirmed, however, by direct experiments involving the use of extracts from these plants.

Dose: CAUTION. See discussion of Tropical Periwinkle above.

PINKROOT
Spigelia marilandica

PARTS USED: Rhizome and roots
OTHER COMMON NAMES: Maryland, Carolina, or Indian Pink; Worm-Grass; Wormweed; American Worm-Root; Star-Bloom

Botanical Description: The Pinkroot is an herbaceous plant with a perennial root, which sends off numerous

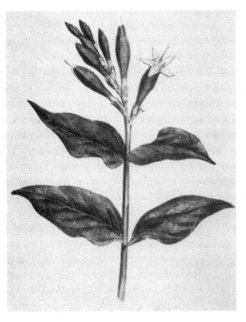

PINKROOT: The principal medicinal use of *Spigelia* is as an anthelminthic, used particularly for expelling roundworms. The roots contain a compound similar to coniine (found in Hemlock) and nicotine.

fibrous branches. The stems, several of which rise from the same root, are simple, erect, 4-sided, nearly smooth, and from 12 to 20 inches high. The leaves are opposite, sessile, ovate-lanceolate, acuminate, entire, and smooth, with the veins and margins slightly pubescent. Each stem terminates in a spike, which leans to one side, and supports from 4 to 12 flowers with very short peduncles. The calyx is persistent, with 5 long, subulate, slightly serrate leaves, reflexed in the ripe fruit. The corolla is funnel-shaped, and much longer than the calyx, with the tube inflated in the middle, and the border divided into 5 acute, spreading segments. It is of a rich carmine color externally, becoming paler at the base, and orange-yellow within. The edges of the segments are slightly tinged with green. The stamens, though apparently very short, and inserted into the upper part of the tube between the segments, may be traced down its internal surface to the base. The anthers are oblong, heart-shaped; the germ superior, ovate; the style about the length of the corolla, and terminating in a linear fringed stigma projecting considerably beyond it. The capsule is double, consisting of two cohering, globular, one-celled portions, and containing many seeds.

The plant is a native of our southern states, being seldom if ever found north of the Potomac. It grows in rich soils on the borders of woods, and flowers from May to July. The root is the part that has been recognized as official by the *U.S. Pharmacopoeia,* although the whole plant has been gathered and dried for sale. (U.S.D.)

Medicinal Uses: Overdose can be fatal, but use of Pinkroot has rarely been reported to produce ill effects so long as it is eliminated. For this reason it is commonly prescribed in combination with Calomel, Senna, or some other cathartic.

The principal medicinal use of *Spigelia* is as an anthelmintic; it is especially valued for its usefulness in the expulsion of the roundworm. White traders learned of this worm remedy from the American Cherokee Indians.

A preparation sold under the name Worm Tea contained Spigelia, Senna, Manna, and Savin. It was mixed in different strengths by the apothecary to suit individual needs.

The roots contain spigeline, which resembles coniine (found in Hemlock) and nicotine, which

153

explains its stimulant effects.

Dose: Not recommended. Requires expertise of a skilled herbalist to be effective yet not toxic.

PIPSISSEWA
Chimaphila umbellata, C. Maculata

PARTS USED: Leaves and herb

OTHER COMMON NAMES: Spotted Wintergreen, Bitter Wintergreen, King's Cure, Ground Holly, Winter, Love, Rheumatism Weed

Botanical Description: *Chimaphila umbellata,* or the Pipsissewa, is a small evergreen plant, with a perennial creeping yellowish root, which gives rise to several simple, erect or semi-procumbent stems, from 4 to 8 inches in height, and ligneous at their base. The leaves are wedge-shaped, somewhat lanceolate, serrate, cori-

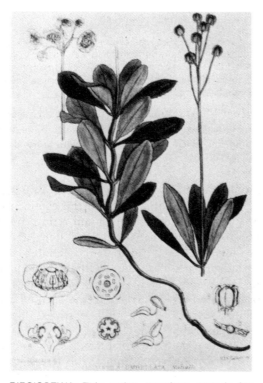

PIPSISSEWA: This native American remedy for rheumatism and scrofula (a type of tuberculosis) was also used by the settlers for the same purposes; both groups also took the plant as a tea to induce sweating.

aceous, smooth, of a shining sap-green color on the upper surface, paler beneath, and supported upon short footstalks, in irregular whorls, of which there are usually 2 on the same stem. The flowers are disposed in a small terminal corymb, and stand upon nodding peduncles. The calyx is small, and divided at its border into 5 teeth or segments. The corolla is composed of 5 roundish, concave, spreading petals, which are of a white color tinged with red, and exhale an agreeable odor. The stamens are 10, with filaments shorter than the petals, and with large, nodding bifurcated, purple anthers. The germ is globular and depressed, supporting a thick and apparently sessile stigma, the style being short and immersed in the germ. The seeds are numerous, linear, chaffy, and enclosed in a roundish, depressed, 5-celled, 5-valved capsule, having the persistent calyx at the base.

This humble but beautiful evergreen is a native of the northern latitudes of America, Europe, and Asia. It is found in all parts of the United States, and extends to the Pacific Ocean. It grows under the shade of woods, and prefers a loose sandy soil, enriched by decaying leaves. The flowers appear in June and July. All parts of the plant are endowed with active properties. The leaves and stems are kept in the shops.

C. maculata, or Spotted Wintergreen, probably possesses virtues similar to those of *C. umbellata.* The character of the leaves of the two plants will serve to distinguish them. Those of the *C. maculata* are lanceolate, rounded at the base, where they are broader than near the summit, and of a deep olive green color, veined with greenish white; those of the *C. umbellata* are broadest near the summit, gradually narrowing to the base, and of a uniform shining green. In drying, with exposure to light, the color fades very much, though it still retains a greenish hue.

Pipsissewa, when fresh and bruised, exhales a peculiar odor. The taste of the leaves is pleasantly bitter, astringent, and sweetish; that of the stems and root unites with these qualities a considerable degree of pungency. Boiling water extracts the active properties of the plant, which are also imparted to alcohol. (U.S.D.)

Medicinal Uses: Why the generic name of these plants is formed of two Greek words for "winter" and "love" remains a mystery, although their use in folk medicine is readily explained. This native

American remedy for rheumatism and scrofula (a type of tuberculosis) was also used by the settlers for the same purposes; both groups also took the plant as a tea to induce sweating. It is credited with tonic, astringent, and diuretic properties, and was administered in the treatment of cystitis and was held to be diuretic and antiseptic to the urinary tract. A decoction was applied externally for blisters and scrofulous sores and swellings, but the Pipsissewa remains a first-rate folk remedy for miscellaneous urinary-tract infections.

Chemically the leaves of this half-shrub contain ericolin, arbutin, chimaphilin, urson, tannin and gallic acid. Chimaphillin, as well as extracts of this plant, show antibacterial properties in test tube experiments. This can explain the use of this plant in scrofula, and in treating cystitis.

Dose: Approximately ½ ounce of leaves or herb to 1 pint of water. Water boiled separately and poured over the plant material and steeped for 5–20 minutes, depending on the desired effect. Drunk hot or warm, 1 to 2 cups per day.

Still, the best method of taking the herb is in the form of fluidextract, which is readily made into a syrup: dose, 2–6 grams.

PLANTAIN
Plantago major, P. lanceolata, and other *Plantago* species

PARTS USED: Leaves and seeds
OTHER COMMON NAMES: Rib Grass, Ribwort, Ripple Grass, Soldier's Herb, Broad-Leaved Plantain, Narrow-Leaved Plantain

Botanical Description: *Plantago major.* The Broad-Leaved Plantain is a stemless, smooth or hairy herb, with leaves 1 to 10 inches long, forming a rosette near the ground. Leaf blades are thick, broad-oval to somewhat heart-shaped, and grooved with five to nine longitudinal veins, and the leaf stems are broad and trough-shaped. Tiny flowers are borne in cylindrical heads at the tip of slender stalks 6 to 24 inches or more long, each flower 4-parted and having 4 long stamens and a superior ovary. Each small fruiting capsule contains 5 to 16 seeds.

Plantago lanceolata. A native of Eurasia, the Narrow-

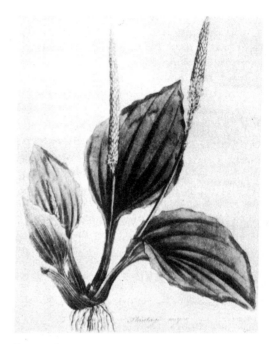

PLANTAIN: Used medicinally since antiquity, this common weed was utilized to relieve thirst and reduce fever, and as an astringent. To treat boils, sores and wounds, the leaves are bruised and applied whole.

Leaved Plantain differs from the preceding species in having narrower, hairy leaves, with 3 to 5 longitudinal veins, and each fruiting capsule with only 2 seeds. (Neal)

Medicinal Uses: Plantain has been used medicinally since antiquity. Formerly this common weed was utilized to relieve thirst and reduce fever, to remove obstructions within the system, and as an astringent. Later it was seldom used internally but remained a popular external stimulant application to boils, sores, and wounds. The leaves were bruised and applied whole to the affected area in poultice form. To relieve bee stings, the fresh leaves are rubbed on.

P. media, the Hoary Plantain, and *P. lanceolata,* the Narrow-Leaved Plantain (Rib Grass), possess the same properties as *P. major* and may be used interchangeably.

A European species, *P. psyllium,* the Fleawort, has seeds which are used medicinally due to their mucilaginous nature. They are demulcent and emollient and were used for the same purposes as Flax seed (see article on Flax).

The seeds of most *Plantago* species contain high concentrations of mucilage, and thus will have a demulcent and emollient effect externally, and will act as a laxative if taken internally due to the swelling of the seeds.

Dose: External—Fresh leaves, bruised and applied whole, directly to skin problems, and wounds.

Internal—Infusion of ½ ounce of leaves to 1 pint of water, steeped for 5 to 20 minutes, drunk hot or warm, 1 to 2 cups per day. Infusion of ½ oz. of seeds to 1 pint of water, steeped for 5–20 minutes; drink 1 tablespoon 3–6 times per day.

PLEURISY ROOT
Asclepias tuberosa

PARTS USED: Root

OTHER COMMON NAMES: Butterfly Weed, Wind Root, Canada Root, Tuber Root

Botanical Description: The root of the Butterfly Weed or Pleurisy Root is perennial, and gives origin to numerous stems, which are erect, ascending, or procumbent, round, hairy, of a green or reddish color, branching at the top, and about 3 feet in height. The leaves are scattered, oblong-lanceolate, very hairy, of a deep rich green color on their upper surface, paler beneath, and supported usually on short footstalks. They differ, however, somewhat in shape according to the variety of the plant. In the variety with decumbent stems, they are almost linear, and in another variety cordate. The flowers are of a beautiful reddish-orange color, and disposed in terminal or lateral corymbose umbels. The fruit is an erect lanceolate follicle, with flat ovate seeds connected to a longitudinal receptacle by long silky hairs.

This plant differs from other species of *Asclepias* in not emitting a milky juice when wounded. It is indigenous, growing throughout the United States from Massachusetts to Georgia, and when in full bloom in the months of June and July, exhibiting a splendid appearance. It is most abundant in the southern states. The root is the only part used in medicine.

This is large, irregularly tuberous, branching, often

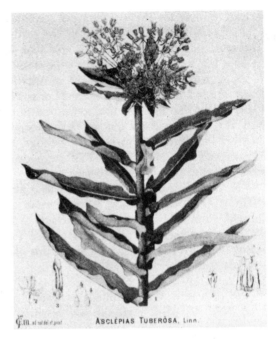

ASCLÉPIAS TUBERÓSA, Linn.

PLEURISY ROOT: This medicinal derives its name from its effectiveness as an expectorant, helping to expel phlegm from the bronchial and nasal passages.

somewhat fusiform, fleshy, externally brown, internally white and striated, and in the recent state of a subacrid nauseous taste. When dried it is easily pulverized, and has a bitter but not otherwise unpleasant taste. It yields its virtues readily to boiling water. (U.S.D.)

Medicinal Uses: The Pleurisy Root derives its name from its effectiveness as an expectorant, helping to expel phlegm from the bronchial and nasal passages; it was used in a variety of respiratory ailments besides pleurisy, including cough, consumption, and bronchitis. Because of its claimed antispasmodic properties, the root, dried and powdered, was administered to cure infant colic. Adults likewise drank an herb tea of the root as an aid in eliminating flatulence.

Pleurisy Root, prior to the advent of synthetic drugs, was widely used by medical practitioners in the United States. Medical journals frequently carried scientific articles on the effectiveness of Pleurisy Root preparations as a diaphoretic, expectorant, emetic, and cathartic, the specific effect being dependent on the amount of the preparation used. The active principles responsible for these effects, however, remain unknown.

Dose: For medicinal use, 1 teaspoonful of the powdered root is used per 1½ pints of boiling water, boiled in a covered container for about ½ hour, at a slow boil. Liquid is allowed to cool slowly in the *closed* container. Drunk cold, 1 swallow or 1 tablespoon at a time, 1 to 2 cups per day.

POMEGRANATE
Punica granatum

PARTS USED: Bark, Rind and Fruit
OTHER COMMON NAMES: Grenadier

Botanical Description: The Pomegranate is a small shrubby tree, attaining in favorable situations the height of 20 feet, with a very unequal trunk, and numerous

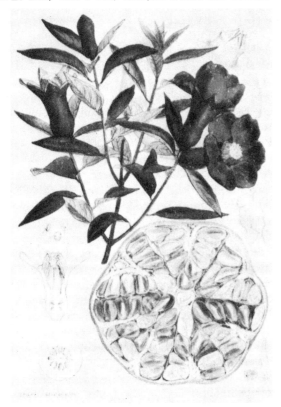

POMEGRANATE: Used to treat tapeworm infestation, this popular fruit has been eaten and cultivated for at least 5,000 years.

branches, which sometimes bear thorns. The leaves are opposite, entire, oblong or lance-shaped, pointed at each end, smooth, shining, of a bright green color, and placed on short footstalks. The flowers are large, of a rich scarlet color, and stand at the end of the young branches. The petals are roundish and wrinkled, and are inserted into the upper part of the tube of the calyx, which is red, thick, and fleshy. The fruit is a globular berry, about the size of an orange, crowned with the calyx, covered with a reddish-yellow, thick, coriaceous rind, and divided internally into many cells, which contain an acidulous pulp, and numerous oblong, angular seeds.

This tree grows wild upon both shores of the Mediterranean, in Arabia, Persia, and Japan, has been introduced into the East and West Indies, and is cultivated in all civilized countries where the climate is sufficiently warm to allow the fruit to ripen. In higher latitudes, where it does not bear fruit, it is raised in gardens and hothouses for the beauty of its flowers, which become double, and acquire increased splendor of coloring by cultivation. Doubts have been entertained as to its original country.

The fruit of the Pomegranate, for which the plant is cultivated in tropical climates, varies much in size and flavor. It is said to attain greater perfection in both these respects in the West Indies than in its native country. The pulp is red, succulent, pleasantly acid, and sweetish; and is used for the same purposes as the orange, though not officinal. It is the rind of the fruit which was principally used in medicine in the United States; other parts of the plant, however, are also used in medicine. (U.S.D.)

Medicinal Uses: The fruit is eaten, and its juice is used to make refreshing drinks, particularly in the Middle East, where the fruit has been cultivated for 5,000 years (Israel). The powdered fruit rind was held to be astringent, and was utilized to treat diarrhea, excessive perspiration, as a gargle for sore throats, for intermittent fevers, and for leucorrhea.

The root bark was administered by the ancients to rid the intestines of worms. This medicinal usage was overlooked by Europeans until 1804, when a practitioner in India who had cured an Englishman of a tapeworm was persuaded to share his secret remedy. Nausea and vomiting some-

157

times accompanied the purgative action of this plant; patients were consequently advised to fast for 12 hours prior to treatment. Two hours after administration of the remedy, a brisk cathartic was given to expedite discharge of the remains of the worm. The remedy was repeated day after day, sometimes as many as four times, until success was achieved.

Of all types of intestinal worm infestations, Pomegranate root bark is most useful in cases of tapeworm. The active principle, discovered in 1878, is the liquid alkaloid pelletierine, which was used in human medicine for a number of years, and then became relegated to veterinary use. Thus, it is well established that root bark preparations of Pomegranate would be effective when used to expel worms from the intestinal tract.

Anyone who has bitten into the peel of a Pomegranate fruit can testify to the highly astringent nature of this material. In fact, it is known that the fruit peel contains about 30 percent of tannin, which is the active astringent substance.

Dose: 1 teaspoon of root bark, chopped small, to 1½ pints of boiling water, boiled in a covered container at a slow boil for about ½ hour. Liquid allowed to cool slowly in the *closed* container. Drunk cold, 1 mouthful at a time, over the day, to a maximum of 1 cup total.

POPLAR
Populus nigra, P. balsamifera

PARTS USED: Leaf buds
OTHER COMMON NAMES: Black Poplar, Balsam Poplar, Balm of Gilead

Botanical Description: *Populus Nigra,* or the Black Poplar, is a tall tree, with dull gray branches and dark furrowed bark on the older trunks. Petioles distinctly flattened. Blades triangular-ovate, abruptly pointed, broadly cuneate to truncate at base, finely and bluntly serrate, 5–10 centimeters long and usually slightly broader, glandless at the base, pubescent when young. Stamens 30 or fewer. Stigmas 2, broadly dilated. Capsules ovoid, 7–9 millimeters long, 2-valved, twice as long as their pedicels.

Native of Eurasia; frequently planted and occasionally

escaped. Commoner and more widely distributed than the species is the horticultural form known as the Lombardy Poplar and variously as *P. italica, P. dilatata,* and *P. nigra* var. *italica,* characterized by strictly erect branches forming a narrowly conic crown; it can scarcely be regarded as a member of our flora, although often reported as escaped.

P. balsamifera, the Balsam Poplar, is a tall tree with dark gray furrowed bark and glabrous twigs. Terminal bud viscid. Petioles terete or nearly so. Blade ovate to ovate-lanceolate, acute or short-acuminate, finely serrate, cuneate to rounded at base, or even subcordate, glabrous, pale beneath. Scales of the catkins long-ciliate. Stamens 12–30. Stigmas 2, nearly sessile, broadly dilated. Capsules ovoid, 2-valved, 5–8 millimeters long, crowded on short pedicels, forming a compact spike-like raceme.

Habitat: Wet woods, river banks, and shores, Labrador to Alaska, south to Connecticut, northern Pennsylvania, northern Indiana, Iowa, Nebraska, Nevada, and Oregon. (B&B)

Medicinal Uses: Poplar leaf buds are covered with a resinous exudate; their smell is balsamic and pleasant, the taste bitterly aromatic.

Poplar buds (from *P. nigra* or *P. balsamifera*) have been used for the same purposes as the Turpentines and other balsams. Macerated in oil, they were applied externally as a liniment for the treatment of rheumatism. A popular salve was made in France of equal parts (100 grams) of Poppy, Belladonna, Henbane, and Black Nightshade, moistened with 400 grams of alcohol, rested for 24 hours, then heated with 4000 grams of lard for 3 hours, after which 800 grams crushed Poplar buds were added and the mixture was heated for 10 more hours, then strained. This anodyne ointment was used to treat painful local afflictions including sores and burns. Known as "Pommade de Bourgeons de Peuplier," it was widely used throughout Europe. There were several different ways to concoct this ointment, using the same plant materials.

In tincture form the buds have been given for chest complaints and in the treatment of inflammation of the kidneys.

Poplar buds are rich in chemical substances having actions similar to aspirin, such as salicin and mixtures of phenolic acids. Thus, Poplar buds taken *internally* would be useful in minor rheumatic pains. The phenolic acids would contribute to the effectiveness of extracts being used for coughs as well. We can find no rationale for the application of Poplar bud extracts externally to relieve rheumatism symptoms, since the active chemicals are not known to be absorbed through the skin.

Dose: A handful of buds, macerated in olive oil, and applied sparingly externally.

PRICKLY ASH
Zanthoxylum americanum (Z. fraxineum)

PARTS USED: Bark and berries
OTHER COMMON NAMES: Toothache Tree,
   Angelica Tree, Suterberry, Pellitory Bark,
   Yellow-Wood, Northern Prickly Ash

Botanical Description: The Prickly Ash is a shrub from 5 to 10 feet in height, with alternate branches, which are covered with strong, sharp, scattered prickles. The leaves are alternate and pinnate, consisting of 4 or 5 pairs of leaflets, and an odd terminal one, with a common footstalk, which is sometimes prickly on the back, sometimes unarmed. The leaflets are nearly sessile, ovate, acute, slightly serrate, and somewhat downy on their under surface. The flowers, which are small and greenish, are disposed in sessile umbels near the origin of the young shoots. The plant is polygamous, some shrubs bearing both male and perfect flowers, others only female. The number of stamens is 5, of the pistils three or four in the perfect flowers, about 5 in the pistillate. Each fruitful flower is followed by as many capsules as it had germs. These capsules are stipitate, oval, punctate, of a greenish-red color, with 2 valves, and 1 oval blackish seed.

This species of *Zanthoxylum* is indigenous, growing in woods and in moist shady places, throughout the northern, middle, and western States. The flowers appear in April and May, before the foliage. The leaves and capsules have an aromatic odor recalling that of the oil of lemons.

The bark, as found in the shops, is in pieces more or less quilled, from one to two lines in thickness, of a whitish color, internally somewhat shining, with an ash-colored epidermis, which in some specimens is partially or wholly removed, and in those derived from the small branches is armed with strong prickles. The bark is very light, brittle, of a farinaceous fracture, nearly or quite inorodous, and of a taste which is at first sweetish and slightly aromatic, then bitterish, and ultimately acrid. The acrimony is imparted to boiling water and alcohol, which extract the virtues of the bark. (U.S.D.)

Medicinal Uses: The bark and berries of Prickly Ash share the same active principles, but the bark is preferred for the uses described below.

This plant is a stimulant and was also used to produce perspiration. It was once a popular remedy for chronic rheumatism, and was used extensively in the United States for this purpose. The bark was simply chewed, raw, or inserted into cavities, as a toothache remedy.

Prickly ash bark was also employed in the treatment of flatulence and diarrhea. The berries are aromatic in addition to the above properties, and were used medicinally only in this connection.

Dose: Women suffering from chronic pelvic diseases used this plant as a counterirritant, applying hot packs of 2–4 ounces of fluidextract *zanthoxylum*, mixed with 1 ounce of tincture of cayenne pepper to 2 quarts of water, to the external pelvic area, to relieve their distress.

A decoction may be prepared using 1 teaspoon of the bark, boiled in a covered container with 1½ pints of water for about ½ hour, at a slow boil. Liquid allowed to cool slowly in the *closed* container. Drunk cold, 1 swallow or 1 tablespoon at a time, 1 to 2 cups per day.

PUMPKIN
Cucurbita pepo

PARTS USED: Seeds
OTHER COMMON NAMES: Melon Pumpkin

Botanical Description: A bristly-hairy annual vine with branched tendrils, probably a native of America, it is grown for its edible fruits, which are commonly used in pies, and are popular for Halloween. Leaves are triangular heart-shaped, to 12 inches long, with pointed,

159

toothed lobes. Flowers are large, yellow, solitary at leaf axils; the fruit large, orange, globose, regularly furrowed, white-seeded. Among varieties are the vegetable marrow, summer squash, scallop squash, and yellow-flowered gourds, the last grown for their small, hard-shelled, variously shaped, ornamental fruits. A bush variety, running little if at all, yields the Italian squash, or zucchini, a green vegetable which looks like a cucumber. (Neal)

Medicinal Uses: Pumpkin seeds have been used in almost every culture in the world for centuries as an aid to remove intestinal worms (vermifuge) from the body, or more specifically, to rid the body of tapeworms (taenifuge).

In 1820 a Cuban physician reported that three ounces of the fresh flesh of the Pumpkin would accomplish the death and expulsion of the tapeworm exactly as does the recommended dose of

1½ ounces of seeds. However, the Pumpkin-flesh dosage had to be repeated to be effective, whereas the treatment with the seeds, following a 12-hour fast, followed in 1 hour by a cup of tea, and by a brisk cathartic an hour after that, and finally by a hearty meal in 2 hours' time, was reportedly effective in expelling the tapeworm without a repetition of the dose. Medicinal knowledge of the Pumpkin was first introduced into this country in 1851 by Richard Soule.

The amount of Pumpkin seeds employed for vermifuge purposes ranges from 10–200 grams per dose in humans. Studies carried out in the People's Republic of China, in the Soviet Union, and elsewhere have shown that Pumpkin seeds are very effective in removing worms from the bodies of both animals and humans.

The active anthelmintic agent in Pumpkin seeds has been known for some time; it is an unusual

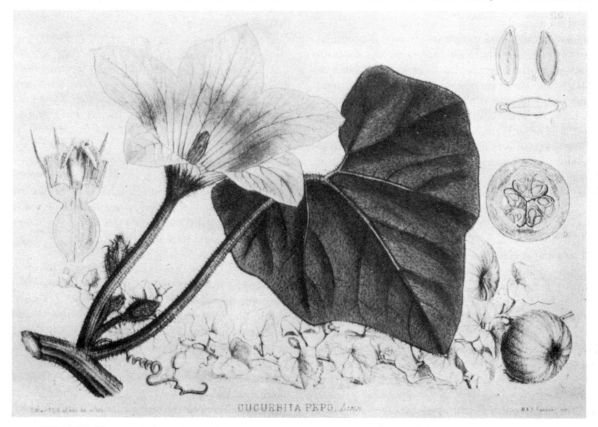

CUCURBITA PEPO. Linn

PUMPKIN: The seeds have been used in almost every culture for centuries as an aid to remove intestinal worms, especially tapeworms.

amino acid known as cucurbitin. Cucurbitin is present in Pumpkin seeds in quantities ranging from 0.18 to 0.66 percent.

Purified cucurbitin was studied in 150 patients with various types of intestinal worm infestations. It was shown to be unusually safe when given by mouth, especially against the beef and pork tapeworm, and pinworms. No contraindications were recommended for the use of cucurbitin as a result of the study. A small number (3 percent) of the patients (5/150) had mild side effects from the drug, including nausea, dizziness and weakness.

Other studies in the United States have shown that when 30–65 grams daily of Pumpkin seeds are taken by mouth, a slight decrease in the amount of urine excreted occurs. On the other hand, daily elimination of urea and uric acid in the urine was increased.

Thus, we can once again point out a rational basis for the use of a centuries-old herbal remedy, based on animal and human studies.

Dose: From 1 to 2 ounces of Pumpkin seeds, as fresh as possible (shelled), beaten to a paste with finely powdered sugar, and diluted with water or milk, when taken; no food to be eaten for 24 hours *prior* to taking this remedy.

Three or four hours afterward, 1 or 2 tablespoonfuls of castor oil should be taken.

The seed oil was also given (as an alternative to the above) in doses of ½ ounce, repeated once or twice at an interval of 2 hours and followed in 2 hours more by a dose of castor oil. (Bentley)

QUASSIA
Picrasma excelsa

PARTS USED: Wood

OTHER COMMON NAMES: Bitter Root, Bitter Ash, Bitter Wood

Botanical Description: *Picrasma excelsa*, as its name implies, is a lofty tree, sometimes attaining the height of not less than 100 feet, with a straight, smooth tapering trunk, which is often 3 feet in diameter near its base, and is covered with a smooth, gray bark. The leaves are pinnate, the leaflets being petiolate and oblong pointed and arranged in opposite pairs, with a single leaflet at

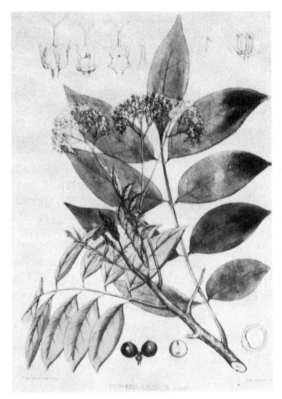

QUASSIA: A powerful simple bitter tonic, this medicinal was widely used in Europe for gastric upsets, as an appetite stimulant, and as a laxative. In overdoses, vomiting results.

the end. The flowers are small, of a yellowish-green color, and disposed in panicles. They are polygamous and pentandrous. The fruit is a small black drupe. This species inhabits Jamaica and the Caribbean Islands, where it is called Bitter Ash. Most of the commercial quassia is obtained from this tree. (U.S.D.)

Medicinal Uses: Quassia was brought to Stockholm in 1756 by a Swede who had purchased it in Surinam from a native healer named Quassi. While the drug soon became popular, the Quassia of Surinam was eventually superseded by *P. excelsa* from the West Indies. A powerful simple bitter tonic, the medicine was widely used in Europe for gastric upsets, as an appetite stimulant, and as a laxative in cases of chronic constipation in convalescents.

In overdoses, quassia causes vomiting. It has been thought by some to possess narcotic proper-

161

ties, since it acts as a narcotic poison on flies, and perhaps on higher animals as well. "Flypaper" used for trapping and killing flies was once made of an infusion of quassia sweetened with sugar.

Quassia wood contains extremely bitter chemical substances known as "quassinoids," the major one being called quassin. These bitter principles are very poorly soluble in water, and for this reason the wood has been used to prepare "Quassia cups." A Quassia cup is filled with hot water and the water is allowed to cool somewhat before being drunk. This results in a liquid that is very bitter and thus acts to stimulate the appetite. Quassia cups can be used in this way for a number of years and will retain an ability to produce a bitter water extract.

We have found no laboratory evidence for the folkloric claim that Quassia preparations will have an expectorant effect.

Dose: The medicinal dose is prepared by using one teaspoon of granulated wood per 1½ pints of boiling water, boiled in a separate container for about ½ hour, at a slow boil. Liquid allowed to cool slowly in the *closed* container. Drunk cold, 1 mouthful at a time, 1 cup per day. When used as a tincture or fluidextract the dose was 0.32 to 0.65 gram.

RASPBERRY, RED
Rubus strigosus

PARTS USED: Root bark and leaves

Botanical Description: Found in dry or moist woods, fields, and roadsides, north to Alaska, south to New England, Pennsylvania, Indiana, Iowa, and in the west to Arizona. Flowers May–July. A variable plant in which have been distinguished 5 varieties and a form; these apparently represent only fluctuating variability. Noteworthy among them is the dwarf form *Egglestonii*, with the floricane leaves all simple, known only from a few stations in Vermont. Hybrids with *R. occidentalis* occur. Plants of Vermont and New York with dark red fruit, the inflorescence of *R. occidentalis* and the foliage of *R. strigosus*, known sometimes as *R. neglectus*, may be hybrids between these species. Our plants are closely related to *R. ideaus*, the European Raspberry, source of our cultivated varieties. This plant has glandless pedicels often armed with stouter, broad-based spines. It is sometimes reported as escaped in our range but does not appear to be established. A glandless form is also known from northern Minnesota, and a few stations outside our range, and is referred to *R. idaeus*.

The Red Raspberry has stems up to 2 meters long, erect, spreading, or even decumbent, sparsely to densely armed with slender-based spines and stiff bristles. Primocane leaflets 3–5, ovate to lanceolate, acuminate, sharply serrate mostly above the middle, softly gray-pubescent beneath; when 5, the intermediate pair inserted close to the terminal one. Inflorescence an umbelliform terminal cluster of 2–5 flowers, often also with 1 or 2 solitary flowers from the upper axils; pedicels stipitate-glandular and more or less bristly, the bristles exceeding the glandular hairs and gland-tipped when young. Sepals soon reflexed. Petals white or greenish white, spatulate to obovate, erect, shorter than the sepals. Fruit usually red, never black, about 1 centimeter in diameter. (B&B)

Medicinal Uses: Red Raspberry leaf or root tea is an excellent astringent remedy for diarrhea, and will also allay nausea and vomiting. The leaf tea is also drunk during pregnancy to facilitate childbirth, and, as indicated above, will help with "morning sickness."

Red Raspberry leaves contain high concentrations of tannin, which is most likely responsible for the antidiarrheal and astringent effects of this plant. We have been unable to find direct experimental evidence in support of the antinauseant and antivomiting effects alleged for this plant; however, folkloric usage for these complaints remains great, especially among pregnant women wishing to avoid these symptoms.

Dose: One teaspoonful of the leaf is used per cup of boiling water. Drunk cold, 1 or 2 cups per day. During pregnancy: ½ ounce steeped with 1 pint of boiling water 3–5 minutes, drunk warm, 1 pint per day.

The root bark is used in the proportion of one teaspoonful of chopped root bark per 1½ pints of water; boil down to 1 pint, and administer 1 to 2 ounces cold, 3 or 4 times per day.

162

RHUBARB
Rheum officinale, and other *Rheum* species

PARTS USED: Root and rhizomes

OTHER COMMON NAMES: Chinese or Turkey Rhubarb

Botanical Description: All the plants of this genus are perennial and herbaceous, with large branching roots, which send forth vigorous stems from 4 to 8 feet or more in height, surrounded at their base with numerous very large petiolate leaves, and terminating in lengthened branching panicles composed of small and very numerous flowers, resembling those of *Rumex*, or the Dock. Without describing the several species minutely, we shall mention those particulars with regard to them by which they are respectively characterized.

Rheum palmatum. The root of this species is large, divided into thick branches, brittle, externally brown, internally of a deep yellow color. The leaves are palmate, with 5 or 7 deeply sinuated pointed segments, are somewhat rough, and stand on long smooth footstalks, which are somewhat channeled on their upper surface, and rounded on the sides. It is said to inhabit China, in the vicinity of the Great Wall.

R. undulatum. The root of *R. undulatum* is large, roundish, externally brown, internally yellow, and divided into numerous ramifications which penetrate

deeply into the soil. The leaves are long, pointed, wavy, and somewhat villous, have at their base on each side a deep sinus, and are supported upon footstalks flat on their upper surface, with acute edges. This species is a native of Siberia, and probably also of China.

R. compactum. This is distinguished by the leaves being very smooth, shining, somewhat lobed, very obtuse, and finely denticulate. The root is thick, divided into many long branches, and internally of a fine reddish-yellow color. The plant is said to be a native of China.

R. australe. The leaves of this species are roundish, cordate, obtuse, rough beneath and on the margin, with the sinus at the base dilated, and with furrowed roundish footstalks. The branches and peduncles are papillose-scabrous; the leaflets of the perianth oval oblong, finely crenate at the apex. The plant grows in the highlands of China and in the Himalaya mountains.

R. rhaponticum. The leaves are very large, cordate, obtuse, smooth, with the veins on the under surface hairy, the sinus at the base dilated, and the footstalks furrowed above and rounded at the edge. The root is large, fleshy, often branching, of a yellow color diversified with red internally, and reddish-brown on the outside. The Rhapontic rhubarb grows on the banks of the Caspian Sea, in the deserts between the Volga and the Urals, and on the mountains of Krasnojar in Siberia. (U.S.D.)

Medicinal Uses: Rhubarb is an unusual medicine in that it combines cathartic with astringent properties; since the purgative effect precedes the astringent, the latter does not interfere with the former. It is for these well-balanced opposite actions that Rhubarb is so valuable as a cathartic gentle enough even for infants in proportionately small dosage. First it relieves constipation, then checks bowel evacuation through its astringent property.

As a tonic and stomachic in small doses, Rhubarb invigorates the powers of digestion. In strong doses, Rhubarb has a tendency to cause painful griping of the bowels; in order to avoid this problem it is often mixed with aromatics such as Anise, Ginger, Peppermint, and Spearmint.

When Rhubarb is roasted or boiled long enough, the purgative property is largely destroyed, while the astringency remains. It is thus

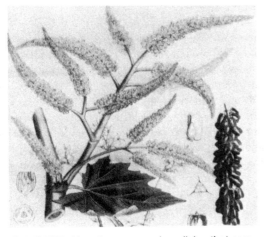

RHUBARB: Here is an unusual medicine that combines cathartic with astringent properties. It first relieves constipation and then checks bowel evacuation through its astringent property. See cautions in text.

163

treated when used as a remedy for diarrhea, when no purging is desired.

Externally, powdered Rhubarb has been applied to indolent and sloughing ulcers.

The leaf-blades, but not the petioles, of the plant are poisonous, containing oxalic acid and oxalates. Several cases of deaths have been reported in humans who have eaten the cooked leaf-blades.

Chemically, the rhizomes and roots of most *Rheum* species contain mixtures of anthraquinones in the free form, and also as sugar derivatives (glycosides). In addition, Rhubarb roots are known to contain high concentrations of astringent tannins.

Rhubarb preparations are used as cathartics, and also to control diarrhea (antidiarrhetic). This paradox deserves an explanation. It is known that when small doses of Rhubarb preparations are taken internally, the predominant action is to produce a laxative effect. This is due to the predominant effect of the anthraquinones and anthraquinone sugar derivatives. However, when large amounts are taken, the action of the astringent tannins in the Rhubarb root predominate. Hence, in large doses, an antidiarrheal effect results.

Rhubarb preparations applied topically to wounds and sloughing ulcers are often beneficial since the tannins afford a covering to the affected area, and the body then proceeds to heal the wound by normal processes.

A word of caution here is required. In the past a favorite method for treating burns was to cover them with an ointment or cream containing tannin or tannic acid. Although this was very effective, there have been reports of severe reactions in some persons undergoing such treatment. These adverse effects are only noted when large areas of the body have been burned, for example, if 40 percent or more of the body surface area is burned. The reason for the toxic effect is that enough of the tannic acid is absorbed by the body through the burned area, enters the bloodstream, and eventually goes to the liver. Tannins are not compatible with the liver, and severe reactions often result. Thus, if one applies Rhubarb, which contains tannins, to small body areas to alleviate

sloughing ulcers, there would be no adverse effects, but application to extensive areas of the body should be avoided.

Dose: The root is prepared for medicinal use in the proportion of 1 teaspoon of granulated root per 1½ pints of boiling water. Drunk cold, 1 cup per day, a mouthful at a time.

See cautions above regarding internal use of the toxic leaf-blades and extensive use of external applications.

ROSE
Rosa gallica

PARTS USED: Unexpanded petals and buds
OTHER COMMON NAMES: Red Rose

Botanical Description: This species is smaller than *R. centifolia*, but resembles it in the character of its foliage. The stem is beset with short bristly prickles. The

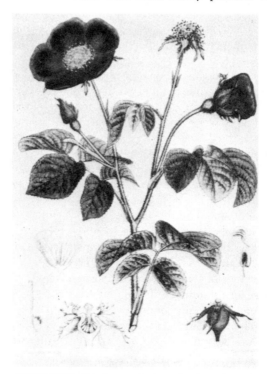

ROSEBUDS: It is known that rosebuds and petals are rich source of vitamin C, astringent tannins, and related phenolic compounds. They are thus used to advantage as tonics and astringents.

flowers are very large, with obcordate widely spreading petals, which are of a rich crimson color, and less numerous than in *R. centifolia*. In the center is a crowd of yellow anthers on threadlike filaments, and as many villose styles bearing papillary stigmas. The fruit is oval, shining, and of a firm consistence. The red rose is a native of the south of Europe, and is cultivated in gardens throughout the United States.

The petals, which are the part employed, should be gathered before the flower has blown, separated from their claws, dried in a warm sun or by the fire, and kept in a dry place. Their odor, which is less fragrant than that of *R. centifolia,* is improved by drying. They have a pleasantly astringent and bitterish taste. Their sensible properties and medical virtues are extracted by boiling water. (U.S.D.)

Medicinal Uses: The use of Rose petals dates from very ancient times; early writers considered them purgative, astringent, and tonic, and used them in chronic catarrhs, hemoptysis, diarrhea, and leucorrhea. Avicenna and other physicians after him recommended the petals in pulmonary phthisis.

The medicinal properties of the petals are generally considered very mild. The buds and petals have a pleasantly astringent and bitterish taste, and were formerly prepared as a simple tonic. Their medicinal application ultimately dropped off entirely, and they remained in use only as an elegant vehicle for tonic and astringent medicines, due to their coloration and flavor qualities.

The essential oil, because of its powerful aroma, has been believed since early times to exert an effect on the nervous system. Hippocrates recommended the oil in diseases of the uterus.

It is known that Rose buds and petals are a rich source of vitamin C, astringent tannins, and related phenolic compounds. They are thus used to advantage as tonics and astringents.

Dose: Approximately ½ ounce of buds and petals to 1 pint of water. Water boiled separately and poured over the plant material and steeped for 5 to 20 minutes, depending on the desired effect. Drunk hot or warm, 1 to 2 cups or more per day, at bedtime and upon arising.

RUE
Ruta graveolens

PARTS USED: Herb

OTHER COMMON NAMES: German Rue, Garden Rue

Botanical Description: Common Rue is a perennial plant, usually 2 or 3 feet high, with several shrubby branching stems, which, near the base, are woody and covered with a rough bark, but in their ultimate ramifications are smooth, green, and herbaceous. The leaves are doubly pinnate, glaucous, with obovate, sessile, obscurely crenate, somewhat thick and fleshy leaflets. The flowers are yellow, and disposed in a terminal branched corymb upon subdividing peduncles. The calyx is persistent, with 4 or 5 acute segments; the corolla consists of 4 or 5 concave petals somewhat sinuate at the margin. The stamens are usually 10, but sometimes only 8 in number. The plant is a native of the

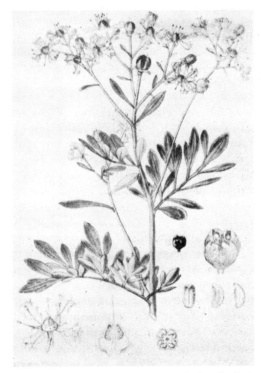

RUE: This is a very popular herbal abortifacient, having been used for this purpose as well as to induce menstruation. The plant contains chemical constituents which make the person who uses it extremely sensitive to sunlight.

south of Europe, but cultivated in our gardens. It flowers from June to September. The whole herbaceous part is active; but the leaves are usually employed.

These have a strong disagreeable odor, especially when rubbed. Their taste is bitter, hot, and acrid. In the recent state, and in full vigor, they have so much acrimony as to inflame and even blister the skin, if much handled, but the acrimony is diminished by drying. Their virtues depend chiefly on a volatile oil which is very abundant, and is contained in glandular vesicles, apparent over the whole surface of the plant. Besides volatile oil, they contain chlorophyll, albumin, an azotized substance, extractive, gum, starch or inulin, malic acid, and lignin. Both alcohol and water extract their active properties. (U.S.D.)

Medicinal Uses: The volatile oil is the source of Rue's medicinal properties, and it is a powerful local irritant. Handling the fresh leaves can cause redness, swelling, and even blistering of the skin. Care should be exercised when using Rue as an internal medicine, as it can cause, in sufficient quantity, violent gastrointestinal pains and vomiting, mental confusion and prostration, as well as convulsive twitching. Large doses may also produce abortion.

In proper amounts, Rue has been valued since the time of the early Greeks for its stimulant properties on the nervous and uterine systems. It has been used to treat hysteria and colic, and to provoke menstruation as well as to correct excessive or protracted menstrual bleeding. It has also been employed as an anthelmintic, and the oil has been used externally as a rubefacient.

For ages Rue was considered beneficial in warding off contagion; even in recent times it has been employed to keep off noxious insects.

Rue is one of the most popular of all herbal abortifacients, having been used for this purpose as well as to induce menstruation in cases of amenorrhea. A number of animal experiments have shown that various types of Rue extracts will cause abortion, and this is probably due to a direct stimulant effect on uterine muscle. The agent responsible for this effect is the furoquinoline alkaloid skimmianine.

However, a number of cases of human poisoning have been reported when Rue extracts were used to induce menses and/or abortion. Apparently, in order to cause these effects, large doses must be taken. It must be that in large doses, some chemical constituent of the plant other than skimmianine has a predominant toxic effect.

There are a number of chemical constituents known to be present in Rue that can cause a person to become extremely sensitive to light. Overexposure to sunlight after taking Rue preparations would result in severe sunburns. Rue also is known to cause severe dermatitis in some individuals.

Thus, even though there is a rational basis for the abortifacient and menstrual inducing effects of Rue, the incidence and potential severity of side effects following its use should be sufficient to warn us to refrain from using it for any prolonged period of time.

Dose: The traditional medicinal dose is 1 teaspoon of the herb, chopped fine, per cup of boiling water, boiled separately and poured over the plant material and steeped for 5 to 20 minutes, depending on the desired effect. Drunk cold, 1 teaspoon at a time, 1 cup per day. Caution should be exercised with the use of this herb.

ST. JOHN'S WORT
Hypericum perforatum

PARTS USED: Tops and Flowers
OTHER COMMON NAMES: Hypericum, Klamath Weed, Goatweed

Botanical Description: Root perennial, ligneous, creeping, tufted, much branched, yellowish brown. Stems erect, 1 to 3 feet high, firm, glabrous, cylindrical, ridged between each joint by 2 opposite angles, continuations of the midrib of each leaf, which render the stem 2-edged. Leaves small, sessile, opposite, each pair crossing those immediately below, oblong or obovate-lanceolate, rather obtuse, entire, glabrous, light green, with numerous pellucid dots; a small simple leafy branch proceeds from the axil of each lower leaf. Flowers in terminal leafy panicles, on dichotomous branches, with oblong, opposite bracts, at the base of each pedicel. Calyx of 5, lanceolate, acute, entire sepals, margined with black glandular dots. Petals 5,

166

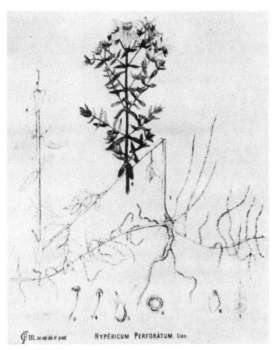

ST. JOHN'S WORT: Internal use of this species should be avoided, since it is firmly established that it contains the phototoxic constituent hypericin.

ovate, acute, bright yellow, entire at one margin, crenate at the other, glandular like the calyx. Stamens numerous, usually in 3 parcels, terminated by yellow, roundish, didymous anthers, each tipped with a dark purple dot or gland. Ovary superior, ovate, glabrous, supporting 3 diverging styles, and contains several small, oblong, shining, blackish brown seeds.

Distribution: Europe (Arctic), Northern Africa, Siberia, western Asia to the Himalayas; introduced into the United States. Frequent in woods, thickets, and hedgebanks in England. Flowers July to September. (B.F.M.)

Medicinal Uses: St. John's Wort was valued by the ancients and continued to enjoy a good reputation among the earlier modern physicians. Although the USFDA has included this plant on their March 1977 "unsafe herb list," it has been used beneficially for thousands of years, especially for wounds and bruises, administered both internally and externally.

It is possible that the employment of St. John's Wort as a remedy for wounds was originally suggested, according to the "doctrine of signatures," by the red juice of its capsules, which was taken as a signature of human blood, and perhaps also by the punctured appearance of the leaves. Externally it has also been claimed useful in scratches, skin irritations, and insect bites, when mixed with olive oil to form an ointment.

Among the peasantry of Europe, there was apparently at one time a superstitious belief that this plant could be used to drive devils out of a person possessed; however, this may have been based on the observation of its usefulness in treating hypochondriasis and insanity. The plant was a popular charm against witchcraft and evil spirits.

Internal use of *Hypericum perforatum* should be avoided, since it has been firmly established that this plant contains the phototoxic constituent hypericin. After taking the plant or its extracts, and following exposure to sunlight, light-skinned individuals will suffer a dermatitis, severe burning, and possibly blistering of the skin. The severity of these effects will depend on the amount of plant consumed and the length of exposure to sunlight.

Dose: Not recommended for internal use.

SAFFLOWER
Carthamus tinctorius

PARTS USED: Flowers
OTHER COMMON NAMES: Bastard Saffron, American Saffron, Dyer's Saffron

Botanical Description: The Dyers' Saffron, or Safflower, is an annual plant, with a smooth erect stem, somewhat branched at top, and a foot or two in height. The leaves are alternate, sessile, ovate, acute, entire, and furnished with spiny teeth. The flowers are compound, in large terminal, solitary heads. The florets are of an orange red color with a funnel-shaped corolla, of which the tube is long, slender, and cylindrical, and the border divided into five equal, lanceolate, narrow segments.

The plant is a native of the Levant and Egypt, but is cultivated in various parts of Europe and America. The florets are the part employed. They are brought to us chiefly from the ports of the Mediterranean. Considera-

167

ble quantities are produced in this country, and sold under the name of American Saffron.

Safflower in mass is of a red color, diversified by the yellowness of the filaments contained within the floret. It has a peculiar slightly aromatic odor, and a scarcely perceptible bitterness. Among its ingredients are two coloring substances, one red, insoluble in water, slightly soluble in alcohol, very soluble in alkaline liquids, and called *carthamite,* the other yellow and soluble in water. It is the former which renders Safflower useful as a dyestuff. Carthamite mixed with finely powdered talc forms the cosmetic powder well known by the name of *rouge.* (U.S.D.)

Medicinal Uses: In large doses Safflower is thought to have laxative value, and when given as a warm infusion to have a diaphoretic effect.

Carthamus flowers are sometimes fraudulently mixed in commerce with much more costly Saffron, which they resemble in color, but they may be distinguished by their tubular form and by the yellowish style and filaments which they enclose. Like Spanish Saffron *(Crocus sativus), Carthamus* is used in treating measles, scarlatina, and other inflammatory eruptions of the skin, including those of viral origin, in order to promote and hasten eruption. Saffron, in addition, was extensively employed by the ancients and by medieval physicians as a highly stimulant antispasmodic and to relieve menstrual cramping and pain.

This annual herb is the source of Safflower oil, much used in recent years for cooking. The fruits are edible and, fried, are used to make chutney.

Dose: The medicinal dose is 1 teaspoon of flowers, granulated, steeped for 5–20 minutes in 1 cup of boiling water. Drunk cold, 1 tablespoon at a time, one cup per day.

SARSAPARILLA
Smilax medica, S. officinalis, S. aristolochiaefolia

PARTS USED: Root
OTHER COMMON NAMES: Mexican Sarsaparilla

Botanical Description: *Smilax aristolochiaefolia* has an angular stem, armed with straight prickles at the joints,

and a few hooked ones in the intervals. The leaves are smooth, bright green on both sides, shortly acuminate, 5-nerved, with the veins prominent beneath. They vary much in form, the lower being cordate, auriculate-hastate, the upper cordate-ovate. In the old leaves the petiole and midrib are armed with straight subulate prickles. The inflorescence is an umbel of from 8 to 12 flowers, with a smooth axillary peduncle and pedicels about 3 lines long.

S. officinalis. In this species the stem is twining, angular, smooth, and prickly; the young shoots are unarmed; the leaves ovate-oblong, acute, cordiform, 5- or 7-nerved, coriaceous, smooth, 12 inches long and 4 or 5 broad, with footstalks an inch long, smooth, and furnished with tendrils. The young leaves are lanceolate-oblong, acuminate, and three-nerved. Large quantities of the root are said to be sent down the Magdalena River.

It is the source of Honduras Sarsaparilla.

The medicinal species of *Smilax* grow in Mexico, Guatemala, and the warm latitudes of South America.

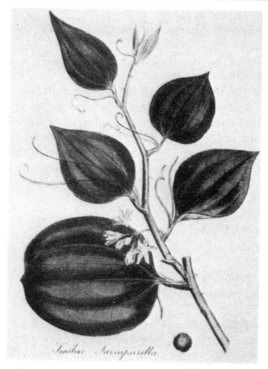

SARSAPARILLA: Commonly regarded as tonic, diaphoretic, and diuretic, this herb in actuality is probably no more than a mild gastric irritant due to its saponin content.

The roots are very long and slender, and originate in great numbers from a common head or rhizome, from which the stems of the plant rise. The whole root with the rhizome is usually dug up, and as brought into market exhibits not unfrequently portions of the stems attached, sometimes several inches in length. The commercial Sarsaparillas are conveniently divided into the mealy and non-mealy Sarsaparillas. The first class comprises especially the Honduran, Guatemalan, and Brazilian varieties; the second the Jamaican, Mexican, and Guayaquil Sarsaparillas. (U.S.D.)

Medicinal Uses: Commonly regarded as tonic, diaphoretic, and diuretic, Sarsaparilla in actuality is probably no more than a mild gastric irritant due to its saponin content. Introduced into European medicine in the mid-sixteenth century as a treatment for syphilis and subsequently discarded for that purpose, Sarsaparilla was thereafter used for many chronic diseases, such as rheumatism and scrofula. The smoke of Sarsaparilla was even inhaled by asthmatic patients.

Mexican Sarsaparilla (*S. aristolochiaefolia*), one of the commerical sources of the "drug," is used extensively in that country. Some Indian tribes use a root decoction to lower fevers, and for kidney troubles, while it is also generally used externally for skin diseases and rheumatism.

Dose: 1 teaspoon of the root, boiled in a covered container of 1½ pints of water for about ½ hour, at a slow boil. Liquid allowed to cool slowly in the *closed* container. Drunk cold, 1 swallow or 1 tablespoon at a time, 1 to 2 cups per day.

SASSAFRAS
Sassafras albidium

PARTS USED: Root bark
OTHER COMMON NAMES: Saxafrax

Botanical Description: This is an indigenous tree of middling size, rising in favorable situations from 30 to 50 feet in height, with a trunk about a foot in diameter. In the southern states it is sometimes larger, and in the northern parts of New England is little more than a shrub. The bark which covers the stem and large branches is rough, deeply furrowed, and grayish; that of

the extreme branches or twigs is smooth and beautifully green. The leaves, which are alternate, petiolate, and downy when young, vary much in their form and size even upon the same tree. Some are oval and entire, others have a lobe on one side; but the greater number are 3-lobed. Their mean length is 4 or 5 inches. The flowers, which are frequently dioecious, are small, of a pale yellowish-green color, and disposed in racemes which spring from the branches below the leaves, and have linear bracts at their base. The corolla is divided into 6 oblong segments. The male flowers have 9 stamens; the hermaphrodite, which are on a different plant, have only 6, with a simple style. The fruit is an oval drupe, about as large as a pea, of a deep blue color when ripe, and supported on a red pedicel, which enlarges at the extremity into a cup for its reception.

The Sassafras is common throughout the United States, and extends into Mexico. It is said also to grow in Brazil and parts of China. In this country it is found both in woods and open places, and is apt to spring up in the

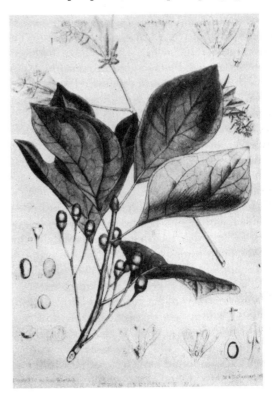

SASSAFRAS: The essential oil from the root bark of this species has been experimentally determined many times to have antiseptic properties.

169

neighborhood of cultivation, and in neglected or abandoned fields. In Pennsylvania and New York it blooms in the beginning of May, but much earlier in the South. The fresh flowers have a slightly fragrant odor, and almost all parts of the plant are more or less aromatic. The wood is porous, light, fragile, whitish in the young tree, reddish in the old, and but feebly endowed with aromatic properties. The root consists of a brownish-white wood, covered with a spongy bark divisible into layers. The latter portion is by far the most active. (U.S.D.)

Medicinal Uses: Generally considered a harmless, gentle, warm aromatic, stimulant, diuretic, diaphoretic, and astringent, Sassafras has rarely been used alone in medicine, and its main use seems to have been to make less agreeable tasting, more efficient medicines more palatable. The root bark, combined with Sarsaparilla and Guaiacum, has been given for chronic rheumatism, skin diseases, and syphilitic affections. Sassafras tea has been a popular "tonic" in domestic medicine, given for high blood pressure and to promote perspiration in colds. The pith, which is mucilaginous and rather gummy, was employed as a soothing application for inflamed eyes and was given to persons suffering from dysentery, catarrhs, and nephritis.

Despite its reputation for gentle action, Sassafras in overdose has been reported to produce narcotic poisoning and accidental abortion, although it was apparently never used as an abortifacient.

The aromatic oil is still used as an antiseptic and as a flavoring agent. The essential oil from the root bark of Sassafras has been experimentally determined many times to have antiseptic properties, and if applied externally would undoubtedly have such an effect, as reported in folkloric use.

Water extracts of Sassafras root bark continue to be used widely, especially in North America, as refreshing aromatic teas. Such teas contain small amounts (about 7–10 milligrams per cup) of a chemical compound known as safrole. In the early 1960s it was found that safrole, when fed to rodents in their diet, resulted in liver damage, and more specifically, liver cancer, in a high percentage of animals. This caused the U.S. Food and Drug Administration to prohibit the sale of safrole-containing materials, such as Sassafras root bark, for use in foods and flavors.

However, despite an official ban, Sassafras root and root bark remain as an item of commerce in the United States, and are still widely used.

Of importance is that safrole itself does not produce cancer in animals. It must be converted by the animal to a substance containing one additional hydroxy group, i.e., 1-hydroxysafrole. The latter substance is termed a proximate carcinogen. The proximate carcinogen 1-hydroxysafrole is well established to be produced by several animal species, including rats, mice and dogs, when safrole is administered orally.

Interestingly enough, in 1977 the result of a study conducted in Switzerland was published in which safrole was taken orally by one human adult, and the proximate carcinogen 1-hydroxysafrole could not be found in the urine of this individual.

It is well known that chemical compounds may be converted differently by different species. If additional confirming experiments are carried out in humans, and it is found that safrole is not changed to a carcinogen, the official ban on the sale of Sassafras root bark may be removed.

Dose: For those who may wish to defy the official ban, it is interesting to note that in former times this plant was very frequently used as a spring tonic. One cup of boiling water was added to a teaspoonful of the granulated rootbark. It was taken cold, a mouthful at a time, to a maximum of 1 cup daily. Useful externally for poison ivy and poison oak.

SAVIN
Juniperus sabina

PARTS USED: Tops of branches and attached leaflets

OTHER COMMON NAMES: Sabina, Savine

Botanical Description: This is an evergreen shrub, rising 3 or 4 feet to 15 feet in height, with numerous erect, pliant branches, very much subdivided. The bark of the young branches is light green, that of the trunk, rough and reddish-brown. The leaves are numerous, small, erect, firm, smooth, pointed, of a dark-green color, glandular in the middle, opposite, imbricated in four rows, and completely invest the younger branches. The flowers are male and female on different trees. The fruit is a blackish-purple berry, of an ovoid shape, marked with tubercles, the remains of the calyx and petals, and containing three seeds.

The Savin is a native of the south of Europe and of the Levant. It is said also to grow wild in the neighborhood of our northwestern lakes. The ends of the branches, and the leaves by which they are invested, are collected for medical use in the spring. When dried they fade very much in color.

There is reason to believe that *Juniperus virginiana*, the common red cedar, is sometimes substituted in the shops for the Savin, to which it bears so close a resemblance as to be with difficulty distinguished. The two species, however, differ in their taste and smell. In

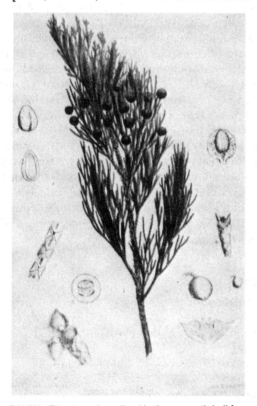

SAVIN: The drug described is the essential oil from the leaves and flowering tops of this Juniper species. Test tube experiments have shown that it will contract uterine tissue.

J. virginiana, moreover, the leaves are sometimes terminate.

The tops and leaves of the Savin have a strong, heavy, disagreeable odor, and a bitter, acrid taste. These properties are owing to a volatile oil which is obtained by distillation with water. They impart their virtues to alcohol and water. (U.S.D.)

Medicinal Uses: Savin (the essential oil from the leaves and flowering tops of *J. sabina*) has many recorded uses, but it must always be employed with caution. Although it is used internally relatively rarely, Savin was given in powdered form to stimulate the menses and also to achieve the seemingly opposite effect of checking uterine hemorrhages. Other uses range from a remedy for worms to a cure for chronic rheumatism as well as chronic gout.

Externally, powdered or infused Savin was applied to warts, ulcers, and psoriasis; some people utilized the juice from fresh leaves for these purposes. Since Savin is highly irritant, these applications seemed to help such skin afflictions by aggravating them, thereby speeding up the natural progression of the disease and effecting a quicker recovery.

Savin has been used in the United States and in Europe as a popular abortifacient, but gained a reputation for toxicity during the 1930s, when a number of deaths were attributed to the use of savin as an abortifacient. However, it was subsequently shown that the toxic material was a synthetic phthalate derivative that was added to the Savin. Thus, it is not clear from literature reports, most of which were published during that period of time, whether Savin itself is really toxic.

It is clear that savin will contract uterine tissue in test tube experiments, and thus could possibly be beneficial in alleviating amenorrhea and atonic menorrhagia, as indicated by its folkloric uses. However, the employment of Savin itself cannot be recommended as a safe aid to alleviate these conditions, since it is a highly concentrated and complex mixture; but a tea prepared from the tops of *J. sabina* could exert a much milder and probably more beneficial effect.

Dose: Approximately ½ ounce of leaves and flowering tops to 1 pint of water. Water boiled separately and poured over the plant material and steeped for 5 to 20 minutes, depending on the desired effect. Drunk hot or warm, 1 to 2 cups per day, at bedtime and upon awakening.

SCULLCAP
Scutellaria laterifolia

PARTS USED: Whole plant

OTHER COMMON NAMES: Skullcap, Hoodword, Mad Weed, Mad Dog, Side-Flowering Scullcap, Blue Pimpernel, Hooded Willow-Herb, Quaker Bonnet

Botanical Description: *Scutellaria laterifolia* is an indigenous, perennial herb, with a stem erect, much branched, quadrangular, smooth, and 1 or 2 feet high. The leaves are ovate, acute, dentate, subcordate upon the stem opposite, and supported upon long petioles. The flowers are small, of a pale blue color, and disposed in long, lateral, 1-sided, leafy racemes. The plant grows in wet shaded places in the United States and Canada.

The dried tops are described as "about 50 centimeters in length, smooth; stem quadrangular, branched; leaves opposite, petiolate, about 5 centimeters in length, ovate-lanceolate or ovate-oblong, serrate; flowers about 6 millimeters in length, in axillary 1-sided racemes, with a pale blue corolla and bilabiate calyx, closed in fruit, the upper lip helmet-shaped. Odor slight; taste slightly bitter. (U.S.D.)

Medicinal Uses: Employed rather commonly as a tonic and general relaxant in times of excitement, Scullcap tea was a very mild and safe nervine. In the Thomsonian system of medicine it was used in the treatment of delirium tremens, St. Vitus' dance, convulsions, lockjaw, tremors, and was given to teething babies.

The sedative and antispasmodic properties of this perennial herb were applied widely in the treatment of rabies, beginning with a series of experiments in 1772. This use earned the plant its nickname "Mad Dog Scullcap."

Dose: One teaspoon of granulated leaves per cup of boiling water. Repeat as often as you like.

172

SENEGA SNAKEROOT
Polygala senega

PARTS USED: Root

OTHER COMMON NAMES: Rattlesnake Root, Mountain Flax, Seneca Root

Botanical Description: This unostentatious plant has a perennial branching root, from which several erect, simple, smooth, round leafy stems annually rise, from 9 inches to 1 foot in height. The stems are occasionally tinged with red or purple in their lower portion, but are green near the top. The leaves are alternate or scattered, lanceolate, pointed, smooth, bright green on the upper surface, paler beneath, and sessile or supported on very short footstalks. The flowers are small, white, and arranged in a close spike at the summit of the stem. The calyx is the most conspicuous part of the flower. It consists of 5 leaflets, 2 of which are wing-shaped, white, and larger than the others. The corolla is small and closed. The capsules are small, much compressed,

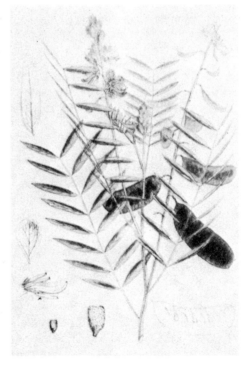

SENNA (INDIAN): The leaflets and pods of this species and of senna itself have the advantage over most other laxatives of being less "harsh," or producing less "intestinal griping."

obcordate, 2-valved, 2-celled, and contain 2 oblong ovate, blackish seeds, pointed at one extremity.

This species of *Polygala*, commonly called Senega Snakeroot, grows wild in all parts of the United States, but most abundantly in the southern and western sections, where the root is collected in great quantities for sale. (U.S.D.)

Medicinal Uses: It is said that Senega was originally introduced into practice as a remedy for rattlesnake bite, but came to be recognized as of questionable value in treating the bites of venomous animals. The primary application of Senega has been as an expectorant, to help the expulsion of mucus from the respiratory tract, in cases of bronchitis, asthma, and, where otherwise indicated, in similar pulmonary conditions. In larger doses the plant has been used as an irritant poison to produce vomiting and purging of the intestinal tract, but this usage was very infrequent, there being more desirable plants available for this purpose.

Extracts of Senega Snakeroot have been shown experimentally to have expectorant properties when administered orally to a variety of animals, including cats, guinea pigs, and rabbits. It is thus reasonable to believe that tea prepared from the roots of this plant would have similar beneficial effect in humans.

Dose: The medicinal dose is 1 teaspoon of granulated root, boiled in a covered container with 1½ pints of water for about ½ hour, at a slow boil. Liquid allowed to cool slowly in the *closed* container. Drunk cold, 1 tablespoon at a time, 1 cup per day. For purging, 1 cup is drunk hot in the morning.

SENNA
Cassia acutifolia (Alexandrian Senna), *C. angustifolia* (Indian Senna)

PARTS USED: Dried leaflets

Botanical Description: The plants which yield Senna belong to the genus *Cassia*, of which several species

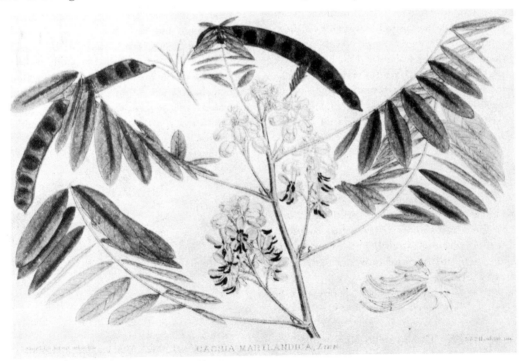

SENNA: Highly valued as a cathartic, working particularly on the lower bowel, where it increases peristaltic movements of the colon, senna is one of our most highly reputed natural laxatives.

173

contribute to furnish the drug. These were confounded together by Linnaeus in a single species, which he named *Cassia senna*. Since his time, the subject has been more thoroughly investigated. Botanists at present distinguish at least three species, *C. acutifolia*, *C. obovata*, and *C. elongata*.

Cassia acutifolia. This is a small undershrub, from 2 to 3 feet high, with a straight, woody, branching, whitish stem. The leaves are pinnate, alternately placed upon the stem, and have at their base 2 small narrow pointed stipules. The leaflets, of which 4 or 5 pairs belong to each leaf, are almost sessile, oval lanceolate, acute, oblique at their base, nerved, from ½ inch to 1 inch in length, and of a yellowish-green color. The flowers are yellow, and arranged in axillary spikes. The fruit is a flat, elliptical, obtuse, membranous, smooth, grayish-brown, bivalvular legume, about 1 inch long and ½ inch broad, scarcely if at all curved, and divided into 6 or 7 cells, each containing a hard, heart-shaped, ash-colored seed. *C. acutifolia* grows wild in great abundance in Upper Egypt, and probably in other parts of Africa having similar qualities of soil and climate. It is this species that furnishes the Tripoli Senna, and the greater part of that variety known in commerce by the title of Alexandria Senna. (U.S.D.)

Medicinal Uses: Senna is an Arabic name, and the first recorded medical uses appear in Arabic writings of the ninth century of the Christian era.

Senna is highly valued as a cathartic, working particularly on the lower bowel, where it increases peristaltic movements of the colon by its local action upon the intestinal wall. It is consequently utilized in cases of chronic constipation.

The leaflets and pods of *Cassia acutifolia* and *C. angustifolia* are very popular laxative preparations, that have the advantage over most other laxatives of being less "harsh," or producing less "intestinal griping." The reason for the laxative effect is that the leaves and pods contain varying amounts of complex anthraquinones known as sennosides (sennoside A and B are the two major active constituents). Many laxative preparations are available that combine the sennosides with a stool softener, but the dual combination has not been proved more effective than the sennosides alone, or extracts of Senna leaves or Senna pods, to the best of our knowledge.

Senna is often combined with aromatics such as Anise, Fennel, Ginger, Nutmeg, Peppermint, and others to reduce still further the tendency to produce intestinal griping. Its nauseous taste can be removed by preparing the plant as an alcoholic extract.

Dose: One teaspoon of the leaves per cup of boiling water; *steeped* (not boiled) for ½ hour. Taken ½ cup at bedtime, or 1 tablespoon 3 times a day.

SHAVE GRASS
Equisetum hiemale, E. arvense

PARTS USED: Whole Plant
OTHER COMMON NAMES: Horsetail, Scouring Rush

Botanical Description: Root perennial, slender, dark brown, creeping, jointed, with numerous capillary fibers. Sterile stems decumbent at the base, 1 to 2 feet high, with undivided, ascending, whorled branches, angular, with about 12 striae, microscopically tuberculate, leafless, but furnished at each articulation with about 12 subulate, erect, dark brown sheaths, membranous at the margin; fertile stems, which appear before the sterile ones, from 6 to 8 inches high, erect, unbranched, leafless, smooth, tubular within, silvery brown externally; sheaths, distant, erect, long, cylindrical, ventricose, striated, incised, and toothed. Fructification terminates the stem in a long, oblong, lanceolate, light brown spike.

Distribution: Europe (Arctic), Northern Africa, northern Asia, Himalayas, North America. Common in England on roadsides, banks, etc. Fructification appears in April. (B.F.M.)

Medicinal Uses: A mild diuretic, Shave Grass was administered to promote urination in dropsical complaints and kidney dysfunctions. Because the diuretic action of Shave Grass is quite weak, it is likely to have been utilized in the cases of very sensitive or weakened patients, or for pregnant women, as there were no deleterious side effects.

The cuticle of the stems contains abrasives which made the plant useful in scouring metal culinary articles; it was widely used by artisans for

174

SHEPHERD'S PURSE
Capsella bursa-pastoris

PARTS USED: Whole Herb
OTHER COMMON NAMES: Shepherd's Heart

Botanical Description: Stem 1–5 decimeters tall, branching, pubescent below, glabrous above; basal leaves in a rosette, usually lyrate-pinnatifid; stem leaves auricled, dentate to entire; flowers in long racemes; petals white, 1.5–2 millimeters long; pedicels slender, spreading at right angles or nearly so, 8–15 millimeters long; siliques obcordate-triangular, 5–8 millimeters long, strongly flattened contrary to the partition; styles less than 0.5 millimeter long; seeds numerous, oblong, orange-yellow, wingless, about 1 millimeter long; cotyledons incumbent. Waste land and street margins in cities and towns, roadsides and fields, February–May; widespread weed occurring in most parts of the world; introduced. (Texas)

Medicinal Uses: Shepherd's Purse was administered for the alarming symptom of blood in the urine (hematuria). This condition can be caused by a lesion of the urinary tract, contamination during menstruation or during the 6 weeks following childbirth, prostate disease, tumors, poisoning, and toxemia.

Shepherd's Purse extracts have been shown to prevent duodenal ulcer formation induced by stress in rats, and to show marked anti-inflammatory activity under a variety of test conditions in animals. Extracts of this plant have also shown significant antitumor activity against several experimental tumor systems in laboratory animals. One study has shown that extracts of this plant do not inhibit the growth of bacteria in test tube experiments. There is also reasonable evidence, in animals and in humans, that this plant has hemostatic properties. To date, high quantities of vitamin C have not been reported present in Shepherd's Purse, and thus, although it has been used as a remedy for scurvy, this antiscorbutic claim may not be warranted.

Dose: 1 teaspoonful of herb per 1 cup of boiling water. Steep 3–5 minutes. Drunk cold, 1 tablespoon at a time, 1 to 2 cups per day.

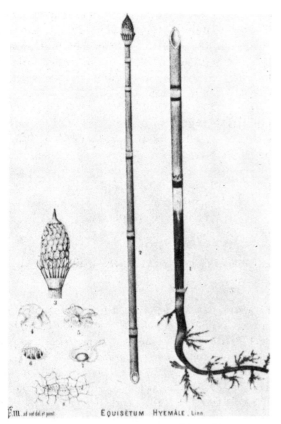

EQUISETUM HYEMALE, Linn.

SHAVE GRASS: A mild diuretic, Shave Grass was administered to promote urination in dropsical complaints and kidney dysfunction.

polishing wood, ivory, brass, and objects of similar materials.

Although diuretic effects are attributed to extracts of *Equisetum hiemale* very frequently in the literature, very few experiments have been carried out to verify this effect. At best, the experiments show a low level of diuretic activity, which is almost entirely attributable to the irritant action of silica that is present in the plant in high concentrations. It is highly questionable whether diuresis should be induced on the basis of a purely irritant effect on the kidneys, in that long-term ramifications of this continuous irritation could be detrimental.

Dose: One teaspoon of plant per cup of boiling water. Drunk cold, 1 to 2 cups per day, 1 tablespoon at a time. (Do not continue usage longer than 3 days.)

175

SKUNK CABBAGE
Symplocarpus foetidus (Spathyema foetida)

PARTS USED: Root, rhizome, and seeds
OTHER COMMON NAMES: Skunk Weed, Pole Cat Weed, Meadow Cabbage, Swamp Cabbage

Botanical Description: The Skunk Cabbage is a very curious plant, the only one of the genus to which it belongs. The root is perennial, large, abrupt, and furnished with numerous fleshy fibers, which penetrate to the depth of 2 feet or more. The spathe, which appears before the leaves, is ovate, acuminate, obliquely depressed at the apex, auriculated at the base, folded inward at the edges, and of a brownish-purple color, varied with spots of red, yellow, and green. Within the spathe, the flowers, which resemble it in color, are placed in great numbers upon a globose, peduncled spadix, for which they form a compact covering. After the spathe has decayed, the spadix continues to grow, and when the fruit is mature, has attained a size exceeding by several fold its original dimensions. The different parts of the flower, with the exception of the anthers, augment in like proportion. At the base of each style is a roundish seed, immersed in the spadix, about the size of a pea, and speckled with purple and yellow. The leaves, which rise from the ground after the flowers, are numerous and crowded, oblong, cordate, acute, smooth, strongly veined, and attached to the root by long petioles, which are hollowed in front, and furnished with colored sheathing stipules. At the beginning of May, when the leaves are fully developed, they are very large, being from 1 to 2 feet in length, and from 9 inches to 1 foot in breadth.

This plant is indigenous, growing abundantly in meadows, swamps, and other wet places, throughout the whole northern and middle sections of this country. Its flowers appear in March and April, and in the lower latitudes often as early as February. The fruit is usually quite ripe, and the leaves decayed, before the end of August. The plant is very conspicuous from its abundance, and from the magnitude of its leaves. All parts of it have a disagreeable fetid odor, thought to resemble that of the offensive animal after which it is named. This odor resides in an extremely volatile principle, which is rapidly dissipated by heat, and diminished by desiccation. The root is the part usually employed in medicine.

It should be collected in autumn, or early in spring, and dried with care.

The acrimony, however, is dissipated by heat, and is entirely lost in decoction. It is also diminished by time and exposure; and the root should not be kept for use longer than a single season. (U.S.D.)

Medicinal Uses: Credited with antispasmodic, emetic, diuretic, and narcotic properties, Skunk Cabbage has been used to treat asthma, chronic dry coughing spells and other upper respiratory problems, chronic rheumatism, nervous affections, muscular spasms and twitchings, hysteria, and dropsy (water retention). Externally, it has been utilized as an ointment or salve for skin irritations.

The roots are an excellent emergency food, especially good baked or fried.

Dose: For medicinal use 1 teaspoon of granulated root is slowly boiled with 1 pint of water, for approximately ½ hour in a covered container. Take 1 tablespoon at a time, 1 cup per day.

SLIPPERY ELM
Ulmus fulva

PARTS USED: Inner Bark
OTHER COMMON NAMES: Indian Elm, Moose Elm, Sweet Elm

Botanical Description: The Slippery Elm is a lofty tree, 50 or 60 feet in height, with a trunk 15 or 20 inches in diameter. The bark of the trunk is brown, that of the branches rough and whitish. The leaves are petiolate, oblong-ovate, acuminate, nearly pubescent, and very rough on both sides. The buds, a fortnight before their development, are covered with a dense russet down. The flowers, which are apetalous, appear before the leaves, are sessile, and in clusters at the extremities of the young shoots. The clusters of flowers are surrounded by scales, which are downy like the buds. The calyx is also downy. The stamens are 5, short, and of a pale-rose color. The fruit is a membranaceous capsule or samara, enclosing in the middle one round seed, destitute of fringe.

Ulmus fulva is indigenous, growing in all parts of the United States north of the Carolinas, but most abundantly west of the Allegheny Mountains. It extends westward to the Dakotas and northward to western Quebec and Lake Huron. It flourishes in open, elevated situations, and requires a firm, dry soil. From the White Elm *(U. americana)* it is distinguished by its rough branches, its larger, thicker, and rougher leaves, its downy buds, and the character of its flowers and seeds. Its period of flowering is in April. (U.S.D.)

Medicinal Uses: The demulcent properties of Slippery Elm bark led to its application in a number of ailments. The pillager Ojibwa tribe of North America made a tea from the inner bark to treat sore throat. The tea is also reportedly helpful for coughs. One pint of warm tea, administered as an enema, was given to babies to soothe the bowels after they had been cured of constipation or colic by repeated enemas. The bark was also eaten after convalescence, both for its soothing effects on the stomach and intestines, and for its nutritional value. Drunk combined with milk, it

was easily digested, assimilated and eliminated. Used as an ointment, Slippery Elm sap was employed in Thomsonian medicine during labor as a lubricant for the midwife's hand when she ascertained the presentation of the infant internally. The Thomsonian system also used a poultice of Slippery Elm, Lobelia, and a little soft soap as a means of bringing abscesses and boils to a head. These were then lanced and drained. Mausert considered this one of the most mild and harmless laxatives for children, causing no pain.

Slippery Elm sticks were used in some North American Indian tribes to provoke abortion by inserting them into the cervix.

All of the effects indicated for Slippery Elm bark are explained on the basis of an abundance of mucilage-containing cells surrounding each fiber of the bark. When the bark, in strips or powdered form, comes into contact with water, the mucilage cells swell enormously and thus produce a lubricating, demulcent, emollient, and/or laxative

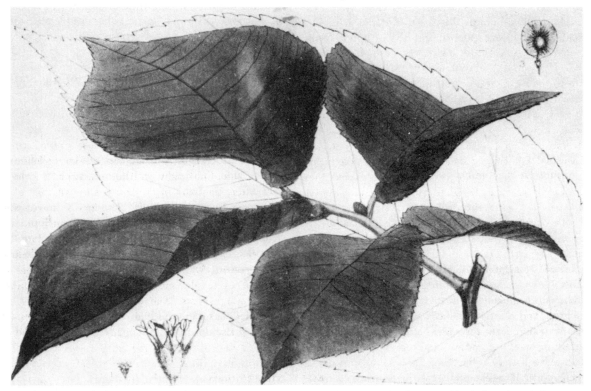

SLIPPERY ELM: Narrow strips of this bark were used to provoke abortion by some North American Indian tribes. Inserted into the cervix the moistened bark often causes hemorrhage and infection.

177

effect when administered locally or by mouth. Powdered Slippery Elm bark is especially useful to soothe sore throats, and it has a pleasant, aromatic odor and taste as well.

Narrow strips of Slippery Elm bark, when soaked in water for a few minutes, become very slippery and pliable. For this reason, it has been reported that some pregnant women have attempted to induce abortion by inserting a long strip of the moistened bark into the cervix in order to mechanically disrupt the fetus and terminate pregnancy. This is an extremely dangerous practice, since many deaths have resulted due to uncontrollable hemorrhaging. Serious infections can also be expected due to the unsanitary conditions under which this type of practice is carried out.

In some states in the United States, the law requires that Slippery Elm bark be broken into pieces no longer than 1.5 inches in length before being sold. The intent of such laws is obviously to discourage the use of Slippery Elm bark for the induction of abortion.

Dose: One teaspoon of the bark, boiled in a covered container with 1½ pints of water for about ½ hour, at a slow boil. Liquid allowed to cool slowly in the *closed* container. Drunk cold, 1 swallow or 1 tablespoon at a time, 1 to 2 cups per day.

SOAPWORT
Saponaria officinalis

PARTS USED: Rhizome, Root and leaves
OTHER COMMON NAMES: Bouncing Bet, Fuller's Herb, Sheep Weed, Saponaire, Bruisewort

Botanical Description: About 30 species of this genus, native to Eurasia and North Africa.

Saponaria officinalis. Plant perennial, stout, erect, glabrous, to 6 decimeters high; stems simple or sparingly branched, leafy; leaves opposite, oval-lanceolate to elliptic or sometimes ovate, subobtuse to acute at apex, narrowed at base to a short broad petiole, to 8 centimeters long and 35 millimeters wide, prominently 2- to 5-nerved; flowers showy, in dense terminal corymbs; bracts foliaceous or much-reduced and narrow; calyx

tube cylindric or nearly so, naked, obscurely nerved, to 2 centimeters long, the 5 lanceolate teeth about 2 millimeters long; petals 5, white or pink, cuneate, notched at apex, well-exserted and spreading, crowned with an appendage at the top of the prominent claw; stamens 10; styles 2; ovary 1-celled or incompletely 2- to 4-celled; capsule included, subcylindric, dehiscent by 4 short apical teeth. In fields and waste places in east Texas, June–September; a native of Europe that is locally naturalized in various places in temperate North America. (Texas)

Medicinal Uses: The name of the Soapwort is derived from the fact that when agitated in water, the rhizomes and roots form a lather, like a solution of soap. The active principle responsible for this lathering effect is saponin, which carries the detergent as well as the medicinal properties of this plant. In 1917 in China there were reportedly eleven species of trees that contained saponin which were utilized in the formation of detergents for the purpose of laundry washing.

Soapwort was prescribed by medieval Arab physicians for leprosy and other skin complaints. The leaves, soaked for a short time, yield an extract which has been used to promote sweating, as a remedy against rheumatism, and to purify the blood.

Dose: Rhizome and root—1 teaspoon of rhizome or root, boiled in a covered container with 1 pint of water for about ½ hour, at a slow boil. Liquid allowed to cool slowly in the *closed* container. Drunk cold, 1 swallow or 1 tablespoon at a time, 1 to 2 cups per day.

Leaves—Approximately ½ ounces of leaves to 1 pint of water. Water boiled separately and poured over the plant material and steeped for 5 to 20 minutes, depending on the desired effect. Drunk hot or warm, 1 to 2 cups per day.

SOLOMON'S SEAL
Polygonatum officinale

PARTS USED: Root
OTHER COMMON NAMES: Sealwort

Botanical Description: The members of *Polygonatum*

are perennial glabrous herbs with horizontal creeping more or less knotty rhizomes and fibrous roots; stem simple, erect or arching, naked below, leafy above; leaves simple, alternate, amplexicaul to sessile or shortly petiolate, typically elliptic; inflorescence axillary consisting of one to several pendulous flowers on deflexed or arcuate peduncles; calyx and corolla united into a cylindric tube, with 6 lobes that are usually shorter than the tube; stamens 6, included, inserted on the perianth tube; filaments filiform or flattened, smooth or roughly papillose; anthers linear-oblong to sagittate, bilobed at base, introrse; ovary 3-celled, with several ovules in each cell; fruit a dark-blue or black globose pulpy several-seeded berry. About 50 species in North Temperate Zone. (Texas)

Medicinal Uses: The root was formerly used for its emetic properties, and externally for bruises, especially near the eyes, as well as for treatment of tumors, wounds, poxes, warts, pimples, etc. It was thought to be effective in assisting the knitting of broken bones, taken internally. In sixteenth-century Italy Solomon's Seal was esteemed as a cosmetic wash which would maintain healthy skin and prevent freckles, sunburn, pimples, and the mottling of old age.

The roots of Solomon's Seal contain allantoin, a substance well known for its healing and anti-inflammatory effects. Extracts of the root of this plant lower blood sugar levels in rabbits, lower blood pressure, and have a cardiotonic action, indicating possible usefulness in heart conditions.

Dose: For external as well as internal use, a decoction is prepared, using 1 teaspoonful of the root, boiled in a covered container with 1½ pints water for about ½ hour, at a slow boil. Liquid allowed to cool slowly in the *closed* container. Drunk cold, 1 swallow or 1 tablespoon at a time, 1 to 2 cups per day, when taken internally.

SPEARMINT
Mentha viridis

PARTS USED: Leaves and flowering tops
OTHER COMMON NAMES: Mint

Botanical Description: Spearmint, sometimes called simply Mint, differs from Peppermint, or *M. piperita*, chiefly in having sessile or nearly sessile, lanceolate, naked leaves; elongated, interrupted, panicled spikes; setaceous bracts; and stamens longer than the tube of the corolla. Like Peppermint, it is a native of England. In the United States it is cultivated in gardens for domestic use; and in some places more largely for the sake of its oil. It also grows wild in low grounds in parts of the country which have been long settled. Its flowering season is August. It should be cut in very dry weather, and, if intended for medical use, just as the flowers appear; if for obtaining the oil, after they have expanded.

The odor of Spearmint is strong and aromatic, the taste warm and slightly bitter, less pungent than that of Peppermint, but considered by some as more agreeable. These properties are retained for some time by the dried plant. They depend on a volatile oil which rises on distillation with water, and is imparted to alcohol and water by maceration. (U.S.D.)

Medicinal Uses: Much the same as Peppermint, without the cooling sensation in the mouth which accompanies the ingestion of that plant, Spearmint is an aromatic stimulant. It is used for mild indigestion, to cure nausea, to relieve spasmodic stomach and bowel pains, help the expulsion of stomach and intestinal gas, and to otherwise remedy the deleterious effects of too much food or an improper diet. Spearmint is also combined with other less palatable medicines to make them more agreeable or to allay their tendencies of producing nausea or griping pain.

The leaves and flowering tops of Spearmint owe their pleasant and aromatic properties, as well as characteristic taste, to a volatile oil. The major active principle in the oil is a simple terpene derivative, carvone.

Dose: Approximately ½ ounce of leaves and flowering tops to 1 pint of water. Water boiled separately and poured over the plant material and steeped for 5 to 20 minutes, depending on the desired effect. Drunk hot or warm, 1 to 2 cups or more per day.

179

SPINDLE TREE (WAHOO)
Evonymus atropurpureus

PARTS USED: Bark, roots, fruit, and seeds
OTHER COMMON NAMES: Priest's Biretta,
Burning-Bush, Indian Arrow-Wood,
Euonymus, Wahoo

Botanical Description: *Evonymus atropurpureus* is a tall, erect shrub, with quadrangular branchlets, and opposite, petiolate, oval-oblong, pointed, serrate leaves. The flowers, which stand in loose cymes on axillary peduncles, are small and dark purple, with sepals and petals commonly in fours. The capsule or pod is smooth and deeply lobed. The plant is indigenous, growing throughout the northern and western states.

The plants belonging to this genus are shrubs or small trees, presenting in the autumn a striking appearance from the rich red color of their fruit, which has obtained for them the name of Burning-Bush. *E. americanus* and *E. europaeus* have been cultivated in gardens as ornamental plants. Two or more of the species have been used in medicine. Their properties are probably similar, if not identical. (U.S.D.)

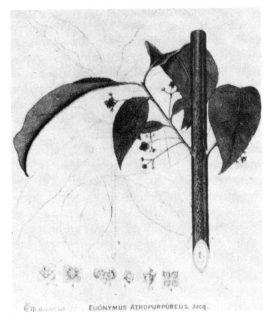

EUÓNYMUS ATROPURPUREUS, Jacq.

SPINDLE TREE: This is one herb which rightly belongs on the FDA's "Unsafe Herb" list. The fruits are powerfully toxic; ingestion of as few as three or four have proven fatal to a child.

Medicinal Uses: This is one plant which deserves its place on the USFDA 1977 unsafe herb list. The fruits are terribly toxic; ingestion of as few as 3 or 4 can prove fatal to a child and can cause an adult extreme pain and discomfort, as they function as a drastic purgative.

Despite its toxicity, all parts of the tree have been employed at one time or another in traditional medicine. Among the many usages were the following: The dried root bark was believed to be stimulant, laxative and diaphoretic (producing sweating); as a result of this latter characteristic it was employed in the treatment of dropsy (water retention). The oil expressed from the seeds was used for its emetic and purgative properties. The fruits were held to be diuretic; however, in light of their toxicity in even small quantity, the dosage must have been minute. The inner bark was utilized in treating eye diseases.

Wahoo fruit and seeds contain cardiac glycosides, which would be expected to produce a diuretic effect in persons with cardiac insufficiency. Large amounts would also be predicted to cause emesis. These cardiac glycosides, however, are not present in other parts of the plant.

Dose: EXTREMELY TOXIC. No dosage is recommended for home use.

SQUAW VINE
Mitchella repens

PARTS USED: Vine
OTHER COMMON NAMES: Partridge Berry,
Winter Clover, Deer Berry, Hive Vine,
Checker Berry, One Berry

Botanical Description: There are two *Mitchella* species, the other being Japanese.

Ours is *Mitchella repens*, a small glabrous trailing evergreen herb forming appressed mats of indefinite size; leaves petioled, opposite, ovate to orbicular, rounded to cordate at base, obtuse at apex, shining, pinnately veined and sometimes variegated with whitish lines, 15–25 millimeters long; stipules triangular-subulate; peduncle short, terminal, bearing 2 flowers at its summit; flowers fragrant, white, often tinged with purple, in pairs with their ovaries united, occasionally

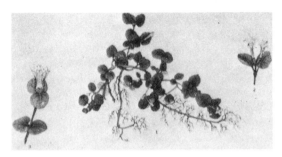

SQUAW VINE: Experimentally, a fluidextract of this interesting evergreen herb has shown no uterine stimulant activity in pregnant guinea pigs. Most likely then, the claims that this plant is useful in facilitating parturition are unfounded.

3- to 6-merous, always dimorphous, all flowers of some individuals have exserted stamens and included stigmas, all flowers of other individuals with included stamens and exserted style; calyx 4-toothed; corolla tube about 13 millimeters long, densely bearded inside, surpassing the oblong spreading lobes; style 1; stigmas 4, linear; drupes edible, 4–6 millimeters in diameter, bright-red or rarely white (f. *leucocarpa*), overwintering, crowned with the calyx teeth of the 2 flowers, with 4 small seedlike bony nutlets to each flower. On dry or moist knolls in woods in east Texas, May–July; from Florida to Texas, north to eastern Canada, Ontario, and Minnesota. (Texas)

Medicinal Uses: Credited with astringent, tonic, and diuretic properties during the period it was included in the National Formulary, Squaw Vine found its principal traditional usage among the American Indians, whose women drank Squaw tea to facilitate childbirth. All aspects of labor, delivery of the child and the afterbirth, stimulation of the uterus, and so forth, were thought to be assisted by drinking tea brewed from this plant. (Pipsissewa and Squaw Vine were thought to have similar properties.)

Experimentally, Squaw Vine fluidextract has been tested for uterine stimulant activity against guinea pig pregnant and nonpregnant uterus, and was without effect. Thus, most likely the claims for this plant to be useful in facilitating parturition are unfounded. The plant contains tannins, which probably account for its beneficial effects as a local astringent. We have found no experimental basis for the use of Squaw Vine as a diuretic.

Dose: One teaspoon of the ground vine is used per cup of boiling water, steeped for 5–10 minutes, and drunk cold, 1 to 2 cups per day, 1 tablespoon at a time.

SQUILL
Urginea maritima (U. scilla)

PARTS USED: Bulbs, divested of outer coats and centers
OTHER COMMON NAMES: Sea Onion, Scilla

Botanical Description: Native to the Mediterranean region, India, and tropical and southern Africa, this is a perennial·herb, with a short, thick, flattened hard axis or rootstock emitting beneath long tough cylindrical roots, and closely set above with very numerous large overlapping scales forming a tunicated bulb which is 4–6 inches long, nearly globular, but slightly produced at the top, the outer scales thin and papery, red, orange-brown, or dirty-white in color, strongly veined with

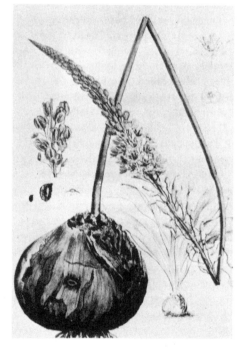

SQUILL: This Mediterranean bulb is a dangerous plant, making an excellent rat poison. When disguised in a mixture with other herbs as an encapsulated medicinal, it may be unintentionally fatal.

numerous parallel nerves, torn and usually truncate, the inner ones smaller, fleshy, closely investing one another, broad and blunt, curved, nerved like the outer ones, yellow or green where exposed to the air. Leaves few, large, 1½–2 feet or more long when fully grown, spreading and recurved, inserted at the base of the flowering stem, and appearing long after the flowers, narrowly oblong-lanceolate, tapering at the base, acute at the apex, variable in width, quite entire, dark glossy green, thick, rather wavy. Flowers numerous, on long slender pedicels, erect in bud, spreading during flowering, and again erect with fruit, each with a small lanceolate-linear, spurred bract at its base, rather laxly arranged in a very long, slender, erect raceme, 1–1½ feet long, the stout, smooth, cylindrical, purplish rachis continuing the bare erect scape of about the same length, which is given off from the axil of one of the leaves. Perianth-leaves 6 in two rows, nearly equal, very slightly connected at the very base, 1 inch long, spreading, persistent, oval, subacute, with a single faint midrib, white with a green tinge. Stamens 6, hypogynous, or very slightly attached to the base of the perianth-leaves, and shorter than them, filaments short, slightly flattened at the base, anthers oblong-oval, versatile, greenish. Ovary ovate-ovoid, sessile, faintly 3-lobed, smooth, shining, 3-celled, with numerous horizontal ovules, style about as long as the ovary, simple, stigma obscurely 3-lobed. Fruit a dry capsule about ½ inch long, on an erect stalk, and surrounded at the base by the shrivelled persistent perianth, oblong, blunt, deeply 3-lobed, 3-celled, pericarp dry and papery, splitting loculicidally, yellow. Seeds about 6 in each cell, ascending, imbricated, about ¼ inch long, flattened, obliquely obovate, testa membranous, dark purple-brown, finely reticulated, extended into a marginal wing, embryo cylindrical, straight in the axis of the fleshy endosperm.

This bulb is found in dry sandy places, expecially the seacoast—to which, however, it is by no means confined—in most parts of the Mediterranean district. Its range also includes the Canary Islands and the Cape of Good Hope. The great bulb is usually half immersed in the sand, and produces the long racemes of flowers in late autumn, the leaves following in early spring. The Squill is grown in many botanical gardens, having been first recorded as cultivated in England in 1629.

It is a variable plant; the bulb differs greatly in size and in color, and the leaves and flowers also present similar varieties, which has led to the formulation of several species. (Bentley)

Medicinal Uses: Squill is quite a dangerous plant, and makes an excellent rat poison. Here is one herb which belongs on the USFDA unsafe herb list, but it is not to be found there.

In small doses Squill reportedly acted as an expectorant and diuretic; in larger doses as an emetic and purgative; and in overdose as an irritant poison. Obviously not for home use, Squill may prove valuable in the hands of the skilled herbalist-physician for its digitalis-like effect on the heart. It can be useful in treating heart disease, but overdose will cause death due to heart paralysis.

When disguised in a mixture with other herbs as an encapsulated medicinal it may be fatal.

That the bulb of Squill has cardiotonic effects was first indicated in the Ebers Papyrus (fourteenth century B.C.), and it was used by Greek physicians to treat dropsy, which is a manifestation of congestive heart failure.

There are two varieties of Squill, a white and a red variety; these should be discussed separately.

White Squill contains active cardiac glycosides similar in structure and action to those present in Foxglove (in Foxglove article, see remarks on *Digitalis purpurea*), the major active substances being named scillaren A and scillaren B. Currently, Squill preparations are used in medical practice in Europe, but not in the United States. Squill has essentially the same effects as *Digitalis* on the heart, and the only advantage over *Digitalis* is that is can be used in those patients who cannot tolerate the latter drug.

Red Squill has been used as a raticide; 250,000 kilograms were imported annually into the United States prior to World War II. It is curiously toxic to rats, other animals either refusing to eat it, or being unaffected by it. That is, if animals other than rats eat Red Squill, they apparently always vomit, and are thus otherwise unaffected by it (unless the herb is "disguised" in a mixture!). Since rats do not vomit, they retain the plant material, and it eventually kills them. Red Squill is 500–1,000 times more toxic to rats than is White

Squill. The active poison in Red Squill is called scilliroside.

Dose: POTENTIALLY LETHAL. No recommended home use dose.

SQUIRTING CUCUMBER
Ecballium elaterium

PARTS USED: Juice sediment from fruit
OTHER COMMON NAMES: Wild Cucumber

Botanical Description: The Wild or Squirting Cucumber is a perennial plant with a large fleshy root, from which rise several round, thick, rough stems, branching and trailing like the common cucumber, but without tendrils. The leaves are petiolate, large, rough, irregularly cordate, and or a grayish-green color. The flowers are yellow and axillary. The fruit has the shape of a small oval cucumber, about 1½ inches long, 1 inch thick, of a greenish or grayish color, and covered with stiff hairs or prickles. When fully ripe, it separates from the peduncle, and throws out its juice and seeds with considerable force through an opening at the base, where it was attached to the footstalk. The name of Squirting Cucumber was derived from this circumstance, and the scientific and official title is supposed to have had a similar origin, though some authors maintain that the term *elaterium* was applied to the drug rather from the mode of its operation upon the bowels than from the projectile property of the fruit. It is a native of the south of Europe, and is cultivated in Great Britain, where, however, it perishes in the winter. (U.S.D.)

Medicinal Uses: The fruit of this perennial vine, shaped like a small oval cucumber, separates from its peduncle when ripe and expels its juice and seeds with considerable force through an opening at the base, where it is attached to the footstalk; hence the plant's name. The sediment from the juice of the fruit, known as elaterium, traces its name back as far as Hippocrates, who used the term to signify any active purge. The plant was known to the ancients for its purgative effects, and was also used by them to stimulate menstruation.

Elaterium has been called the most powerful hydragogue cathartic known, effective in extremely small doses. The fruit juice of the Squirt-

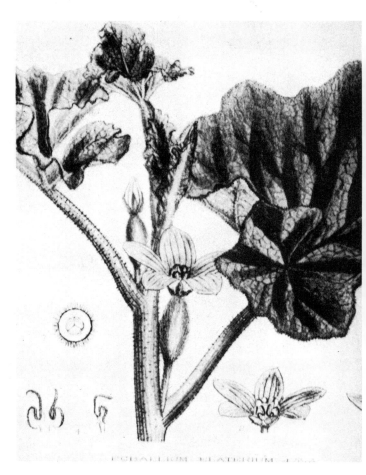

SQUIRTING CUCUMBER: Ecballine, a compound derived from the fruits, is used in treating baldness as well as scalp diseases.

ing Cucumber is well known to cause a powerful hydragogue cathartic effect in humans. This effect is caused by the major principles in the juice, a mixture of compounds referred to as cucurbitacins.

There is evidence, in animals, that the juice of the Squirting Cucumber has an effect on the heart that would suggest a useful application in humans to treat dropsy (congestive heart failure). However, human experiments are lacking to support this contention. Further, the toxicity of the cucurbitacins must be taken into account when considering the use of Squirting Cucumber for any condition requiring long-term use, such as in dropsy.

We have found no experimental evidence that this plant would be useful in treating mania and melancholy, as reported by some herbalists. In large doses it would probably have an emetic effect due to the cucurbitacins, but experimental evidence to support this is lacking.

183

Ecballine, a compound derived from the fruits, is used in treating baldness as well as a cure against scalp diseases.

Dose: This plant is not recommended for home use, due to its toxicity in accidental overdose.

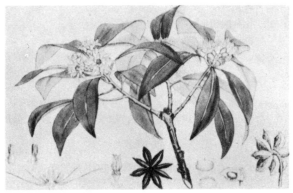

STAR ANISE: Employed in Chinese medicine for centuries to cure rheumatism and lumbago, the seeds and oil have known stimulant effects.

STAR ANISE
Illicium verum

PARTS USED: Fruit

OTHER COMMON NAMES: Chinese Anise, Chinese Star Anise, Yellow-Flowered Starry Aniseed Tree

Botanical Description: *Illicium anisatum* (Japanese Star Anise). A native of Asia and North America, this small tree reaches 20 feet high, much branched, with smooth, round branches, young twigs marked with the scars of fallen leaves and spotted with brown. Leaves evergreen, alternate, rather crowded, without stipules, stalked, lanceolate or oblong-lanceolate, tapering and pointed at both ends, quite entire, smooth, shining, thick, with minute pellucid dots, the lateral veins scarcely visible, 2–3 inches long, on the young shoots much larger, 5–6 inches long. Flowers on the young shoots of the year apparently terminal, afterwards axillary, and sometimes coming from the old wood, solitary, or in clusters of threes, shortly stalked, the pedicel surrounded at the base with about six rounded, slightly ciliated bracts, faintly sweet-scented, Sepals 3–6, roundish, caducous, membranous, petaloid, imbricated. Petals about 24 (but varying in number), imbricated in three or more series, spreading, narrow-oblong, blunt,

gradually smaller toward the center, deciduous, pale greenish-yellow. Stamens indefinite (often about 16 or 20) in several rows, hypogynous; filaments thick, short, dilated; anthers adnate, introrse, dehiscing laterally. Carpels 5–15 (often 8) in a single whorl, free, erect, compressed, 1-celled; style slender, short, slightly recurved, with the brownish stigma on its ventral surface. Fruit consisting of 8 or more coriaceous-woody, wrinkled, boat-shaped, more or less beaked, orange-brown follicles arranged in a radiated, spreading circle, and attached by their bases to a central axis, dehiscing along their ventral (upper) margin by a broad chink, internally bright yellow and shining. Seed solitary, in a cavity scooped out in the lower part of the carpel, attached to the axis, ovoid, compressed, polished and shining, hilum large, embryo very small, immersed in the abundant endosperm near the hilum.

It produces abundance of its pretty scented blossoms from January to April, and sometimes also in the autumn. (Bentley)

Medicinal Uses: The fruit of the Chinese Star Anise is remarkable among the herbal remedies for its unusual appearance and its characteristic aroma. If we were to stumble upon this plant without being aware of its medicinal virtues we would undoubtedly try it out. It has been employed in Chinese medicine for centuries, particularly to cure rheumatism and lumbago. The seeds and oil have stimulant, carminative, diuretic, and digestive properties; Star Anise is also used to soothe inflamed mucous membranes of the nasal passages. The fruit is now popularly employed in several commercial brands of herbal tea.

In China the seeds are applied locally to treat toothache, while the essential oil is given for colic in children. Experimentally, alcoholic extracts of the fruit were effective against gram-positive and gram-negative bacteria and against twelve species of fungi.

Star Anise owes much of its therapeutic effect to the essential oil present in the fruits. About 90 percent or more of the essential oil is comprised of anethole, which produces a carminative and mild internal stimulant effect, if taken internally. Thus, there is ample justification for the use of Star Anise infusions or decoctions as a carminative or mild stimulant.

Dose: An infusion of the dried fruit is made using 1 teaspoon to 1 cup of boiling water.

STRAWBERRY
Fragaria vesca

PARTS USED: Whole herb

Botanical Description: Root perennial, cylindrical, scaly, fibrous, sending out numerous creeping stolons, or runners, which throw out fibers from the base, and produce new plants. Stem herbaceous, erect, simple, pubescent, about 6 inches high. Leaves ternate, on long petioles, with 2 lanceolate acute stipules at the base; leaflets ovate, obtuse, inciso-serrate, smooth above, glaucous, nerved, and clothed with silky hairs beneath. Flowers axillary, solitary, on long drooping naked peduncles. Calyx 10-cleft, spreading; persistent, and at length reflexed; 5 of the segments ovate, mucronate; the alternate 5 lanceolate, acute exterior. Petals 5, white, roundish obovate, obtuse, repand, spreading, inserted into the calyx. Stamens numerous, with rather short subulate filaments inserted into the calyx, tipped with cordate erect anthers. Ovaries numerous, ovate, obtuse, aggregated on a roundish receptacle; styles rather thick, short, proceeding laterally from the ovaries, tipped with truncate stigmas. Fruit, commonly called a berry, roundish, obtuse, scarlet, rarely white, consisting of a fleshy succulent substance (the enlarged receptacle), upon the surface of which are scattered the pericarps or carpels (usually called seeds). Carpels small, shining, ovate, somewhat compressed, deciduous, containing a single pendulous seed.

Distribution: Europe (Arctic), Northern Africa, Siberia, western Asia to the Himalayas, eastern and western North America. Abundant in shady places, in woods and thickets, in England. Flowers April and May. (B.F.M.)

Medicinal Uses: Much used as a dessert fruit, Strawberry Leaf tea has long been, and continues to be, a very widely employed and popular tonic beverage for convalescents and children. It is slightly astringent, and quite refreshing. Many pharmaceutical preparations use Strawberry syrup as a base.

Dose: The tea is prepared by using 1 teaspoon of powdered herb per cup of boiling water. It is drunk cold, slowly, 1 to 2 cups per day. For alkalizing the system, Mausert highly recommends the tea.

STROPHANTHUS
Strophanthus kombe, S. hispidus

PARTS USED: Seeds

Botanical Description: Calyx of 5 imbricate sepals which are sometimes foliaceous. Corolla funnel-shaped or campanulate; tube cylindric, with paired appendages in the mouth alternating with the lobes; lobes 5, acuminate, or produced into very long filiform tails. Stamens inserted at the upper end of the cylindric portion of the corolla-tube; anthers conniving in a cone, acuminate, or sometimes produced into a long bristle, shortly sagittate at the base; foot of the connective with a central tuft of closely packed hairs in the upper part and a more or less hairy longitudinal crest below it. Disc, zero. Carpels 2, free, with numerous ovules in each ovary; stigma capitate, 5-grooved with a membranous reflexed frill at the base and a minutely bifid apiculus. Mericarps follicular, oblong or spindle-shaped. Seeds spindle-shaped, slightly compressed, with an apical plumose awn and a deciduous basal coma.

Shrubs often scandent; leaves opposite, rarely ternate; axillary stipules zero; axillary glands subulate or conical, 2–6, rarely more, at the base of each petiole; inflorescence terminal, often on the ends of short branches, corymbose, many- or few-flowered, or reduced to solitary flowers; flowers mostly showy.

Species about 45, natives of Africa and tropical Asia; 3 species in South Africa, extending from Delagoa Bay, Zululand, and Natal to the Bedford District. (So. Africa)

Medicinal Uses: Originally used by natives in the region of Lakes Tanganyika and Nyasa for arrow poison, Strophanthus is formally recognized as a cardiac stimulant. Its action is very similar to that of digitalis, but it exerts its effect more rapidly, diminishes its action in less time, and does not reduce the pulse rate to the same levels as does digitalis.

All parts of these two species, but particularly the seeds, are known to contain cardiac glycosides quite similar in chemical structure and also in their effects on the body to the *Digitalis* glycosides. Strophanthus preparations thus exert a strengthening action on the heart by causing it to slow down and function with stronger force. This confirms the usage long reported in folklore.

Strophanthus is less dependable than digitalis due to its irregular absorption through the intestinal tract. A reported side effect of Strophanthus is diarrhea, produced by increased peristalsis of the intestines. The plant was also felt to be diuretic and has therefore been widely used in cases of chronic heart weakness coupled with dropsy (water retention).

Because it functions more rapidly than digitalis, Strophanthus is of great benefit during an emergency heart failure; in such cases it has been administered intravenously, by injection.

Dose: Not recommended. Too variable in effects for home use.

SUMAC
Rhus glabra

PARTS USED: Bark and fruit

OTHER COMMON NAMES: Sumach, Smooth Sumac, Upland Sumac

Botanical Description: Of this genus there are several species which possess poisonous properties, and should be carefully distinguished from that here described.

This species of *Rhus,* called variously Smooth Sumac, Pennsylvania Sumac, and Upland Sumac, is an indigenous shrub from 4 to 12 feet high, with a stem usually more or less bent, and divided into straggling branches, covered with a smooth light gray or somewhat reddish bark. The leaves are upon smooth petioles, and consist of many pairs of opposite leaflets, with an odd one at the extremity, all of which are lanceolate, acuminate, acutely serrate, glabrous, green on their upper surface, and whitish beneath. In the autumn their color changes to a beautiful red. The flowers are greenish-red, and disposed in large, erect, terminal, compound thyrses, which are succeeded by clusters of small crimson berries covered with a silky down.

The shrub is found in almost all parts of the United States, growing in old neglected fields, along fences,

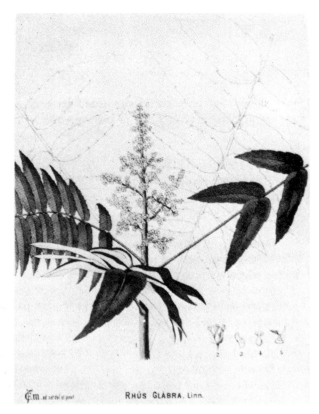

RHÚS GLÁBRA, Linn.

SUMAC: The berries, in decoction, were popular as a gargle for throat irritations. The root was chewed by some North American Indians for mouth sores.

and on the borders of woods. The flowers appear in July, and the fruit ripens in the early part of autumn. (U.S.D.)

Medicinal Uses: Used for their astringent and refrigerant effects, Sumac berries given as a gargle in decoction form were believed helpful during attacks of anginal pain. The decoction was also gargled for throat irritations, or by persons suffering from any inability to breathe easily, such as asthmatics. The high tannin content of the bitter berries made them valuable in the alleviation of diarrheas. The root was chewed by some North American Indians for mouth sores.

Sumac berries contain high concentrations of tannins, which as indicated previously have an astringent effect on mucous membranes. Thus, when water extracts of Sumac berries are used as a gargle, or applied to other mucous membranes, the medicinal effect that is experienced has a rational explanation.

Dose: 1 teaspoon of the berries, boiled in a covered container with 1½ pints of water for about ½ hour, at a slow boil. Liquid allowed to cool slowly in the *closed* container. Drunk cold, 1 swallow or 1 tablespoon at a time, 1 to 2 cups per day.

SWEET FERN
Polypodium vulgare

PARTS USED: Root
OTHER COMMON NAMES: Wood Licorice, Common Polypody, Rock Polypod, Female Fern, Fern Root, Rock Brake

Botanical Description: Rhizome creeping, ligneous, horizontal, dark brown externally, greenish internally, covered with reddish membranous scales, and furnished with dark-colored fibers. Fronds about a foot long, deeply bipinnatifid, with linear-lanceolate, alternate, parallel, obtuse segments, somewhat crenulate at the margin, gradually decreasing in size upwards, and supported on a long, cylindrical, smooth footstalk. Fructification of small yellowish-brown masses, called *sori,* arrounded in a single series on each side the midrib of the leaflets; sometimes so numerous as to be confluent. Sori naked, i.e., not covered by any tegument or involucre, and consist of numerous capsules or conceptacles; each of which is pedicellate, 1-celled, and ejecting the numerous minute spores.

Distribution: Europe, Northern and Southern Africa, Siberia, Dahuria, Japan, western Asia, North America. Frequently on old walls, banks, and stumps of trees in England. In fructification from June to September. (B.F.M.)

Medicinal Uses: Not surprisingly, the taste of this fern is sweet; the rhizome is somewhat reminiscent of the Licorice root in shape. The medicinal virtues of this plant are rather mild, although it was praised lavishly by the ancients for its usefulness in melancholic conditions and visceral obstructions. While the resin is considered anthelmintic, Sweet Fern is also a useful purgative. It possesses demulcent properties as well, which prevent it from being a strong medicine. A very strong decoction is necessary for the expulsion of taenia worms and other intestinal parasitic worms. Sweet Fern is also reportedly useful in alleviating coughs and other chest complaints, and

is a useful tonic in dyspepsia and loss of appetite.

Dose: 1 teaspoon of the root, boiled in a covered container with 1½ pints of water for about ½ hour, at a slow boil. Liquid allowed to cool slowly in the *closed* container. Drunk cold, 1 swallow or 1 tablespoon at a time, 1 to 2 cups per day.

SWEET FLAG
Acorus calamus

PARTS USED: Oil and root
OTHER COMMON NAMES: Calamus, Sweet Root, Sweet Cane, Sweet Sedge

Botanical Description: The Sweet Flag, or Calamus, has a perennial, horizontal, jointed, somewhat compressed root, from ½ inch to 1 inch thick, sometimes several feet in length, sending off numerous round and yellowish or whitish fibers from its base, and bunches of

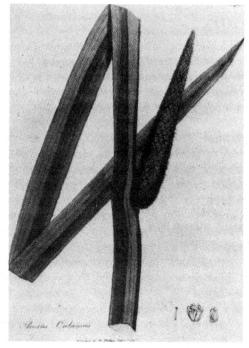

SWEET FLAG: In a two-year rodent feeding study, using the essential oil of this root, cancerous lesions were found in a significant number of the test animals. Only the Indian variety was tested, so no conclusions can be drawn for varieties from other parts of the world.

187

brown fibers resembling coarse hair from its joints, internally white and spongy, externally whitish with a tinge of green, variegated with triangular shades of light brown and rose color. The leaves are all radical, sheathing at the base, long, sword-shaped, smooth, green above, but of a red color variegated with green and white near their origin from the root. The scape or flower-stem resembles the leaves, but is longer, and from one side, near the middle of its length, sends out a cylindrical spadix, tapering at each end, about 2 inches in length, and crowded with greenish-yellow flowers. These are without calyx, and have 6 small, concave, membranous, truncated petals. The fruit is an oblong capsule, divided into 3 cells, and containing numerous oval seeds.

This is an indigenous plant, growing abundantly throughout the United States, in low, wet, swampy places, and along the sides of ditches and streams, and flowering in May and June. It is also a native of Europe and western Asia; and a variety of the same species is found in India. The European plant differs from the American in some unimportant particulars. The leaves as well as root have an aromatic odor; but the latter only is used in medicine. After removal from the ground, the roots are washed, freed from their numerous fibers, and dried with a moderate heat. By the process of drying they lose nearly one half their diameter, but are improved in odor and taste. (U.S.D.)

Medicinal Uses: The medicinal virtues of the root were known to ancient Greek and Arabian physicians, and Calamus has been valued for centuries by the native practitioners of India and elsewhere, as a feeble aromatic aiding digestion and regular elimination. The root is used in powdered form in India and Ceylon as a remedy for expelling parasitic worms from the intestines, and the candied fresh root is chewed in Turkey and India as a treatment for dyspepsia and as a preservative against epidemic diseases. In European countries the root was masticated to clear the voice, and the Plains Indians chewed it for toothache. An insecticide is produced from the essential oil.

The efficacious nature of Sweet Flag decoction or infusion as a carminative and aromatic is well established, based on animal and human experiments. If highly concentrated amounts of the active principles in this plant are taken, effects other than those indicated could be unpleasant.

Even though the use of Sweet Flag has a rational basis of action, it has been disapproved for human use in any form because of studies reported in 1968 by the U.S. Food and Drug Administration. In a two-year rodent feeding study, using *Acorus calamus* essential oil, cancerous lesions were found in a significant number of the test animals. However, only the Jammu (Indian) variety of *Acorus calamus* oil was tested, and it is known that varieties of *A. calamus* from other parts of the world than India are significantly different in their chemical composition.

In view of this, the FDA has banned the use of all varieties of *A. calamus* intended for human use, until such time as it has been determined that varieties other than the one from Jammu do not cause this carcinogenic effect. Since 1968, no reports have been published regarding this problem.

Dose: Essential oil not recommended, pending further scientific investigations. Root infusion made by using 1 teaspoonful to 1½ pints of water. Drunk warm, 1–2 cups per day.

TAMARIND
Tamarindus indica

PARTS USED: Fruit

Botanical Description: The Tamarind tree is the only species of this genus. It rises to a great height, sends off numerous spreading branches, and has a beautiful appearance. The trunk is erect, thick, and covered with a rough, ash-colored bark. The leaves are alternate and pinnate, composed of many pairs of opposite leaflets, which are almost sessile, entire, oblong, obtuse, unequal at their base, about ½ inch long, ⅙ inch broad, and of a yellowish-green color. The flowers, which are in small lateral racemes, have a yellowish calyx, and petals which are also yellow, but beautifully variegated with red veins. The fruit is a broad, compressed, reddish ash-colored pod, very much curved, from two to six inches long, and with numerous brown, flat, quadrangular seeds, contained in cells formed by a tough membrane. Exterior to this shell are several tough

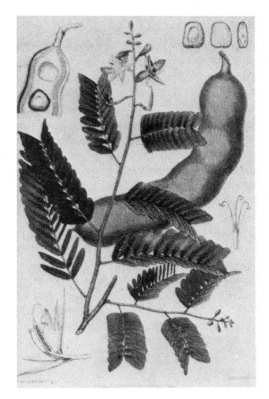

TAMARIND: The fruits owe their laxative effects almost totally to a high sugar concentration. Most of the sugars are not absorbed in the intestinal tract. The resulting bowel movement is usually nonirritating.

ligneous strings, running from the stem to the extremity of the pod, the attachment of which they serve to strengthen. The shells are very fragile, and easily separated. (U.S.D.)

Medicinal Uses: Mildly cathartic, Tamarinds are a beneficial addition to the convalescent diet, and mixed with Senna and chocolate, administered to infants when a gentle cathartic is necessary. The pulp of the fruit contains citric, tartaric, and malic acids, which give it cooling properties; Tamarind is therefore a useful drink in feverish conditions, as well as being a popular cooling beverage in hot countries.

The medicinal properties of Tamarinds were first discovered by Arab physicians. It was also the Arabs who imported Tamarind stock from India to Europe, where it became extensively cultivated.

The fruit of Tamarind owes its laxative, mild

cathartic and refrigerant effects almost totally to a high sugar concentration. The types of sugars are not absorbed to a high degree, when in the intestinal tract. Because of this, they cause water to migrate from the surrounding tissues into the lumen of the intestines. This causes the intestines to expand, which results in a nonirritant type of bowel movement.

Dose: The fruit is eaten as needed.

TANSY
Tanacetum vulgare

PARTS USED: Herb
OTHER COMMON NAMES: Bitter Buttons, Parsley Fern

Botanical Description: This is a perennial herbaceous plant, rising 2 or 3 feet in height. The stems are strong, erect, obscurely hexagonal, striated, often reddish, branched toward the summit, and furnished with alternate, doubly pinnatifid leaves, the divisions of which are notched or deeply serrate. The flowers are yellow, and

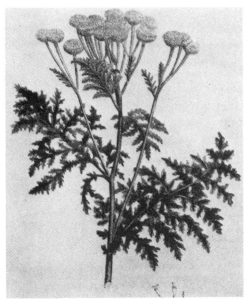

TANSY: At one time an infusion of this plant was rubbed on corpses and wrapped in the shrouds of the dead to repel the onslaught of worms after burial. Externally, the plant is a useful home remedy to kill fleas and lice.

189

in dense terminal corymbs. Each flower is composed of numerous florets, of which those constituting the disk are perfect and 5-cleft, those of the ray very few, pistillate, and trifid. The calyx consists of small, imbricated, lanceolate leaflets, having a dry scaly margin. The seeds are small, oblong, with 5 or 6 ribs, and crowned by a membranous pappus.

Tansy is cultivated in our gardens, and grows wild in the roads and old fields; but was introduced from Europe, where it is indigenous. It is in flower from July to September.

There is a variety of the plant with curled leaves, which is said to be more grateful to the stomach than that above described, but has less of the peculiar sensible properties of the herb, and is probably less active as a medicine.

The odor of Tansy is strong, peculiar, and fragrant, but much diminished by drying; the taste is warm, bitter, somewhat acrid, and aromatic. These properties are imparted to water and alcohol. The medical virtues of the plant depend on a bitter extractive and a volatile oil. The latter, when separated by distillation, has a greenish-yellow color, and deposits camphor upon standing. The seeds contain the largest proportion of the bitter principle, and the least of volatile oil. (U.S.D.)

Medicinal Uses: The principal use of Tansy has been to expel worms from the intestines. At one time Tansy was rubbed on corpses as well as wrapped in the shrouds of the dead to repel the onslaught of worms after burial. Externally, the plant is a useful home remedy to kill fleas and lice.

This herb has also been used as a sudorific (to promote perspiration) and to generate a comfortable internal feeling. When Tansy was introduced from Europe, the American Indians began to use it to induce abortion. Conversely, it was also an old folk remedy for the prevention of miscarriage.

The active constituent of Tansy, tanacetin, is toxic to animals, and in overdoses to man. Among the striking symptoms of poisoning in humans are convulsions, spasms, frothing at the mouth, dilated pupils, rapid and feeble pulse. Its usage as a home remedy is absolutely to be avoided.

The plant contains an essential oil, borneol, thujone, camphor, and resins. Experimentally, various plant parts exhibit much biological ac-

tivity, as follows: antiseptic (flower volatile oil); antibacterial (flowers, roots, and root stocks); antifungal (volatile oil); liver functions (whole plant); and bile stimulation (leaves, flowers and stems).

Dose: There is no recommended medicinal dose for internal use. For external use, as a flea and lice killer, prepare by adding 1 pint of boiling water to 1 teaspoonful of the herb. Apply locally when cold, by soaking cloth or towels in the infusion.

THYME
Thymus vulgaris

PARTS USED: Herb

Botanical Description: A native of the Mediterranean region, this is a small, much-branched shrub, scarcely a

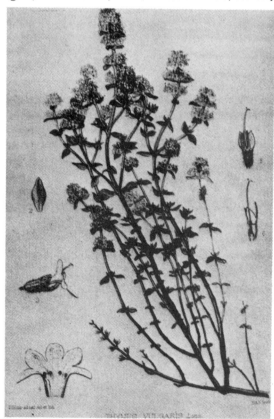

THYME: Thymol has been shown to have antiseptic value, as well as expectorant and bronchodilator effects, in animal as well as human experiments.

foot high, the branches ascending, opposite, slender, very bluntly quadrangular, with a pale-brown bark, the young shoots purplish-red, pubescent with very short stiff white hairs. Leaves opposite, sessile, ¼–⅝ inch long, oval or oval-lanceolate, blunt, entire with the margin revolute, thick, smooth, dotted with numerous oil-glands, paler beneath. Flowers polygamous, numerous, on slender stalks arranged in small shortly stalked cymes in the axils of the uppermost leaves and forming terminal rounded capitate heads, often with a few whorls below. Calyx bilabiate, hairy externally, dotted with glands, the upper lip flat of 3 very short triangular teeth, the lower of 2 stiff curved subulate teeth about as long as the tube, which has a ring of dense white hair at its mouth within. Corolla small, the tube not much exceeding the calyx, cylindrical, smooth within, the limb nearly flat, spreading, the upper lip emarginate, the lower with three blunt rounded lobes, faintly veined. Stamens four inserted in the tube of the corolla, with very short equal filaments and small rounded anthers in the female flowers, in the bisexual flowers with long exserted filaments and the 2 lateral much the longest; anthers kidney-shaped with a wide connective, violet-colored. Style exserted, longer in the female than in the bisexual flowers, bifid. Achenes elevated on a gynophore, perfectly smooth, brown. (Bentley)

Medicinal Uses: Thyme has been used as a medicinal since ancient times. The Greeks Pliny, Dioscorides, and Theophrastus all make reference to this tasty herb.

It has been used for coughs, bronchitis, asthma, and whooping cough; for flatulence, colic in infants, to produce sweating to break a fever, for anemia, and for all kinds of stomach upsets.

The oil, applied locally to carious teeth, has been used as a means of relieving toothache. The herb has also been employed as an antiseptic against tooth decay; the active principle, a simple terpene thymol or thymic acid, has been shown to have disinfectant properties equal to those of carbolic acid. Externally the leaves have been applied in fomentation (cloth or towels dipped in infusion or decoction and applied locally) for aches and pains.

Thymol has been shown to have antiseptic value, expectorant and bronchodilator effects, in animal as well as human experiments.

Thymol additionally releases entrapped gas in the stomach and relaxes the smooth muscle of that organ. This explains the use of Thyme to alleviate the symptoms of colic and flatulence.

Externally, thymol and thymol-containing plants act as rubefacients. That is, thymol causes an increased blood flow to the area of application, which then results in relief of inflammation and pain.

Dose: Approximately ½ ounce of herb to 1 pint of water. Water boiled separately and poured over the plant material and steeped for 5 to 20 minutes, depending on the desired effect. Drunk hot or warm, 1 to 2 cups per day, at bedtime and upon awakening.

TOADFLAX
Linaria vulgaris

PARTS USED: Herb, Leaves
OTHER COMMON NAMES: Yellow Toadflax, Snap Dragon, Butter and Eggs, Ramsted

Botanical Description: Root perennial, woody, tortuous, creeping, whitish, fibrous. Stem erect, cylindrical, glandular, light-green, tough, leafy above, simply, or slightly branched toward the summit, 1 to 3 feet high. Leaves sessile, erectly spreading, numerous, scattered, crowded toward the summit of the stem, linear-lanceolate, acute, entire, somewhat revolute at the margin, pale glaucous green. Flowers in a terminal erect raceme; each flower on a short peduncle, with a linear, acute, reflexed bract at the base. Calyx monophyllous, glabrous, 5-parted, with ovate oblong, acute, erect segments. Corolla large, pale yellow, with an ample ventricose tube, terminating at the base in a conical-subulate spur; limb bilabiate, ringent, upper lip erect, bifid, with the segments rounded, reflexed at the margin; lower lip 3-lobed, the side lobes spreading, somewhat concave, middle lobe much smaller, nearly round; palate formate, prominent, saffron colored, clothed with silky hairs. Stamens 4, furnished with whitish subulate filaments, the 2 longer attached to the lower lip, clavate and villous at the base; anthers oval, yellow, connivent by their parietes. Ovary ovate, subcompressed, glabrous, with a subulate style as long as the shorter stamens, terminated by a capitate truncated stigma. Fruit an ovate-oblong, emarginate, 2-celled capsule opening at the end, subtended by the persistent calyx. Seeds numerous, orbicular, brownish black.

Distribution: Europe (Arctic), excluding Turkey; Siberia; Dahuria. Introduced in North America. Waste ground in some parts of England and Scotland; rarer in Ireland. Flowers July to October. (B.F.M.)

Medicinal Uses: A very common herb, Toadflax was valued for its external and internal usages. To treat hemorrhoids a poultice, or fomentation of the fresh plant was applied locally. This same method was used on various skin diseases. In addition, the flowers were sometimes mixed with vegetable oils to make a liniment.

Taken internally, an infusion of the leaves was used to eliminate kidney stones, the effects being diuretic and cathartic. This remedy was often given to treat dropsy and jaundice, being a favored herb for disorders of the pneumo-gastric region.

Dose: Approximately ½ ounce of leaves or whole herb to 1 pint of water. Water boiled separately and poured over the plant material and steeped for 5–20 minutes, depending on the desired effect. Drunk hot or warm, 1 to 2 cups per day, at bedtime and upon awakening.

TORMENTIL
Potentilla tormentilla, P. erectus

PARTS USED: Root

Botanical Description: This perennial herb is a native of temperate and colder regions of the northern hemisphere. Rootstock short, nearly cylindrical, solid, about ½ inch or more in diameter, branched, truncate below, abruptly tapering above, giving off long cylindrical roots below, the upper part with reddish brown chaffy scales; dark brown externally, bright blood-red in the center. Stems numerous, from the axils of the chaffy scales, very slender, cylindrical, 1 foot or more long, widely spreading or prostrate, pale-green or reddish, shortly hairy, much branched in the upper part. Leaves alternate and shortly stalked below, usually opposite and nearly or quite sessile above, all with lanceolate or oval, entire or palmately toothed stipules, trifoliate, leaflets small, sessile, obovate- or lanceolate-wedge-shaped, entire

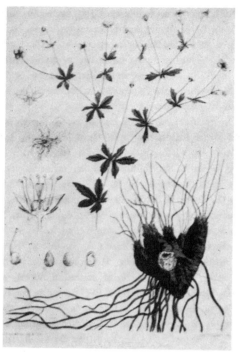

TORMENTIL: In Europe a tincture is frequently utilized for intestinal disorders and in brandy for stomach disorders. The antidysenteric effects of this herb are due to the mildly antiseptic and astringent action of its tannins.

and tapering below, with a few large teeth above, hairy on both surfaces, silky on the veins beneath, dark green, paler below. Flowers small, scarcely ½ inch wide, on long slender stalks terminating the stems and branches (the lower ones apparently coming off opposite the alternate leaves), which repeatedly dichotomize at the opposite leaves, the whole forming a very lax divaricate cyme. Calyx very deeply cut into 4 lanceolate, acute, pale green, hairy, valvate segments, outside of which and alternating with them are 4 other ones about half as long (epicalyx). Petals 4, roundish, with a very short claw, spreading, lemon yellow with the base orange, soon falling. Stamens about 16, inserted on the perigynous rim (disk) of the calyx, which is covered with white hairs, filaments slender, shorter than the petals, yellow, anthers short, rounded. Carpels few, about 6–8, distinct; ovary small, tumid, glabrous; styles lateral, erect, yellow, thickened above. Achenia somewhat kidney-shaped, keeled on the back, smooth, brown, with ridged reticulation when dry. Seed solitary, pendulous, radicle superior, no endosperm.

192

Habitat: A very common plant in all parts of England, especially on heaths, dry fields, roadsides, and woods, flowering from July till late in the autumn. It is also found throughout the continent of Europe and extends into the arctic regions, Siberia, and Iceland, but does not reach North America. (Bentley)

Medicinal Uses: Tormentil is a powerful astringent, and has been used principally to treat diarrhea and hemorrhages. Additionally, it was considered by the ancients to promote sweating and was thought helpful in curing plague. It was administered to treat syphilis, fevers, smallpox, measles, and a vast list of other disorders. As a treatment for warts, a piece of linen was soaked in a strong decoction of Tormentil, placed on the wart, and repeated frequently until success was achieved. The decoction was also gargled to cure mouth ulcers and spongy gums.

The herbalists Gerard and Culpepper both used Tormentil for toothache, comparing it favorably with Cloves. In Europe a tincture is frequently utilized for intestinal disorders and in brandy for stomach disorders.

The root was also utilized, as is the case with most strong astringents, for tanning leather in the Orkney Islands of Scotland. The masticated root was used to dye leather red by the Laplanders.

The dried root contains chinovin, tormentillic acid, and chinova acid. However, the antidiarrhetic and antidysenteric effect of this perennial herb is due to the astringent and mildly antiseptic action of the tannins present in the rhizomes of virtually all *Potentilla* species.

Dose: 1 teaspoon, boiled in a covered container of 1½ pints of water for about ½ hour, at a slow boil. Liquid allowed to cool slowly in the *closed* container. Drunk cold, 1 swallow or 1 tablespoon at a time, 1 to 2 cups per day.

Note: Brew stronger for external, weaker for internal usage.

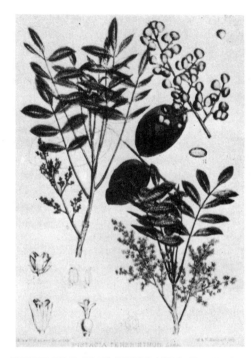

TURPENTINE TREE (TEREBINTH): Terebinth, or Chian Turpentine, was derived from a small tree, and often adulterated with the less costly coniferous turpentines.

TURPENTINE TREE
Pistacia terebinthus, Pinus, Abies, and *Larix* spp.

PARTS USED: Sap
OTHER COMMON NAMES: Terebinth

Botanical Description: The term *turpentine* is now generally applied to certain vegetable juices, liquid or concrete, which consist of resin combined with a peculiar essential oil, called oil of turpentine. They are generally procured from different species of Pine, though other trees afford products known by the same general title, as for instance, *Pistacia terebinthus*, which yields the Chian turpentine. Some of the French writers extend the name of turpentine to other juices consisting of resin and essential oil, as copaiba, balm of Gilead, etc.

Pistacia terebinthus. This is the Terebinth, a small tree with numerous spreading branches, bearing alternate, pinnate leaves, which consist of 3 or 4 pairs of ovate lanceolate, entire, acute, smooth, and shining leaflets with an odd one at the end. The male and female flowers are dioecious, small, and in branching racemes. It is a native of Greece, and flourishes in the islands of Cyprus and Chio, the latter of which has given its name to the turpentine obtained from the tree.

Chian turpentine was collected chiefly in the island of Chio or Scio, by incisions made during the summer in the bark of *Pistacia terebinthus*. The juice flowing from the wounds fell upon smooth stones placed at the foot of the tree, from which it was scraped with small sticks, and allowed to drop into bottles. The annual product of each tree is very small; and the turpentine, therefore, commanded a high price even in the place where it was procured. Very little of it reached this country. It is said to be frequently adulterated with other turpentines. It is a thick, tenacious, pellucid liquid, of a slightly yellowish color, a peculiar penetrating odor more agreeable than that of the other substances of the same class, and a mild taste with little bitterness. On exposure to the air it speedily thickens, and ultimately becomes concrete and hard, in consequence of the loss of its volatile oil.

White turpentine. The common American, or white, turpentine (Terebintha of the *U.S. Pharmacopoeia*), is procured chiefly from *Pinus palustris*, partly also from *Pinus taeda*, and perhaps some other species inhabiting the southern states. In former times, large quantities were collected in New England; but more recently, the Turpentine Trees of that area being largely exhausted, other parts of the country have been the source of supply.

During the winter months, excavations of the capacity of about three pints are made in the trunk of the tree 3 or 4 inches from the ground. Into these the juice begins to flow about the middle of March, and continues to flow throughout the warm season, slowly at first, rapidly in the middle of summer, and more slowly again in the autumn months. The liquid is removed from these excavations as they fill, and transferred into casks, where it gradually thickens, and ultimately acquires a soft solid consistence.

White turpentine, as found in our shops, has a peculiar, somewhat aromatic odor, a warm pungent bitterish taste, and a white color tinged with yellow. It is somewhat translucent, and of a consistence which varies with the temperature. In the middle of summer it is almost semifluid and very adhesive, though brittle; in

the winter it is often so firm and hard as to be incapable of being made into pills without heat. Exposed to the air it ultimately becomes perfectly hard and dry. In the recent state it affords about 17 percent of essential oil. (U.S.D.)

Other turpentines are derived from the American Silver Fir *(Pinus balsamea)*, the European Larch *(Larch europaea)*, and other Pines and Larches.

Medicinal Uses: Terebinth, or Chian turpentine, was derived from a small tree, and often adulterated with the less costly coniferous Turpentines.

"Spirits of turpentine" is the volatile oil distilled with water from the concrete oleoresin. This oil (or "spirits") is locally irritant and feebly antiseptic. It was commonly employed as a stimulating expectorant; as it irritated the mucous membranes it helped to expel phlegm and was a useful treatment in bronchitis. It is a stimulant to kidney function and was sometimes used in mild doses as a diuretic; in larger doses, it is dangerous to the kidneys. It was also used as a carminative, and was considered one of the most valuable remedies in cases of flatulent colic. Terebinth was also used to treat chronic diarrhea and dysentery, typhoid fever, internal hemorrhages, purpureal fever and bleeding, helminthiasis, leucorrhea, and amenorrhea.

Turpentine baths, arranged in such a way that the vapors were not inhaled by the patient, were given in cases of chronic rheumatism. It was also administered in enema form to treat intractable constipation. Applied externally as a liniment or ointment, it has been used in rheumatic ailments such as lumbago, arthritis, and neuralgias. It was also used as a local application to treat and promote the healing of burns and to heal parasitic skin diseases.

Dose: As an enema, ½ to 1 ounce of oil to 1 pint of warm soapsuds.

194

VALERIAN
Valeriana officinalis

PARTS USED: Root

Botanical Description: Valerian is a large handsome herbaceous plant, with a perennial root, and an erect, round, channeled stem, terminating in flowering branches. The leaves of the stem are attached by short broad sheaths, the radical leaves are larger and stand on long footstalks. In the former the leaflets are lanceolate and partially dentate, in the latter elliptical and deeply serrate. The flowers are small, white or rose-colored, odorous, and disposed in terminal corymbs, interspersed with spear-shaped pointed bracts. The number of stamens in this species is 3. The fruit is a capsule containing one oblong ovate, compressed seed.

The plant is a native of Europe, where it grows either in damp woods and meadows or on dry elevated grounds. As found in these different situations, it presents characters so distinct as to have induced some botanists to make 2 varieties. That which affects a dry soil is not more than two feet high, and is distinguished by its narrow leaves. It is superior to the other variety in medicinal virtue.

The root, which is the officinal portion, is collected in spring before the stem begins to shoot, or in the autumn when the leaves decay. It should be dried quickly, and kept in a dry place. It consists of numerous long, slender, cylindrical fibers, issuing from a tuberculated head. As brought to this country it frequently has portions of the stems attached. (U.S.D.)

Medicinal Uses: In an age of anxiety, when tranquilizing agents reign supreme, it may be wise to reconsider the natural sedatives, the nervines used with great success since antiquity. Of the many plants employed to calm nervous patients, quiet hysteria, or allay the fears of hypochondriacs, none seems to come forward with such recommendations as this root.

Valerian root has been used since ancient times in the treatment of epilepsy, particularly when the seizures are brought on by emotions such as fear and anger. It has been employed as a stimulant and antispasmodic in more recent times. Combined with Cinchona it has also been given to treat intermittent fevers.

Valerian is clearly a nonnarcotic, perfectly safe herbal sedative, highly recommended in anxiety states. It is all too tempting to observe the present frequency of tranquillizer use as indicative of doomed, exhausted populations finally crushed by machine civilization. Surely the pace and noise of present life create tension in biological man, but what do you make of this curious entry, recorded in agricultural 1831, by Samuel Thomson, a practicing botanic family physician: "This powder [Valerian] is the best nervine known; I have made great use of it, and have always found it to produce the most beneficial effects, in all cases of nervous affection, and in hysterical symptoms; in fact, *it would be difficult to get along with my practice in many cases without this important article.*"

Apparently, even then, nervousness was a complaint all too frequently brought before the attention of healers.

Thomson recommended half a teaspoon in hot water, sweetened, to promote sleep and leave the patient at ease.

While the unground, dried root is presently available in most herb stores, and very popular (the powdered root is much more potent than the chipped bark), most users are experiencing only a trace, or a remnant of the effects of the fresh root, which is far more potent.

The roots of Valerian contain a complex mixture of substances known as valepotriates, which are known to have sedative and tranquillizing properties. Other important chemical constituents, known as esters, are unstable and are lost during the drying process. For this reason the drug's effects vary considerably, so much so that physicians largely abandoned it by the end of the nineteenth century.

A far more potent action is had by using the juice of the fresh root, in dosages of 1 to 3 tablespoonfuls. Of course, in Europe, Valerian tincture is freely available and a very popular natural "tranquillizer."

As expected, a remedy so strong in ancient and recent usage has proven itself under the sometimes too caustic rituals of the modern pharmacologist. Petkov and associates in Bulgaria recently demonstrated that an extract of the root has central nervous system sedative effects and the ability to steady an arrhythmic heart in lab animals. Perhaps more interesting is Cavazzuti's work in Italy, which demonstrated that a mixture of Valerian, Passionflower, Chamomile, Hawthorn (fluidextracts), sucrose, and orange essence was effective in treating children, "one- to twelve-year-olds with psychomotor agitation and non-adaptation disorders." By the all too infrequently applied double-blind method (rarely applied in evaluating herbs), this herbal mixture displayed genuine effects in treating hyperactivity and insomnia.

Dose: Use *fresh* material! One teaspoonful to 1 cup of boiling water.

VIRGINIA SNAKEROOT
Aristolochia serpentaria

PARTS USED: Rhizome and root

OTHER COMMON NAMES: Serpentaria, Snagrel, Texas Snakeroot

Botanical Description: We have within the limits of the United States 4 species, of which 3—*A. serpentaria*, *A. tomentosa*, and *A. hastata*—contribute indiscriminately to furnish the Snakeroot of the shops. *Aristolochia serpentaria* is an herbaceous plant with a perennial root, which consists of numerous slender fibers proceeding from a short horizontal caudex. Several stems usually rise from the same root. They are about 8 or 10 inches in height, slender, round, flexuose, jointed at irregular distances, and frequently of a reddish or purple color at the base. The leaves are oblong cordate, acuminate, entire, of a pale yellowish-green color, and supported on short petioles at the joints of the stem. The flowers proceed from the joints near the root, and stand singly on long, slender, round, jointed peduncles, which are sometimes furnished with 1 or 2 small scales, and bend downward so as nearly to bury the flower in the earth or decayed leaves. There is no calyx. The corolla is of a purple color, monopetalous, tubular, swelling at the base, contracted and curved in the middle, and terminating in a labiate border with lanceolate lips. The anthers—6 or 12 in number—are sessile, attached to the under part of the stigma, which is roundish, divided into 6 parts, and supported by a short fleshy style upon an oblong, angular, hairy, inferior germ. The fruit is a

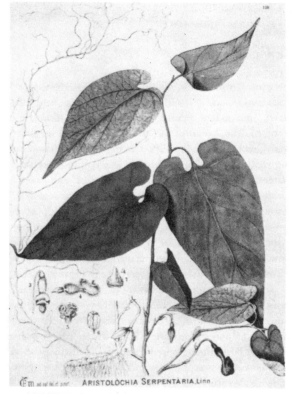

ARISTOLOCHIA SERPENTARIA, Linn.

VIRGINIA SNAKEROOT: This plant was the most famous of the American Indian remedies for the bites of poisonous snakes.

hexangular, 6-celled capsule, containing several small flat seeds.

The plant grows in rich, shady woods, throughout the Midwest, South, and West, abounding in the valley of the Ohio, and in the mountainous regions of our interior. It flowers in May and June. The root is collected in western Pennsylvania and Virginia, in Ohio, Indiana, and Kentucky. (U.S.D.)

Medicinal Uses: This plant was the greatest of the American Indian treatments for the bites of poisonous snakes, and its reputation spread rapidly among the European settlers. Although it was originally introduced into regular medicine for this purpose, its efficacy against snakebite has never been conclusively demonstrated, and the most valuable application of Serpentaria seems to have been as a tonic for persons suffering from intermittent fevers, such as malaria. For this purpose it was often utilized as an adjunct to quinine (Cinchona). Another usage was in the treatment of dyspepsia and indigestion arising from other disease conditions.

In larger doses the plant can cause nausea, vomiting, griping bowel pain, and dysenteric tenesmus. However, in the proper dosage it may be beneficial. In addition to the usages already listed, it is known to be an appetite stimulant.

Virtually all the many species of *Aristolochia* that have been chemically investigated contain two materials in common. The first is an essential oil that holds a number of antiseptic compounds; the second common constituent is a toxic material known as aristolochic acid. Aristolochic acid has been carefully studied in human subjects and is known to be extremely toxic to the kidneys and liver. Undoubtedly, the aristolochic acid content of these plants accounts for most of the uses alleged for them. However, it cannot be recommended that *Aristolochia* species be used for any purpose, primarily on the basis of potential severe toxic reactions that could result.

Dose: The medicinal dose was generally 1 teaspoon of the granulated root per pint of boiling water, steeped for ½ hour. One tablespoon, 3 to 6 times per day, was the dosage. However, the potential toxicity noted above recommends against use of the plant for self-medication.

WALL GERMANDER
Teucrium chamaedrys

PARTS USED: Tops and leaves
OTHER COMMON NAMES: Germander

Botanical Description: Root perennial, slender, yellowish, somewhat creeping, furnished with short, delicate fibers. Stems branched, decumbent at the base, then ascending, simple, obsoletely 4-sided, hairy, 9 inches to 1 foot high. Leaves opposite, shortly petiolate, obtuse, spreading, ovate, approaching to wedge-shaped, smooth, pubescent, veined, bright green above, paler beneath, deeply serrate at the margin and sometimes slightly lobed. Flowers on short peduncles, and are placed 2 or 3 together in the axils of the upper leaves, of which the uppermost, or bracts, are nearly entire at the margin. Calyx angular, hairy, ovate-turbinate, with 5, nearly equal, ovate-acuminate, ciliate teeth, purplish. Corolla reddish purple, much longer than the calyx, with a short curved tube, and divided at the limb into 2 lips, the upper short and bipartite, the lower 3-lobed, the middle lobe large, roundish. Stamens didynamous, much protruded, with slender white filaments, terminated by simple anthers, with 2 confluent, spreading cells. Ovary 4-parted; style filiform, longer than the stamens, surmounted by a bifid stigma. Fruit composed of four achenia, or small nuts, each containing a single seed, enclosed in the persistent calyx.

Distribution: Europe, from Holland southward, western Asia. Found on old walls in England, Scotland, and in sandy fields in Ireland; but rare, and is considered to be a garden escape. Flowers July to September. (B.F.M.)

Medicinal Uses: At one time this herb was part of a popular patent medicine for the treatment of gout and arthritis, known as Portland Powder, which contained equal parts *Aristolochia rotunda* root, *Gentiana lutea* root, tops and leaves of Germander and *Erythroea centaurium,* and leaves of *Ajuga chamoepitys,* the Ground Pine.

The Wall Germander was recommended by ancient herbalists for its vulnerary properties (ability to heal wounds), and continues to be a folk remedy for ulcers and sores. It is also recommended for general use as a tonic for digestion. Other ailments that have reportedly been treated with this plant are anemia, asthma, bronchitis, and other chronic respiratory diseases.

It is astringent, antiseptic, diuretic, and stimulant, and has been used in the treatment of jaundice, dropsy, gout, and ailments of the spleen. The Egyptians used the plant in treating intermittent fevers; interestingly, it was given as a preventative, the dose being taken one hour in advance of the paroxysm which was known to reoccur at four hour intervals.

Dose: Approximately ½ ounce of tops or leaves to 1 pint of water. Water boiled separately and poured over the plant material and steeped for 5–20 minutes, depending on the desired effect. Drunk hot or warm, 1 to 2 cups per day.

WATER LILY
Nymphaea alba, and other *Nymphaea* spp.

PARTS USED: Rhizome

OTHER COMMON NAMES: Water Rose, Nenuphar, Candock

Botanical Description: Among the most beautiful, profuse, and showy flowers borne by aquatic plants are water lilies. *Nymphaea* cultivated in pools has white, red, pink, blue, yellow, or lavender flowers, which are cup-shaped, several inches in diameter, and composed of many overlapping petals. Some are fragrant. They float on top of the water or rise above it, each flower lasting 1 to 7 days or nights, opening later and closing earlier the first time than the following times. The wilted flower either bends over or, in deep water, its stem coils, and the flower descends into the water, where the seed ripens. Six to ten weeks later, the ripened pod bursts, seeds rise to the surface, float awhile, and finally sink. Well-developed plants have rootstocks or tubers rooting in mud over which the water may be 3 inches to 6 feet deep. The round or ovate, leathery leaves, which are several inches in diameter and ordinarily deeply cut at the base, are attached by long stems to the roots and either float on the water or, if crowded, rise a few inches above it. As the different kinds of pond lilies cross readily, many hybrids are formed, and these are what are commonly cultivated. (Neal)

Medicinal Uses: Although all colors of Water Lilies were employed in folk medicine, the white Water Lily in particular was valued, due to its purity, rising out of the often murky marsh, stream or pond.

It was used as an anaphrodisiac, to depress the sexual function. This concept likely originated with the romantic notion of the purity of the flower rising from the muck, more than any true folkloric belief in such abilities. This power was likely attributed only to the white *Nymphaea*.

Externally, white and yellow Water Lilies were used to treat various skin disorders, such as boils, inflammations, tumors, and ulcers. The rootstocks contain much starch, useful as a food in emergencies.

Dose: To depress the sexual function, seek out a white Water Lily and meditate on its purity.

WHITE WILLOW
Salix alba

PARTS USED: Bark

Botanical Description: This is a very extensive genus, comprising not less than 130 species, which, with very few exceptions, are natives of Europe and of the northern and temperate parts of North America. Though they are all probably possessed of similar medical properties, only 3 were admitted to the rank of officinal plants by the British Colleges, viz., *S. alba, S. caprea,* and *S. fragilis.* Of these species, *Salix alba* is the only one which has been introduced into this country, and was recognized in our *Pharmacopoeia.*

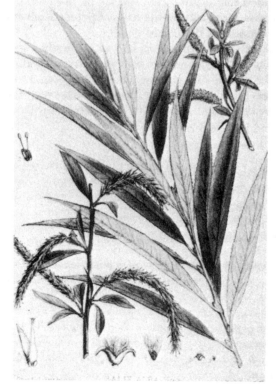

WHITE WILLOW: The bark has a major constituent known as salicin, which is closely related to aspirin. It will produce effects similar to, although weaker than those of aspirin.

Many native species are in all probability equally active; but they have not been sufficiently tried in regular practice to admit of a positive decision in relation to them.

Salix alba. The common European or White Willow is a tree 25 or 30 feet in height, with numerous round spreading branches, the younger of which are silky. The bark of the trunk is cracked and brown, that of the smaller branches smooth and greenish. The leaves are alternate, upon short petioles, lanceolate, pointed, acutely serrate with the lower serratures glandular, pubescent on both sides, and silky beneath. There are no stipules. The flowers appear at the same time with the leaves. The *amenta* are terminal, cylindrical, and elongated, with elliptical, lanceolate, brown, pubescent scales. The stamens are 2 in number, yellow, and somewhat longer than the scales; the style is short; the stigmas 2-parted and thick. The capsule is nearly sessile, ovate, and smooth.

The White Willow has been introduced into this country from Europe, and is now very common. It flowers in April and May; and the bark is easily separable throughout the summer.

That obtained from the branches rolls up when dried into the form of a quill, has a brown epidermis, is flexible, fibrous, and of difficult pulverization. Willow bark has a feebly aromatic odor, and a peculiar bitter astringent taste. It yields its active properties to water, with which it forms a reddish-brown decoction. (U.S.D.)

Medicinal Uses: Dioscorides, the ancient Greek physician (lived at about A.D. 60), was one of the first writers to describe the pain-relieving and fever-lowering properties of the Willows. In the mid-1700s the bark was a popular fever remedy in colonial America. Willow bark has a major constituent known as salicin, which is closely related to aspirin which produces similar, although weaker effects.

The Black Willow (*S. nigra*), a tree with dark brown bark, occurring along streams, was promoted by eclectic practitioners as "a very active sexual depressant." The floral buds were used "in all forms of sexual excitement, and in the nervous disturbances of the menstrual period." Spermatorrhea, defined as "abnormally frequent, involuntary loss of semen without orgasm," was also

treated with this bitter bark. Between 1.3 and 1.8 milliliters of the fluidextract was give 4 times a day.

Dose: 1 teaspoon of White Willow bark, boiled in a covered container of 1½ pints of water for about ½ hour, at a slow boil. Liquid allowed to cool slowly in the *closed* container. Drunk cold, 1 swallow or 1 tablespoon at a time, as needed to promote sweating in chills and fever.

WILD CHERRY
Prunus virginiana

PARTS USED: Stem Bark

Botanical Description: The Wild Cherry tree is one of the largest of the American forest; individuals have been

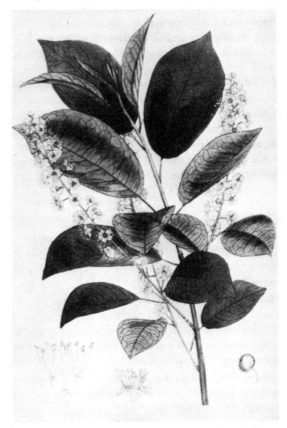

WILD CHERRY: Widely used as a cough sedative, the bark is used as a tonic and to calm irritation while diminishing nervous excitability.

seen on the banks of the Ohio from 80 to 100 feet high, with trunks from 12 to 15 feet in circumference, and undivided to the height of 25 or 30 feet. But as usually met with in the Atlantic states, the tree is of much smaller dimensions. In the open fields it is less elevated than in forests, but sends out more numerous branches, which expand into an elegant oval summit. The trunk is regularly shaped, and covered with a rough blackish bark, which detaches itself semicircularly in thick narrow plates, and by this peculiar characteristic serves as a distinguishing mark of the tree when the foliage is too high for inspection. The leaves are oval oblong, acuminate, unequally serrate, smooth on both sides, of a beautiful brilliant green, and supported alternately upon petioles, which are furnished with from 2 to 4 reddish glands. The flowers are small, white, and collected in long erect racemes. They appear in May, and are followed by globular drupes about the size of a pea, and when ripe of a shining blackish-purple color.

This species of *Prunus* grows throughout the United States, flourishing most in those parts where the soil is fertile and the climate temperate, and abounding in the Middle Atlantic states, and in those which border on the Ohio. The fruit has a sweetish, astringent, bitter taste; and is much employed in some parts of the country to impart flavor to spiritous liquors. The inner bark is the part employed in medicine, and is obtained indiscriminately from all parts of the tree, though that of the roots is most active. It should be preferred recently dried, as it deteriorates by keeping. (U.S.D.)

Medicinal Uses: The most widespread popular use of Wild Cherry bark is as a cough sedative. It acts as a tonic and calms irritation, diminishing nervous excitability. It has been employed in the treatment of bronchitis, and because it slows heart action, has been used in heart disease characterized by frequent, irregular, or feeble pulse. It has also been considered a good remedy for weakness of the stomach or of the system coupled with general or local irritation.

The *Prunus* genus includes the plums, almonds, peaches, apricots, and cherries. All these possess to some degree the glycoside amygdalin, which when combined with water reacts to form hydrocyanic acid. The cancer treatment *laetrile*, currently employed with repeated success in Mex-

ico and Germany and seeking acceptance today in the U.S., contains amygdalin.

Hydrocyanic acid is toxic in sufficient dose, and there are many reports of animals being poisoned fatally by eating the leaves or fruits of many *Prunus* species. The degree of toxicity depends on a number of factors, and it is generally agreed that the wilted leaves are the most toxic.

Both hydrocyanic acid and benzaldehyde, formed during the water extraction of the bark, contribute to the pleasant characteristic odor of Wild Cherry preparations. It should be pointed out that heat should be avoided during the preparation of Wild Cherry extracts, since both hydrocyanic acid and benzaldehyde are very volatile, and would be lost if heat is applied.

Dose: Decoction interferes with the action of the bark. Never boil. For medicinal purposes, prepare an infusion (steeping in just-boiled water), using one teaspoon of the bark per cup of water.

WINTERGREEN
Gaultheria procumbens

PARTS USED: Whole Plant
OTHER COMMON NAMES: Periwinkle, Spice Berry, Tea Berry, Deerberry, Partridge Berry

Botanical Description: This is a small, indigenous, shrubby, evergreen plant, with a long, creeping, horizontal root, which sends up at intervals 1 and sometimes 2 erect, slender, round, reddish stems. These are naked below, leafy at the summit, and usually less than a span in height. The leaves are ovate or obovate, acute, revolute at the edges with a few mucronate serratures, coriaceous, shining, bright green upon the upper surface, paler beneath, of unequal size, and supported irregularly on short red petioles. The calyx is white, 5-toothed, and furnished at its base with 2 concave cordate bracts, which are by some authors described as an outer calyx. The corolla is white, ovate or urceolate, contracted at its mouth, and divided at its border into 5 small acute segments. The stamens consist of curved, plumose filaments, and oblong orange-colored anthers, opening on the outside. The germ, which rests upon a ring having 10 teeth alternating with the 10 stamens, is roundish, depressed, and surmounted by an erect

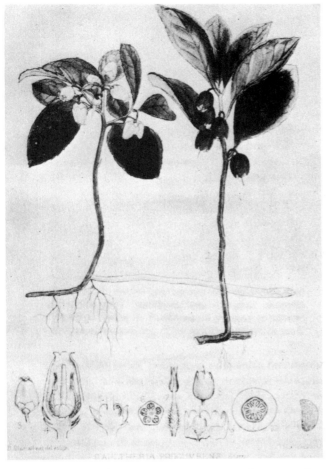

WINTERGREEN: Some of the medicinal actions of this tea can be explained by the methyl salicylate contained in the oil. The compound is closely related to aspirin.

filiform style, terminating in an obtuse stigma. The fruit is a small, 5-celled, many-seeded capsule, enclosed in a fleshy covering, formed by the enlarged calyx, and presenting the appearance of a bright scarlet berry.

The plant extends from Canada to Georgia, growing in large beds in mountainous tracts, or in dry barrens and sandy plains, beneath the shade of shrubs and trees, particularly of other evergreens, as the Kalmiae and Rhododendra. It is abundant in the pine barrens of New Jersey. In different parts of the country it is known by the various names of Partridge Berry, Deerberry, Tea Berry, and Mountain Tea. The flowers appear from May to September, and the fruit ripens at corresponding periods. Though the leaves only are officinal, all parts of the plant are endowed with the peculiar flavor for which these are employed, and which is found in several other plants, particularly in the bark of *Betula lenta*, or Sweet Birch. The fruit possesses it in a high degree, and being at the same time sweetish, is much relished by some

persons, and forms a favorite article of food with partridges, deer, and other wild animals.

To the very peculiar and agreeably aromatic odor and taste which belong to the whole plant, the leaves add a marked astringency, dependent on the presence of tannin. The aromatic properties reside in a volatile oil, which may be separated by distillation. (U.S.D.)

Medicinal Uses: An old favorite, Wintergreen tea is diuretic in small doses; large doses are emetic. It is an aromatic stimulant with astringent properties, and consequently is of assistance in cases of chronic diarrhea. It has been used to promote menstruation and increase milk production in nursing mothers. Oil of Wintergreen has been used as an external application, in the form of cloths soaked in the aromatic liquid and tied to the painful part, in the treatment of body aches and pains.

Some of the medicinal actions can be explained on the basis of the methyl salicylate contained in the oil, which is closely related to acetylsalicylic acid, or aspirin.

Dose: One teaspoon of the plant to 1 cup of boiling water, steeped for 5 to 20 minutes and drunk cold, 1 cup per day, 1 mouthful at a time.

WITCH HAZEL
Hamamelis virginiana

PARTS USED: Bark, twigs, and leaves
OTHER COMMON NAMES: Spotted Hazel, Snapping Hazel, Winterbloom

Botanical Description: Witch Hazel is an indigenous shrub, from 5 to 15 feet tall, growing in almost all sections of the United States, usually on hills or in stony places, and often on the banks of streams.

It is a shrub, up to 5 meters tall, with scurfy or glabrous twigs. Leaves broadly obovate or obovate-oblong, obtuse or acute, with several to many rounded teeth, inequilateral at the broadly rounded or subcordate base, green on both sides, glabrous or stellate-pubescent beneath. Petals bright yellow or suffused with red, spreading, 1.5–2 centimeters long. Sepals dull yellowish brown within. Fruit ovoid or thickly ellipsoid

201

before dehiscence, 1–1.5 centimeters long, the hypanthium often bearing the persistent sepals. (B&B)

Medicinal Uses: The North American Indians used this shrub as a sedative application to external inflammations, and so we inherited yet another valuable gift of nature from the indigenous American. Witch Hazel is utilized today largely as described above, and as a liniment for body aches and pains.

Internally, it was at one time recommended as a fluidextract in the treatment of varicose veins and internal bleeding. Itching hemorrhoids were treated with a soothing ointment made of lard and a decoction of Apple tree bark, Witch Hazel bark, and White Oak bark.

Witch Hazel extracts contain astringent tannins that explain the beneficial effects of water extract in reducing inflammation when applied externally. Commercially available "witch hazel extract," however, does not contain tannins. When the extract is prepared the plant is mixed with water and distilled. The distillate is a clear, colorless liquid having an aromatic odor. It contains a mixture of aromatic substances that have not been well studied. Yet, that this extract is soothing and refreshing when applied externally can be verified by anyone who has used it.

Dose: 1 teaspoon of leaves or bark, granulated, to 1 cup boiling water. Applied cold or gargled as a mouthwash.

WOLFSBANE
Aconitum napellus

PARTS USED: Root

OTHER COMMON NAMES: Monkshood, Aconite, Wolfroot

Botanical Description: This is a perennial herbaceous plant, with a turnip-shaped or fusiform root, and an erect, round, smooth, leafy stem, which is usually simple, and rises from 2 to 4 feet, sometimes even 6 or 8 feet in height. The leaves are alternate, petiolate, divided almost to the base, from 2 to 4 inches in diameter, deep green upon their upper surface, light-green beneath, somewhat rigid, and more or less

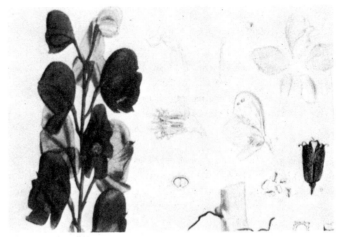

WOLFSBANE: The leaves are known to be an effective sedative and painkiller. The amount needed to produce these effects, however, is very close to the amount that will cause serious poisoning.

smooth and shining on both sides. Those on the lower part of the stem have long footstalks and 5 or 7 divisions, the upper, short footstalks and 3 or 5 divisions. The divisions are narrow at their base, but widen in the form of a wedge toward their summit, and present 2 or 3 lobes, which extend nearly or quite to the middle. The lobes are cleft or toothed, and the lacinae or teeth are linear or linear-lanceolate and pointed. The flowers are of a dark violet-blue color, large and beautiful, and are borne at the summit of the stem upon a thick, simple, straight, erect, spike-like raceme, beneath which, in the cultivated plant, several smaller racemes rise from the axils of the upper leaves. Though without calyx, they have two small calycinal stipules situated on the peduncle within a few lines of the flower. The petals are 5, the upper helmet-shaped and beaked, nearly hemispherical, open or closed, the 2 lateral roundish and internally hairy, the 2 lower oblong-oval. They enclose 2 pedicelled nectaries, of which the spur is capitate, and the lip bifid and revolute. The fruit consists of 3, 4, or 5 podlike capsules.

The plant is abundant in the mountainous forests of France, Switzerland, and Germany. It is also cultivated in the gardens of Europe, and has been introduced into this country as an ornamental flower. All parts of it are acrid and poisonous; but the leaves only are officinal. They should be collected when the flowers begin to appear, or shortly before. (U.S.D.)

Medicinal Uses: Aconite possess sedative,

anodyne, diuretic, and inflammation-reducing properties, but in overdose it and all its relatives are swift and fatal poisons. Nevertheless, in 1762 a Viennese physician, Baron Störck, published experiments proving the value of this plant in the materia medica, claiming success in treating gout, rheumatism, intermittent fevers, and scrofulous swellings.

By the time the twentieth edition of the *U.S. Dispensatory* was issued (1918), Aconite was recognized as a valuable circulatory sedative in heart problems, since it reduced excessive heart action and decreased arterial tension. Concomitant with the reduction of blood pressure Aconite was also noted for its ability to induce sweating.

The plant is a very highly valued homeopathic remedy; in fact, it was originally taken over into regular medicine from homeopathic practice as a substitute for the widespread and undoubtedly sometimes fatal practice of bloodletting that prevailed through the nineteenth century. Homeopathic practitioners also used Aconite in the treatment of pains, to promote a sense of calm, and, parallel to the observations of the *U.S. Dispensatory*, to produce and increase perspiration.

The active principle is aconitine, discovered in 1833. Although it is exceedingly toxic in even very small quantities, there have been reports of people being able to eat the boiled leaves without harm. We cannot substantiate, however, that boiling destroys the fatally dangerous principle, and it should be noted that a decoction of this herb was used to execute the condemned, in early times.

Used externally as a liniment, the plant has proved useful in the treatment of neuralgic and rheumatic pains.

It is well known that the leaves and roots of Wolfsbane contain very potent alkaloids that have been studied in animals and are known to produce sedative and painkilling effects. However, the amount of these alkaloids that will produce these effects is nearly the same as the amount that will produce serious poisonous effects. Thus, one must be cautioned that Wolfsbane is a potentially dangerous plant when considered for any use in humans. An overdose will cause adverse effects on the heart (fibrillations).

Dose: DANGEROUS. Avoid internal use.

WOOD BETONY
Stachys officinalis

PARTS USED: Leaves and root

OTHER COMMON NAMES: Betony, Lousewort

Botanical Description: Root perennial, woody, twisted, brownish, furnished with long white fibers. Stem simple, upright, quadrangular, rough with deflexed hairs, about 1½ feet high. Lower leaves cordate-oblong, furnished with long footstalks; upper ones opposite, oblong, and nearly sessile; the whole deep green, obtuse and crenate. Flowers in terminal oblong spikes, rather short and interrupted, with 2 linear, lanceolate, reflexed bracts at the base. Calyx monophyllous, tubular, 10-ribbed, divided at the border into 5-toothed acute segments. Corolla monopetalous, bilabiate, purple, with a cylindrical curved tube; upper lip plane, entire, and obtuse; lower one large and divided in 3 lobes, the middle lobe larger, roundish, and slightly notched. Stamens 4, didynamous; filaments awl-shaped, inclined toward the upper lip; anthers globose, 2-lobed. Ovary superior, rounded, 4-lobed, supporting a simple filiform style, terminated by a bifid stigma. Fruit consists of 4 oval, brown seeds, situated in the bottom of the persistent calyx.

Distribution: Europe, Northern Africa, Western Siberia; in shady places in woods and meadows in England; rare in Scotland and Ireland. Flowers June to August. (B.F.M.)

Medicinal Uses: Highly esteemed by the ancients, Betony was extolled as a remedy for a wide variety of ailments. The root is both emetic and purgative. The leaves are quite mild, possessing aperient (mildly laxative), cordial, aromatic, and astringent properties, but not to a degree that makes them a valuable medical remedy compared with other plants with similar attributes. A tea brewed from the plant has been used in the treatment of stomach disorders, gout, headaches, and disorders of the spleen.

Betony's major use today is not as a medicinal

but as a flavoring agent in herbal tea blending. It is thought to be a valuable nervine by some people in the herb tea industry.

Dose: Leaves—Approximately 1 ounce to 1 pint of water. Water boiled separately and poured over the leaves and steeped for 5 to 20 minutes, depending on the desired effect. Drunk hot or warm, 1 to 2 cups or more per day.

Root—1 teaspoonful powdered or ground root boiled in 1½ pints of water in uncovered container for ½ hour; boiled down to 1 pint. Drunk cold, 1 cup per day, 1 to 2 tablespoons at a time.

WORMWOOD
Artemisia absinthium

PARTS USED: Leaves and flowering tops
OTHER COMMON NAMES: Absinthium, Absinth, Madderwort

Botanical Description: Wormwood is a perennial plant, with herbaceous, branching, round and striated or furrowed stems, which rise 2 or 3 feet in height, and are panicled at their summit. The radical leaves are triply pinnatifid, with lanceolate, obtuse, dentate divisions; those of the stem doubly or simply pinnatifid, with lanceolate, somewhat acute divisions; the floral leaves are lanceolate; all are hoary. The flowers are of a brownish-yellow color, hemispherical, pedicelled, nodding, and in erect racemes. The florets of the disc are numerous, those of the ray few.

This plant is a native of Europe, where it is also cultivated for medical use. It is among our garden herbs, and has been naturalized in the mountainous districts of New England. The leaves and flowering summits are the parts employed, the larger parts of the stalks being rejected. They should be gathered in July or August, when the plant is in flower.

Wormwood has a strong odor, and an intensely bitter, nauseous taste, which it imparts to water and alcohol. A dark-green volatile oil, upon which the odor depends, is obtained by distillation. The constituents are a very bitter, and an almost insipid azotized matter, an excessively bitter resinous substance, a green volatile oil, chlorophyll, albumen, starch, saline matters, and lignin. (U.S.D.)

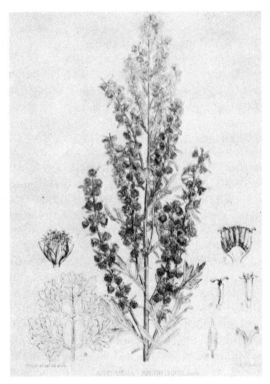

WORMWOOD: Absinthe was made from the poisonous oil of wormwood, giving this plant a bad reputation. Wormwood has been used to make an herbal tea containing only a very small amount of absinthe in the final beverage. The practice is a bad risk.

Medicinal Uses: The volatile oil of Wormwood is an active narcotic poison. The liqueur absinthe, made from oils of Wormwood, Angelica, Anise, and Marjoram, was finally barred from entry into the United States due to the dangers of absinthism. Unlike ordinary alcoholism, Absinthism additionally produces "restlessness at night, with disturbing dreams, nausea and vomiting in the morning with great trembling of the hands and tongue, vertigo and a tendency to epileptiform convulsions."

Wormwood was formerly utilized in several ways, the most important being as an anthelmintic (to expel tapeworms and other intestinal worms)—hence the common name for the plant. It was considered a powerful local anesthetic, and has been applied externally to relieve rheumatic pains, as well as for sprains, bruises and local

204

irritations. Taken internally, it was additionally utilized as a tonic and cathartic. Before the introduction of quinine (Cinchona bark), it was highly regarded as a remedy in intermittent fevers.

Near relatives, *A. indica* and *A. chinensis*, were used in China to produce moxas. These agents are small combustible masses used to cause sloughing following cauterization. They are caustics, used in skin diseases, to destroy infected tissue and to counteract the bites of animals and insects.

(Another relative, *A. vulgaris*, is treated separately in the Mugwort article.)

Wormwood has gained an unfavorable reputation among many as an herbal remedy because of the toxicity of the essential oil prepared by distilling the above-ground portions of the plant. Absinthe contains a high concentration of thujone, which is a convulsant poison and narcotic when taken in large amounts. The use of absinthe is banned in virtually every country in the world.

Wormwood has been used to make an herbal tea, however, containing only a very small amount of absinthe, and hence thujone, in the final beverage. Thujone has a very low water-solubility; thus it would be difficult to experience the adverse effects of absinthe when the plant is used in the form of a normally brewed herbal tea.

We have been unable to find experimental evidence to corroborate the anthelmintic effect of Wormwood but water extracts given to animals by mouth have been shown to produce a cathartic action. A tea of Wormwood would be bitter, and most bitter substances act as tonics by increasing gastric secretion. Mausert prescribed this herb for liver complaints, since it promoted the flow of bile. As a worming agent it is also excellent. Being an active Medicinal, it must be carefully dosed.

Dose: For medicinal use, 1 teaspoon of ground tops and leaves was used per cup of boiling water. It was drunk cold, one cup per day, only a large mouthful at a time.

YAM, WILD
Dioscorea spp.

PARTS USED: Rhizome

OTHER COMMON NAMES: Colic Root, Rheumatism Root, Chinese Yam, Bitter Yam, Wild Yam

Botanical Description: The Yam family includes 10 genera and more than 200 species from temperate and tropical regions. They are herbaceous or shrubby climbers with tuberous or thick underground stems; leaves opposite or alternate, entire and heart-shaped or palmately about 3 parted; flowers not showy, greenish, small, in narrow clusters, commonly unisexual, the 2 sexes on the same plant or, more commonly, on separate plants, otherwise much as in the amaryllis family; seeds flat or winged, in 3-angled or 3-lobed capsules. Roots of some species yield edible tubers or yams. Some forms of sweet potatoes, which belong to the Morning Glory family, are also called yams.

Chinese Yam, *Dioscorea batatas*, is a smooth, high climber with a somewhat angled, twisted stem, a native of China. The ovate, triangular, or more or less 3-lobed leaves are shiny and are alternate, paired, or 3 together, 2 to 3 inches long and wide, have 7 to none distinct longitudinal veins and many fine cross-veins. Minute cinnamon-scented male flowers are borne on 1 or 2 narrow spikes at leaf axils, where small tubers may also develop. The root is perennial and the vine quickly covers its support with foliage. The Japanese Yam (*D. japonica*) is like the Chinese Yam but has long, narrow, heart-shaped leaves. The Yam commonly grown for food in islands of the Pacific, *D. alata*, and looked for in Hawaii by Captain Cook as a food supply, has square, more or less winged stems and ovate or heart-shaped, opposite leaves, 3 to 6 inches long, without aerial tubers at their axils. It may have originated in southeast Asia. The Bitter Yam, *D. bulbifera* or *D. sativa*, has a cylindrical stem, leaves similar to those of the *D. alata*, and often bears tubers at the leaf axils. It is a native of tropics of the Eastern Hemisphere. (Neal)

Medicinal Uses: As the common names clearly indicate, the Yam has been considered a remedy for bilious colic, and Southern blacks once used it as a treatment for rheumatism. The root is diuretic and expectorant, but only in large doses. It is also antispasmodic, which would explain its efficacy in treating bilious colic.

All species of Wild Yam examined to date contain varying amounts of a steroid-like material known as diosgenin. Diosgenin has been shown experimentally to inhibit inflammation in laboratory animals, and thus the Wild Yam could have beneficial effects in rheumatism, as claimed in folklore.

Dose: 2–4 milliliters, given either in the form of a decoction or a fluidextract.

YARROW
Achillea millefolium

PARTS USED: Flowering tops and leaves
OTHER COMMON NAMES: Milfoil

Botanical Description: Yarrow is a perennial herb, very common both in Europe and America. It is from 1 foot to 18 inches in height, and is specifically distinguished by its doubly pinnate, downy, minutely divided leaves, with linear, dentate, mucronate divisions, from which it derived the name of Milfoil, by its furrowed stem and involucre, and by its dense corymbs of whitish flowers, which appear throughout the summer, from June to September. The whole herb has medicinal properties.

Both the flowers and leaves of *A. millefolium* have an agreeable, though feeble, aromatic odor, which continues after drying, and a bitterish, astringent, pungent taste. The aromatic properties are strongest in the flowers, the astringency in the leaves. (U.S.D.)

Medicinal Uses: Yarrow was known to the Greeks as a styptic, vulnerary, and astringent, and hence was used in hemorrhagic complaints. The American Indians used the plant externally to treat burns, wounds, cuts, and bruises. The genus name, *Achillea,* is derived from the name of the Greek warrior Achilles, who according to tradition healed the wounds of his comrades-in-arms with a relative of this plant.

Yarrow has been used both locally and internally in the treatment of hemorrhoids, and has also been given for bladder conditions such as involuntary urination in children. In weak doses, it has been employed as a mild aromatic, sudorific,

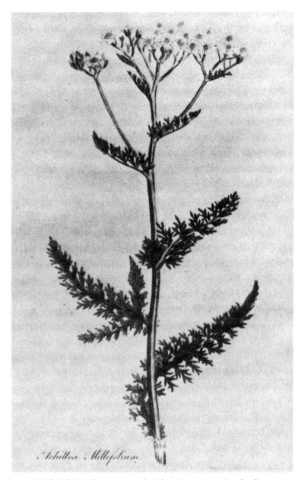

Achillea Millefolium

YARROW: Extracts of this common herb have been shown to reduce inflammation and to induce a calming effect. Antibiotic properties demonstrated in test tube experiments indicate the effectiveness of Yarrow in treating boils or other microbial infections of a minor nature.

tonic and astringent, the leaves being employed for the latter purpose. Its most noteworthy usage was in menstrual irregularities. It is also useful externally for hemorrhoids.

In the Scandinavian countries Yarrow was at one time used as a substitute for the Hop and was probably felt to have sedative properties.

The use of decoctions or infusions of Yarrow flowers as a tonic has been studied experimentally in humans, and it has been confirmed that gastric juices are stimulated by the oral ingestion of extracts of this plant. This would lead to a tonic effect with improved digestion of foods. The effect is due to the presence of bitter principles (azulenes, sesquiterpenes) in the flowers.

Animal studies have shown that extracts of Yarrow can reduce inflammation, and that they have a calming effect. Thus, the use of the juice of this plant for the treatment of ulcers and hemorrhoids has a rational basis. Extracts of Yarrow are also known to have antibiotic effects when evaluated in test tubes. Thus, at least for external application, one would expect that a person suffering from boils or other microbial infections of a minor nature would receive beneficial results by the external application of Yarrow preparations.

Dose: Approximately ½ ounce of the leaves or flowering tops to 1 pint of water. Water boiled separately and poured over the plant material and steeped for 5 to 20 minutes, depending on the desired effect. Drunk hot or warm, 1 to 2 cups per day, at bedtime and upon awakening.

Externally, as needed.

YELLOW DOCK
Rumex crispus

PARTS USED: Root and leaves
OTHER COMMON NAMES: Sorrel, Curled Dock, Dock Root

Botanical Description: General characteristics of *Rumex* genus: Calyx 6-parted, persistent, the 3 interior divisions petaloid, connivent. Seed 1, 3-sided, superior, naked. Stigmata multifid.

Rumex crispus has a yellow, spindle-shaped root, with a smooth furrowed stem two or three feet high, and lanceolate, waved, pointed leaves. The valves are ovate, entire, and all graniferous. It is a native of Europe, and grows wild in this country. It is common in our dry fields and pastures, and about barnyards, and flowers in June and July.

Dock Root, from whatever species derived, has an astringent bitter taste, with little or no smell. It readily yields its virtues to water by decoction. (U.S.D.)

Medicinal Uses: The roots reputedly have an unusual ability to take up whatever iron is present in the soil, and consequently Yellow Dock root has

long been a valued remedy for anemia. The root is also laxative, tonic, and astringent; and has been recommended in skin conditions. When the gums are spongy the powdered root is a recommended dentifrice.

The leaves were valued as a cure for scurvy; however, they contain oxalic acid, and there are reported cases of death due to oxalic acid poisoning from the ingestion of the leaves. Caution is therefore advised concerning the use of too many leaves, since there are far safer sources of vitamin C to be found.

The roots are rich in a complex mixture of anthraquinones and anthaquinone glycosides, similar to the types of chemical found in Cascara bark and Frangula berries. It is these anthraquinone derivatives that produce the laxative effect characteristic of the roots of Yellow Dock.

The roots of Yellow Dock are also rich in tannins, which are responsible for the astringent effect of preparations from this plant when applied externally. Thus, external applications for various skin conditions have a valid scientific basis.

Dose: Dock root is given in powder or decoction. Two ounces of the fresh root, bruised, or 1 ounce of the dried, may be boiled in a pint of water, of which 2 fluid ounces may be given as a dose, repeated as the patient can bear it. Avoid the leaves because of their toxicity.

Externally, apply powder as needed.

YERBA SANTA
Eriodictyon californicum

PARTS USED: Leaves
OTHER COMMON NAMES: Mountain Balm, Consumptive's Weed, Bear's Weed, Gum Bush

Botanical Description: *Eriodictyon californicum* is a low evergreen shrub growing abundantly upon dry hills in California. It is glabrous, resinous, having short petiolate, long lanceolate leaves, irregularly more or less serrate, sometimes entire, whitened beneath, between the reticulations, by a minute and close tomentum, above glabrous. The corolla is tubular funnel-form; the calyx being sparsely hirsute.

207

E. tomentosum, which grows often along with *E. californicum,* especially in the southern part of California, is readily distinguished by its dense coat of short villous hairs, whitish or rusty-colored with age. It is also a larger shrub than *E. californicum,* has its corolla somewhat salverform and its leaves oblong or oval, and obtuse. (U.S.D.)

Medicinal Uses: The leaves of this shrub have been used as a bitter tonic, and to disguise the bitterness of quinine. They were particularly valued for their expectorant properties, which made this a very popular remedy for asthma, chronic bronchitis, and colds. Yerba Santa was also felt to be helpful in cases of chronic genito-urinary inflammations. For treating respiratory ailments, the leaves were sometimes smoked, but they could also be administered as an infusion as described below.

The "Holy Herb" contains a resin, pentatriacontane, and cerotonic acid.

Dose: 1 teaspoon of the leaves in a cup of boiling water, steeped for ½ hour. Drunk warm, one-half cup before retiring, or a mouthful 3 times per day.

YOHIMBE
Corynanthe yohimbe (Pausinystalia yohimba)

PARTS USED: Bark

Botanical Description: This a tree of the family *Rubiaceae,* native to tropical West Africa.

Medicinal Uses: Yohimbe bark is one of the most frequently sought out aphrodisiacs that the world has ever known, and is still used for this purpose today, particularly in Cameroon. We have carried out an exhaustive search of the scientific literature for publications describing the effects of Yohimbe bark extracts on animals or humans in order to confirm or deny this effect. To our surprise, we were unable to find a single scientific paper that describes any type of effect for this plant in animals or in humans. However, many papers have been published by scientists attempting to relate the results of experiments in animals with yohimbine to the alleged aphrodisiac effect of decoctions or infusions of the bark, in man.

To summarize these findings, very clearly Yohimbine causes a dilation of the blood vessels in animals and in man, including those in the genitalia. Thus, in man, an increased flow of blood is routed to the penis, which theoretically should result in an erection, following the administration of yohimbine (and also Yohimbe bark, from which yohimbine is derived). Unfortunately, yohimbine in doses required to attain this effect also acts as a powerful agent in reducing normal blood pressure, due to the dilatory effect on the blood vessels. As would be expected, a person with extremely low blood pressure would no longer have the physical strength to enter into a vigorous sexual experience that would be anticipated as a reason for taking Yohimbe bark, and thus the effect would be nullified.

Yohimbine, and also Yohimbe bark, are powerful drugs. The effective dose is very close to the toxic dose, and thus one should not experiment with either of them out of curiosity. A person with normal low blood pressure should completely avoid the use of either of these two substances.

Some investigators have studied yohimbine in animals in order to ascertain whether or not this material affects ejaculation time and/or frequency, and it was found to do neither.

We have never found reference to the use of Yohimbe bark as an aphrodisiac in females, which tends to point out the long-standing male-chauvinistic attitudes in scientific work. Presumably, Yohimbe bark would also have an aphrodisiac effect in females, since it would cause an increased blood flow to the genitalia.

Dose: CAUTION. Although Yohimbine is on the USFDA unsafe herb list of March 1977, many people will no doubt continue to use it. Safer aphrodisiacs are available.

BIBLIOGRAPHY

Barton, B. H., and Castle, T. *The British Flora Medica*. London: Chatto and Windus, 1877.

Bentley, R., and Trimen, H. *Medicinal Plants*, vols. 1–4. London: J. & A. Churchill, 1880.

Bianchini, F., and Corbetta, F. *Health Plants of the World*. London: Cassell & Co., 1977.

Correll, D. S., and Johnston, M. C. *Manual of the Vascular Plants of Texas*. Renner, Texas: Texas Research Foundation, 1970.

Dyer, T. F. T. *The Folk-Lore of Plants*. New York: Appleton & Co., 1889.

Gleason, H. A. *The New Britton and Brown Illustrated Flora*, vols. 1–3. New York: Botanical Garden, 1952.

Meyer, Joseph E. *The Herbalist*. New York: Sterling, 1968.

Neal, M. C. *In Gardens of Hawaii*. Honolulu: B. P. Bishop Museum, 1965.

National Academy of Sciences. *Herbal Pharmacology in the People's Republic of China*. Washington, D.C.: NAS, 1975.

Phillips, E. P. *The Genera of South African Flowering Plants*. Cape Town: Government Printers, 1926.

Rhind, W. *The Vegetable Kingdom*. London: Blackie & Sons, 1868.

Stephenson, J., and Churchill, J. M. *Medical Botany*, vols. 1–3. London: J. Churchill, 1834.

Steyermark, J. A. *Flora of Missouri*. Ames, Iowa: Iowa Státe University Press, n.d.

Taber, C. W. *Taber's Cyclopedic Medical Dictionary*, 11th ed. Philadelphia: F. A. Davis Co., 1969.

Wood, G. B., and Bache, F. *United States Dispensatory*, 20th ed., Philadelphia: Lippincott Co., 1918.

Uphof, J. C. T. H. *Dictionary of Economic Plants*. Verlag J. Cramer, 1968.

Weiner, M. A. *Earth Medicine—Earth Foods*. New York: Macmillan, 1972.

Wellcome's Excerpta Therapeutica. New York: Burroughs Wellcome & Co. *ca.* 1908

PLANT INDEX

English/Latin

211

Latin/English

General Index

MEDICINAL PLANTS
EXPANDED SECTION

A-Z

MEDICINAL PLANTS EXPANDED SECTION

INTRODUCTION

BULLISH ON HERBS

The future of herbal medicine in America is very bright. People have rediscovered plant remedies and are once again looking to nature for solutions to the ills that flesh is heir to.

This is a natural progression when we consider that the ethno-medical folklore of preindustrial cultures (so called, "primitive") consists of prescriptions for treating most physical ailments. Taken together with the fact that the main active ingredient of approximately 25% of all prescription drugs sold in the U.S. was derived from plants, we can see why folklore has given life to the new scientific interest in herbs.

Not since the two principle anti-cancer drugs, vinscristine and vinblastine, were isolated from the "Madagascar Periwinkle" *(Catharanthus roseus)* in the 1960's have we seen so much interest in the promise of herbal medicine. These powerful plant-derived drugs arrest cell division so dramatically that one of them, vincristine, is used for the treatment of acute leukemia, especially in children. With other drugs these plant-derived compounds are usd to treat other cancers including Hodgkin's disease.

This great success story stimulated a world-wide investigation of centuries old folk medicine and the consumer usage of herbal preparations, mainly teas, in the United States.

In the late 1970's, the interest in herbs seemed to have waned. A new decade was beginning, one that would lead mankind into the new century, a century of high technology, and herbs were assigned an archaic aura. The new President ushered in a glittering decade. Hippies were dead. "Natural"was passé and all that glittered was thought to be golden.

As the 1980's matured, and the romance with surface realities reevaluated, people once again wondered if nature, that most unfickle phenomenon, might not yet hold some answers for mankind's infirmities.

In 1990, we see a new and wonderful outcry to preserve our natural environment. There is a realization that the rainforests are a repository of hundreds if not thousands of potential medicines. Herbal preparations are being tried, for the first time by some, again by many.

AIDS will not go away.

The virus keeps changing form too adeptly for the chemists who create synthetic drugs. Yet here again nature may hold an answer in the form of an apparently remarkable compound derived from an herb, a type of Chinese cucumber (see entry pg. 237).

Herbs in the 21st Century

While estimates of the percent of new prescriptions in the U.S. which contain an active ingredient originating in nature run between 25 and 40 percent, these compounds represent a very short list with very wide usage. Very few new compounds derived from nature have entered the American pharmaceutical marketplace in the past 20 years. The same few developed years ago reappear in new permutations and combinations.

The lack of patent protection, not the lack of effiacy, keeps the pharmaceutical giants in the United States from investing in the development of drugs from plants. Herb companies and smaller pharmaceutical firms have been and will continue to meet the growing consumer demand for nature's remedies, however. In Japan, France and some developing nations, drugs from herbs will become big business.

This is not to create the mistaken idea that the United States will not take part in the coming herb-based revolution in medicine. Currently, pharmaceuticals derived from plants are a $10 billion business in the U.S. and this is just a baseline for medicine from botanicals. By the middle of the next decade, we can expect vast new markets for this class of products, because over 200 research groups worldwide are engaged in creating new medicinals from nature. Surprisingly, the largest number of these research groups are based in the U.S. (97 out of a total 209 world wide research groups are U.S. based).

Europeans have long been able to purchase herbal-based medicinal preparations on an OTC ("over-the-counter") basis. These remedies are utilized as a second-line treatment immediately following alterations in diet, a first-line approach. Such herbal preparations are tried before people turn to physicians for third-line treatments, the potent pharmaceuticals.

In America, our first and second-lines of treating common ailments have largely disappeared. People have been taught to "see a doctor" for the smallest ache, often coming home with a potent pharmaceutical "prescription" just as likely to cause harm as to effect a cure.

With the growth of the herbal industry Americans will join the Europeans in taking charge of their own health-care. The wildly escalating costs of medical care and the legion of tragic iatrogenic effects of prescription drugs have given new meaning to the old saying, "Physician, heal thyself!"

When I was younger, an older, wiser man said to me, "If you don't know how to take care of your health by the time you're forty, you deserve the doctors!"

Herbal remedies are coming of age in America, and none too soon.

Where the Breakthroughs Hide

Owing to their great history of usage of natural products, we can expect China and India to produce many of our future herbal pharmaceuticals. India has three principle systems of traditional medicine: the Ayurveda, Unani, and Siddha. The herbal treatments utilized by adherents in their native India are attracting the attentions of pharmaceutical firms world wide. The government of India is actively investing in the analysis of traditional herbal remedies while Japanese, European, and U.S. corporations are reaching research agreements with Indian and Chinese drug companies to try to capitalize on the commercial potential of these plants.

The hundreds of plants with medicinal properties from India and the additional hundreds from China add up to a powerful starting position for corporations investing in this new interest in traditional herbal medicine. This new interest is based, in part, on the advent of biotechnology. Until these new technologies were evolved in research laboratories only seven major drugs could be synthesized for less cost than they could be extracted from wild plants. Biotechnology companies having failed in the large part to produce sufficient new compounds to justify their immense start up costs, have suddenly "discovered" natural products. Medicinal plants as employed in traditional medical systems offer almost unlimited commercial potential, particularly for biotechnology companies with the proper expertise.

But, it is important to also remember the vast flora of the United States and the traditional Amerind usage of many of these plants for medicinal purposes. Hundreds of plants of North America have potential medicinal value. By reviewing the traditional ethno-pharmacology of Native Americans and subjecting the top 20 candidates to intense pharmaceutical screening, we might expect to discover several new plant medicines of potential benefit to world medicine.

Bali Hai

Our quest for healing plants will inevitably take us to the world's tropical rainforests. Seen by some as the alveoli of Earth's atmosphere, the forest giants reach upwards of several hundred feet, exchanging molecules with low passing clouds.

Thousands of novel medicinal compounds have been isolated from species of the tropics. Rainforests are but one repository of species of potential medicinal value. The low creepers found along seashores, trees and shrubs which live half-way submerged in swamps, such as the mangrove, may also hold promising compounds. Shrubs and vines of the dry inland valleys are not to be overlooked, many have adapted to their environmental niche producing interesting alkaloids, glycosides and saponins.

I remember accidentally slashing my thumb with

a machete on a plant-hunting expedition to Viti Levu, Fiji in 1975. My guide immediately gathered a handful of common "weed," chewed it for a moment and applied it to my fast-bleeding finger. In a matter of seconds the bleeding was arrested. The pain was also eliminated and the wound healed without infection or scarring.

Here we have a "weed" with almost amazing properties and with almost unlimited commercial application. It had long been used to treat wounds in Fiji and, as I later discovered, has similar pantropical applications.

Being constantly wet the rainforest ecosystem is an ideal place for fungi. The people suffer their share of fungal infections and have developed remedies with which to counter them. *Candida* is a common infection of newborn infants, in the form of thrush. Native Fijian practitioners have long utilized a hot water infusion of leaves of *Terminalia* species (tropical almond) also known as Mathake and with great success.

Perhaps this and other species found only on tropical islands hold future breakthroughs which will parallel those forthcoming from Asia, India and the Americas.

The Question of "Standarized Herbs"

There's a potency war brewing. The bottom-line, however, may prove that the 1970's aphorism "small is beautiful" or "less is more," is the answer. Simply upping the percentage content of an active constituent in an herbal preparation may yet prove harmful.

For now, the answer, from the editor's point of view, is to welcome standardization and to proceed with caution—making standardized herbal extracts *only* from plants which have been subjected to safety and efficacy studies. Examples include herbs such as ginseng, ginkgo, ginger, milk thistle, echinaces, turmeric, essential oil of orange (d-limonene), valerian, St. John's Wort, horsetail, bilberry, and others with good efficacy and safety data.

Standardization was introduced to counter the negative effects of poor quality control which plagued the herb industry in the 1970's. With standardized herbs we can reliably count on receiving the same quantity of one or more active constituents per unit taken. Thus, one capsule of milk thistle said to contain 80% silymarin—the chief active principle—can be reliably assumed to contain this consistent quantity.

In nature, herbs vary in their content of active constituents. Soils, climates, harvesting methods, processing, packaging and storage circumstances all affect the relative potency of a finished herbal product. When an active principle in the finished product is so identified on the label, the miscellaneous subjective effects can be objectively controlled, and the consumer can rely upon receiving a stated quantity and balance of activity.

A reasonable course of action, at this stage of knowledge, would be to proceed cautiously, as stated above, standardizing active constituents of herbs with well-established safety and efficacy. By also including the whole plant in the final product, some measure of the inherent natural "checks and balances" or synergism will be retained. With this method, we see an *enhancement* of natural medicinal activity rather than an imbalanced drug-effect.

Increased control of active ingredients, and a general increase in sophistication throughout the industry, coupled with greatly rising demand for herbal products at the consumer level, leads me to conclude that *being bullish on herbs is a very safe course, indeed.*

ALOE VERA
(Aloe vera)

***Wound Healing: Oral & Topical Activity of
Aloe Vera. R. H. Davis, et al.*** Journal of the American Podiatric Medical Assoc., 79(11):559-562, Nov.
1989.:

Ever since the age of Cleopatra, when Aloe was
used to treat burns, this remarkable plant has enjoyed
popular acclaim and wide usage. I first learned of this
plant's properties in 1968 when I read it was being
utilized to treat radiation burns by a research group
at the University of Pennsylvania. Subsequent trials
of my own demonstrated what folklore had long told,
Aloe was an effective, safe, inexpensive treatment for
burns and wounds. The authors' write that *A. vera*
improves wound healing when administered either
orally or topically. "It not only contributes to a
decrease in wound diameter, but also leads to better
vascularity and healthier granulation tissue. The fact
that Aloe is effective orally suggests that it is not broken down by the gastrointestinal tract and is absorbed
into the blood. Aloe possibly improves wound healing by increasing the availability of oxygen and by
increasing the synthesis and the strength of collagen.
Aloe vera has become a subject of scientific study
concerning inflammation and wound healing. As
knowledge about Aloe increases, significant benefits
of a practical nature in the management of healing
wounds can be expected." This ancient healing plant
should remain forever one of humankind's most
important frontline remedies against wounds.

***An Anti-Complementary Polysaccharide with
Immunological Adjuvant Activity from the Leaf
Parenchyma Gel of*** Aloe vera. *L. A.'t Hart, Al J.
J. van den Berg, L. Kuis, H. van Dijk, and R. P.
Labadie.:*

In another study on *Aloe* by a group of researchers
in the Netherlands, immune-enhancing activity was
discovered. Beginning with the traditional medical
usages for this plant, these workers purified an aqueous gel-extract. A "highly active polysaccharide fraction was isolated" from the *Aloe* gel. This component
proved active in the production of antibodies and also
stimulated another aspect of the immune response
(i.e., complementary activity). The authors compare
the effectiveness of this gel fraction of *Aloe* with *dex-*

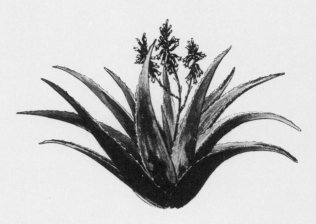

Aloe Vera

tran sulphate, a sulphated polysaccharide found
principally in certain seaweeds. (For about 40 years
Japanese researchers have been testing dextran sulphate and ably demonstrating its anti-tumor and
anti-clotting properties.) The known healing effects
of *Aloe vera* on infected wounds are thought to be
explained by the local activation of complement
which is thought to lead to an influx of monocytes and
PMN's to the injured area.

ANGELICA
(Angelica sinensis) A. acutiloba

***Yamada H, Komiyama K, Kiyohara H, Cyong J-
C, Hirakawa Y & Otsuka Y. Structural characterization and antitumor activity of a pectic polysaccharide from the roots of*** Angelica acutiloba.:
Planta Medica 56: 182-186, 1990.

Angelica acutiloba is also known in plant therapy
circles as *Angelica sinensis*, commonly referred to as
Dong Quai. The root is a broadly recognized medicinal extract used in the management of gynecological
disease in Sino-Japanese herbal medicine. The polysaccharide fraction from *A. acutiloba* has received a
large amount of research attention. A polysaccharide
is a large chain composed of single sugar units, of
either the same or different chemical structure. Crude
polysaccharide fractions from *A. acutiloba* also contain small amounts of protein, and have demon-

strated immunostimulating activities. These include the induction of interferon production, stimulation of immune cell proliferation, antitumor activity, and anti-complementary activity. The recurrent question in these studies has been whether all of these immunomodulating activities can be ascribed to a single, or to a class of polysaccharide fractions. In the current investigations, Yamada et al. sought to purify and characterize a polysaccharide fraction with anti-tumor activity.

The authors performed an initial hot water extraction step upon dried *A. acutiloba* roots, yielding an extract that was 41% of the weight of the original dried plant material. Further extraction with methanol and ethanol, dissolution in water, and dialysis produced a crude polysaccharide fraction yield that was 5% of the dried root weight. This crude fraction was identified as AR-1.

AR-1 was further fractionated into three additional fractions, leading to a total of four fractions (AR-1, AR-2, AR-3, and AR-4). The major fraction was AR-2, which also possessed the lowest protein content.

The anti-tumor activity of the polysaccharide fractions of A. acutiloba was evaluated. Injection of AR-1 into tumor-bearing animals led to significant increases in life span in a number of different tumor types. Comparison among the 4 polysaccharide fractions for antitumor activity in one tumor type indicated the AR-4 fraction to possess the greatest potency. In a previous study, Yamada et al. showed that the AR-4 fraction also possessed the greatest interferon-producing capacity of the 4 polysaccharide fractions tested, with only the AR-4 fraction producing any increase in interferon levels in culture. However, the concentration required to achieve an elevation in interferon levels was quite high. (Yamada H, et al. Studies on polysaccharides from *Angelica acutiloba. Planta Medica 1984. 163- 167).* Additional fractionation of AR-4 was performed in the current study, producing 7 subfractions (AR-4A - AR-4G). Of these seven fractions, AR-4E showed the most potent anti-tumor activity, measured by per cent increase in life span.

Complement is a family of serum proteins involved in the binding and destruction of foreign substances (antigens) that have been recognized by the immune system. Complement is fixed to an antigen, which

then facilitates its destruction (lysis). The ability of *A. acutiloba* polysaccharide subfractions to inhibit complementary activity was greatest with AR-4B, with AR-4E being intermediate. This revealed a disparity between anti-tumor activity and anti-complementary activity.

A third subfractionation was performed, using AR-4E as the parent fraction. This step produced four more subfractions (AR-4E1 - AR-4E4), with AR-4E2 having the greatest anti-tumor potential. This third generation fraction was composed of 87% hexose-type sugars e.g. galactose, arabinose, and rhamnose. The authors performed extensive analysis of the chemical properties of this latter fraction, leading them to conclude that the structure of the side chain of the polysaccharide fraction determines its anti-tumor activity, but not its anti-complementary activity.

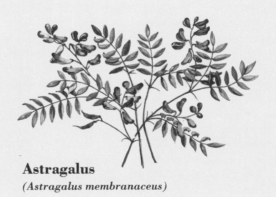

Astragalus
(Astragalus membranaceus)

ASTRAGALUS
(Astragalus membranaceus)

Chu, D-T, Wong WL & Mavligit GM.
Immunotherapy with Chinese medicinal herbs I.
Immune restoration of local xenogeneic graft-versus-host reaction in cancer patients by fractionated Astragalus membranaceus in vitro. Journal of Clinical and Laboratory Immunology 25: 119, 1988.:

Astragalus is another commonly used traditional herb in Chinese medicine. Certain species of Astraga-

230

lus are the source of the widely used food additive, tragacanth gum. *Astragalus membranaceus* has been screened for its immunomodulating activity, and found to augment the proliferation of mononuclear (MNC) white blood cells (macrophages and lymphocytes) *in vitro*. Recent studies originating out of the M.D. Anderson Hospital and Tumor Institute in Houston, Texas have yielded a stronger focus on the immunomodulating scope of *Astragalus membranaceus*.

As with many plant extracts, certain fractions may possess biological activities that are in direct contrast with those of other fractions. Chu et al. performed several extraction procedures and manipulations on air-dried roots of A. membranaceus, ultimately producing 8 different fractions, fraction 7 being the original crude extract.

The authors used a testing model developed in their laboratory, designed to evaluate the competence of human T-lymphocytes in attacking foreign cells (rat skin). The animals were rendered immunosuppressed, due to the administration of cyclophosphamide, a potent immunosuppressive agent routinely used in human organ transplantation procedures. This minimized the influence of the animal's immune system upon the actions of the implanted human cells.

Individuals with various types of cancer, and "normal" controls served as blood donors for MNC's. MNC's were treated with one of the eight fractions derived from the original roots of *A. mamgranaceus*. Fractions 2, 3, 7, and 8 displayed significant immunomodulating activity in cells from controls in this system. Fractions 3, 7 (the original crude extract) and 8 all produced a significant increase in the immunocompetence of the animals. However, fraction 2 led to a further reduction of immune function, indicating this fraction to have *immunosuppressive* actions. The remaining fractions had no observable immunorestorative effects.

The treatment of MNC's from cancer patients revealed additional striking results. Only fractions 3, 7, and 8 were used in this part of the study. Five of the 13 cancer patients' MNC's experienced immune restoration in their T-cell activity. The MNC's from the remaining 8 patients had intact T-cell function before incubation with the fractions; following incubation, T-cell function was actually increased.

The authors continue by pointing out that the immune responsivity seen in most of the Astragalus-treated cells from cancer patients was greater than that observed in the cells from untreated normal donors. Cancer patients' cells treated with fractions 3 and 8 displayed the greatest degree of immune restoration, being significantly greater than that of untreated normal control values. Treatment with fraction 7 did not produce a significantly greater response.

Comparison of the stimulating effects of fractions 3, 7, and 8 on MNC's from both cancer and normal donors revealed fraction 3 to possess a higher stimulating activity in cancer patients than in normals. No difference existed between the two groups for the other two fractions. Fraction 3 also proved to have superior immunorestorative actions in cancer patients alone, relative to the crude extract (7), and the extract derivative (8).

A companion study evaluated the ability of immunosupressed animals treated with fraction 3 to generate an immune response against untreated human MNC's (Chu D-T, et al. **Immunotherapy with Chinese medicinal herbs. II. Reversal of cyclophosphamide-induced immune suppression by administration of fractionated *Astragalus membranaceus* in vivo. Journal of Clinical and Laboratory Immunology 25: 125-129, 1988).** This is similar to a reversal of the previous experiments, where the animals T-cells are tested in their capacity to attack human T-cells. They found fraction 3 to completely reverse the effects of cyclophosphamide-induced immunosuppression upon their test system. Although fraction 3 was administered intravenously, it is very likely that oral administration of a carefully fractionated Astragalus preparation would also exert significant immunorestorative activity in such conditions as cancer and AIDS.

BILBERRY
(Vaccinium Myrtillus)

Here is a common fruit with quite uncommon benefits. The "European Blueberry," "Whortleberry" or just plain "Blueberry" (in Europe) is eaten fresh or cooked. Even a wine is made from the berries, "Heidelbeerwein" or "Heidelbeersekt."

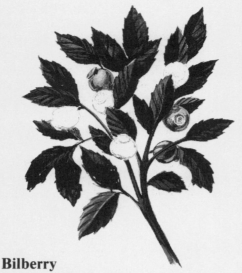

Bilberry
(Vaccinium Myrtillus)

Few people realized that these delicious fruits improved night-time visual acuity until tests with extracts were conducted. Folklore, of course, supported this claim, and another writer on herbs reports that "RAF pilots swore that the intake of bilberry jam prior to night missions significantly improved dark adaptation and visual acuity" (Mowry, 1989).

What does improved vision have to do with the theme of inflammation? In a nutshell it has been discovered that the anthocyanins contained in bilberry act to prevent capillary fragility and inhibit platelet aggregation. This is so because the anthocyanins affect prostaglandins (Morazzoni, 1986). Interestingly, the endothelial layer of our blood vessels is generated from prostaglandin endoperoxides which may be an *unstable* prostacyclin (PGI$_2$). This compound inhibits platelet aggregation and is so thought to prevent the first step in the formation of a thrombus or blood clot. In experiments with rats, it was found that bilberry extracts given orally actually *increased* such PGI$_2$ activity released from arterial tissue. This finding coincides with a previous discovery that these anthocyanins stimulate the release of vasodilator prostaglandin *in vitro*. What this boils down to is that as well as preventing platelets from sticking together these compounds from bilberry have "potential for the prevention of thrombosis" (Timberlake, 1988, in Cody, 1988).

This may be of interest to diabetics who often suffer from thickened capillaries caused by increased collagen. Lagrue *et al.* (1979) ran a chemical trial on 54 diabetic patients and found that 500 to 600 mg of bilberry extract per day, for 8 to 33 months, almost totally normalized this collagen thickening. The same extract proved to exert a "significant preventative and curative anti-ulcer activity" when given to rats (Cristoni & Magistretti, 1987). Apparently, bilberry anthocyanosides have multiple beneficial effects; they act on blood capillaries to increase their resistance and reduce their permeability. They speed up the regeneration of retinal purple and adaptation to darkness when given by injection in tests on rabbits (Alfieri & Sole, 1964).

Many clinical tests have shown that bilberry anthocyanosides given orally to humans improve vision in healthy people and also help treat people with eye diseases such as pigmentary retinitis (Fiorini *et al.*, 1965; Jüneman, 1968; and others).

Toxicology reports are especially promising regarding the anthocyanins. Tests in rats, mice and rabbits showed *no* abnormalities or toxicity (Omori, 1973, and others). Even pregnant women who were given extracts of bilberry (and vitamin E) were seen to have fewer varices and various blood problems. The study author concluded that the extract "was well tolerated and no side effects were found in either the mother or the infant" (Bastide, 1968).

BUPLEURUM (SHOSAIKOTO)
(Bupleurum falcatum)

Amagaya S & Ogihara Y. Effects of Shosaikoto, an Oriental herbal medicinal mixture, on restraint-stressed mice. **Journal of Ethnopharmacology 28: 357, 1990.:**

Stress can be of a non-specific origin, or can involve specific physical or psychological factors capable of producing a disease state. The ability of stress to cause disease may be related to its ability to suppress the immune system. Numerous plant extracts have been described as having powerful anti-stress activity (adaptogenic).

In Oriental traditional medicine, certain herbal mixtures containing the plant *Bupleurum falcatum*

(Bupf) are used for the treatment of chronic inflammatory and autoimmune diseases, and in the management of certain neurological disorders. Shosaikoto is a Bupf-containing (29% by weight) extract reported previously by these authors to possess immunomodulating activity, stimulating immune cell activity in immune suppressed or normal mice, and suppressing immune responsivity in hyperimmune rats. The formula also includes *Piniella ternata (21%)*, *Scutellaria baicalensis*, *Zizyphus vulgaris*, and Korean ginseng (12.5% each), licorice root (8%), and ginger root (4%). The current study sought to evaluate the effects of Shosaikoto on stress-induced immunosuppression in mice.

Adrenal gland enlargement is one of the hallmarks of continuous exposure to a significant stressor. Indeed, adrenal glands from stressed rats in this study increased in weight by approximately 13%. However, two different Shosaikoto oral dosing schedules (equivalent to two and ten times the normal human dose) had no effect upon adrenal gland weight. These authors cite some of their previous work, which found that Shosaikoto stimulated the pituitary-adrenal cortex axis, leading to elevations in blood corticosterone levels and *increases* in adrenal gland weight, in normal mice. Diazepam (Valium™), a powerful anti-anxiety drug, also had no effect upon adrenal gland weight.

Shosaikoto was able to restore the immunosuppression resultant to the physical stress, although only at the lower dosage. These animals showed a significantly enhanced immune response to foreign red blood cells, relative to the untreated or high dose Shosaikato groups. Conversely, only the higher dosage of the plant extract combination was able to restore rectal temperature to normal following the final exposure to the stress. The authors conclude that Shosaikoto may act as an immunorestorative agent via its direct immunomodulating and/or anti-stress activities. Additionally, they suggest that Shosaikoto also acts upon the central nervous system in a manner similar to that of Valium.

A companion paper by the same authors tested the effects of Shosaikoto upon age-induced amnesia in rats (Amagaya S, et al. **Effects of Shosaikato, an Oriental herbal medicinal mixture, on age-induced amnesia in rats.** *Journal of Ethnopharmacology 28: 349-356, 1990).* Besides mitigating the age-related increases in body weight seen in control animals, aged animals fed a Shosaikoto-enriched diet also displayed higher kidney weights, equal to those seen in the young animals. Shosaikoto-treated animals also displayed learning response times significantly lesser than those of the control old animals, and equal to those of the young animals. Additionally, Shosaikoto appeared to reduce age-related memory loss, preserving memory function virtually identical to that seen in the young animals.

Analysis of neurochemicals from the brains of the various groups indicated that Shosaikato-treated animals had higher levels of dopamine, found to be low within the brains of Alzheimer's disease patients. The authors suggest in their conclusion that the reputed beneficial effects of Shosaikoto in Alzheimer's may be due to its abililty to elevate brain dopamine levels, possibly leading to improved memory and cognitive processing. A detail meriting attention is the amount of Shosaikoto fed to the animals in this study. These animals received only half of the low dose, and one-tenth of the high dose, of Shosaikoto given to the animals in the stress study described above. The effects of higher doses upon neurological function/chemistry warrants further investigation.

Combining the results of these two papers, it appears justified to state that the components of Shosaikoto act as biological response modifiers in the immune and central nervous systems. Their promise as immunomodulating and neuroactivating agents awaits further studies.

These structure-activity relationship studies are crucial to the understanding of the specific component(s) responsible for the biological effects of a given plant extract, and in the development of powerful plant drug extracts with a high degree of specificity. Reducing a plant extract to a single molecule or compound does indeed lead one into the world of conventional medicine, as many drugs currently used were once derived from plant sources. However, this process also provides a marker, or series of markers, whereby crude plant extracts can be objectively assessed for their content of active principles.

BUTCHER'S BROOM
(Ruscus aculeatus)

Oral contraceptives are made from steroids derived in large part from the plant kingdom. So too are other important steroids, such as cortisone, testosterone and estradiol. Thanks to the pioneering efforts of many scientists who investigated the plant world for starter compounds these synthetic drugs are now available at very low prices.

The saponin glycosides found in some plants are the basis for the production of many useful steroid pharmaceuticals. During the course of investigations into finding new saponins, two new sapogenins were discovered in the rhizomes of butcher's broom. These were named Ruscogenin and Neo-ruscogenin and are chemically similar to diosgenin, the principle steroid starter compound found in Mexican yams (various species of *Dioscorea*) (Caujolle *et al.*, 1953; Moscarella, 1953).

This member of the Lily family has very active chemical constituents, saponins, similar to those found in licorice and sarsaparilla. That this evergreen shrub, native to the Mediterranean region, has been found to contain highly active chemical constituents would not come as a surprise to ancient peoples. While the stiff, leaf-like twigs were once used by butchers to whisk scraps from their cutting blocks, ancient Mediterranean healers utilized the rhizome for a wide variety of circulatory and inflammatory disorders. Varicose veins were cured with this species according to the Roman scholar Pliny (c. 60 A.D.), while in more ancient years Greek doctors reported curing "swelling" with "the miracle herb." Horse-chestnut is also effective for varicose veins and edema of the legs.

Relatively recent pharmacological findings indicate vasoconstrictive and anti-inflammatory properties (Tyler, 1988; Caujolle, 1953; Cahn, 1964; Capra, 1972). Tests conducted on animals by Capra (above reference) showed that the Ruscogenins have good anti-inflammatory activity. As for toxicity, tests in the mouse and rat showed that when administered orally, these compounds from Butcher's broom were well tolerated (Capra, 1972).

The saponins it contains constricts the veins and decreases the permeability of capillaries. Consequently several writers state that this so-called "phle-

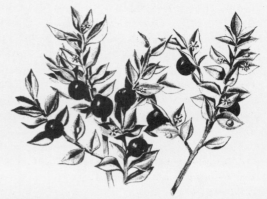

Butcher's Broom
(Ruscus aculeatus)

botherapeutic agent" (Tyler, 1988) is utilized to treat disorders of circulation, such as varicose veins and hemorrhoids (Chabanon, 1976; Marcelon, 1983).

Beneath the stiff twigs of this plant long employed for mundane purposes courses chemical constituents with profound effects.

CACAO
(Theobroma cacao)

Theobroma, the Latin name for the chocolate plant, means "food of the Gods." Montezuma, the Aztec emperor, so loved the chocolate beverage prepared from the seeds of this small tree that he drank fifty jars of it a day. The royal beverage was flavored with vanilla and other spices, then beaten to a foam and served in gold goblets.

During the Spanish occupation of Mexico, bags of cacao beans were a recognized form of currency. The Spaniards spread this fabled product throughout the West Indies and later brought it to Africa and the Orient. Cacao was introduced to Europe about the same time as tea and coffee and at first was considered a great luxury to be enjoyed only by the wealthy.

Cacao trees are often found growing wild beneath larger trees along riverbanks. When cultivated, they are grown directly from seeds planted in the ground. Pods appear on the trunk and lower branches in the fourth year. Inside each of these pods are about forty nutritious and flavorful seeds from which chocolate and cocoa are produced. They contain up to 50 percent oil, known as cocoa butter, 15 percent starch, 15 percent protein, and theobromine, a mild stimulant.

To produce milk chocolate, the beans are fermented, roasted and ground; then sugar, milk, vanilla and extra cocoa butter are added. Cocoa is made by pressing out most of the cocoa butter after roasting the seeds. Chocolate is rich and sweet because it contains cocoa butter and sugar, while cocoa is dry and bitter.

Chocolate is produced and exported mainly by Ghana and Nigeria, and some of the world's commercial crop originates in Brazil and other parts of South America. Tropical regions in Asia and the Pacific contribute a small amount as well.

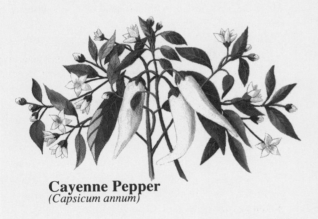

Cayenne Pepper
(Capsicum annum)

CAYENNE
(Capsicum frutescens)

The stimulant effect of the common chili pepper is reflected in its use as a condiment in foods, with a resulting promotion of digestion. As a medicine, cayenne pepper is a general stimulant, and has been reported of value in the treatment of dyspepsia, diarrhea, and prostration. It has been used as a remedy for nausea from seasickness. As a gargle, the seeds are valued as a treatment for sore throat and hoarseness. In the treatment of ague (painful swelling of the face due to decayed or ulcerated teeth or a cold), inhalation of the steam of Cayenne and vinegar, coupled with a small mouth poultice containing one teaspoon of cayenne pepper, will reportedly afford relief by producing a free discharge of saliva.

Cayenne pepper acts as a rubefacient when applied externally, and as a stimulant internally, due to the presence of *capsaicin*, which is the "hot principle" in the fruits of this plant. Oleoresin of *Capsicum* is still used in the preparation of a number of popular proprietary products to be applied locally for the relief of sore muscles, and produces the desired effect by mildly irritating the surface of the skin, which causes an increased blood flow to the area of application. The increased blood flow results in reduced inflammation of the affected area. In a recent letter to *The Lancet*, it was reported that topical applications of *capsaicin* (a phenol present in hot peppers) cream was successfully used to completely alleviate the severe stump pain experienced by a middle-aged female diabetic. This double-amputee patient subsequently underwent a placebo trial, where it was proved that this cream completely relieved the pain, the placebo having no effect. Given the successful outcome of this extreme example, it would be reasonable to expect *capsaicin* creams to yield beneficial topical results when applied to various painful neuropathies. (Rayner, *et al.*, 1989).

Further information regarding the anti-inflammatory property of capsaicin is revealed in the paper, "Direct Evidence for Neurogenic Inflammation and its Prevention by Denervation and by Pretreatment with Capsaicin." (Jancs, 1967), as quoted in Dr. Garcia-Leme's book, *Hormones and Inflammation*, 1989. In studies with rats given capsaicin systemically, the results proved, "sensory nerve endings became insensitive to chemical pain stimuli for a long time. Neurogenic inflammation cannot be elicited in animals pretreated with capsaicin." Additionally, two Indian scientists recently reported, "Long-term treatment with capsaicin 'desensitizes' the membrane against various gaseous irritant-induced free radical damage." (De & Ghosh, 1989). They found that this compound from chili peppers protects lung tissue (in experiments with rats) by increasing superoxide dismutase (SOD), catalase (CAT) and peroxidase (POD) activities. In as yet unpublished studies by the same authors, pretreatment with capsaicin also protects the lung of rats from nitrogen dioxide and formaldehyde-induced free radical damage.

It must be noted that the above reported *protective* effects of capsaicin only occurs with *short-term treatment*. Whether this implies that capsaicin should be used sparingly and intermittently will only be known when human studies are conducted.

Interestingly, both cayenne pepper preparations and the active principle *capsaicin* have been shown in humans and in animals to stimulate the production of gastric juices, resulting in improved digestion.

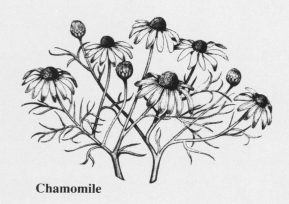

Chamomile

CHAMOMILE
(Anthemis nobilis)

Schreiber A, Carle R & Reinhard E. On the accumulation of apigenin in chamomile flowers. Planta Medica 56: 179-181, 1990.:

Chamomile flowers are a time-tested plant remedy with calming and anti-inflammatory actions. Current research directions in the manufacturing of plant extracts are focusing upon the production of a consistent preparation of known composition. Chamomile flowers contain a wide variety of flavonoids that have received a great deal of research attention.

A principal flavonoid found in chamomile flowers is apigenin. As with virtually all flavonoids, apigenin may be present in the native plant as both the free flavonoid (aglycone), and as a flavonoid linked to different sugar molecules (glycosides) at varying positions on its chemical structure.

Previous studies designed to evaluate the apigenins in chamomile flowers were performed on samples of dried chamomile plants. Usually chamomile flowers are *dried* after harvesting and before extraction at a temperature of 40° C (104° F). Even careful drying changes the original flavonoid pattern in the plant.

In the current study, Schreiber et al. have attempted to measure the effect of different handling procedures on the formation of apigenin-family compounds in post-harvest treated *fresh* chamomile flowers. Using different combinations of shock freezing in liquid nitrogen, slow cooling, thawing, drying at various temperatures, and storing under different conditions, they found a great variance in the flavonoid makeup of chamomile flowers.

The salient finding from their studies is that free apigenin does not occur in the living flower, as previously suggested from studies using dried flowers. This applies to both the flower heads AND the ligulate florets. Conversely, fresh flowers that were shock frozen in liquid nitrogen, and then thawed and kept at 50° C (122° F) for 2 hours, displayed remarkable increases in the content of the aglycone. Drying alone (40° C) proved to be a suitable, albeit weak method of inducing the production of free apigenin, confirming the results of previous studies which had spuriously suggested the occurrence of free apigenin in the native flower parts.

Apigenin does appear to be one of the principal pharmacologically active compounds found in chamomile. However, Schreiber et al. state that the amount of apigenin present within a commercial preparation is not of clinical nor economical significance; due to the ability of the intestinal tract to produce the aglycone from apigenin glycosides. They refer to classical studies performed in the 1960's which defined the prominent role of the intestinal microflora in breaking the glycosidic bonds between a flavonoid and a sugar molecule. This microflora-mediated cleavage yields the free aglycone, and its glycoside. Schreiber et al. conclude that apigenin glycosides are bioactive precursors to the flavonoid apigenin, which is released by human intestinal microbial enzymes specific for apigenin-glycoside bonds. Additionally, they state that a product possessing a low apigenin content indicates a higher quality extract.

The use of chamomile as an apigenin precursor source expands the classical application of this plant as a medicinal agent. Apigenin is a nontoxic and non-mutagenic flavonoid also found in certain vegetables, with significant potential as being a cancer preventive agent *(Wei H, Tye L, Bresnick E & Birt DF. Inhibitory effect of apigenin, a plant flavonoid, on epidermal orntihine decarboxylase and skin tumor promotion in mice. Cancer Res 50: 499-502, 1990).* Further studies detailing the bioavailability of apigenin from chamomile flower extracts of varying apigenin glycoside content, and its chemopreventive effects, will undoubtedly reveal practical and exciting directions to apply in the future.

CHINESE CUCUMBER
(Trichosanthes Kirilowii)

The Source of Compound Q Chinese Cucumber *(Trichosanthes Kirilowii)* Anti-AIDS: Hope or Hype?

The hottest herb of the past 40 years is a species of Chinese cucumber which is the source of the drug GLQ223. Not since *Rauwolfia* (Indian snakeroot) was introduced from Ayurvedic medicine as an anti-hypertensive in the 1950's under the name reserpine has an herbal remedy generated so much hope and hype.

Now it is true that the plant itself is not being tested for anti-AIDS activity. The drug, GLQ223, is a highly purified version of trichosanthin, which is a protein isolated from root tubers of *T. Kirilowii* from southern China.

Exciting preliminary results show that this plant extract, "Compound Q," selectively destroys macrophages infected with the human immunodeficiency virus type 1 (HIV-1). Infected T cells are thought to be the major sites of the virus in the human body. In addition, the CD4+T cells have been found to be a reservoir for latent HIV-1 viruses.

When Michael McGrath, M.D., at San Francisco General Hospital, first tested the drug he thought it might destroy all T cells in the body. Nevertheless, he deemed this radical treatment worth the risk. Then, quite by chance Dr. McGrath discovered that this remarkable plant derived drug killed *only* infected T-cells!

Here we had a *selective* agent to try against AIDS.

In China trichosanthin is used to bring about mid-trimester abortion *(abortifacient).* It achieves this by selectively killing specialized cells found in the uterus. This drug is also used (again in China) as a treatment for choriocarcinoma, a cancer of these cells found in the uterus. Apparently, trichosanthin is either selectively absorbed by these cancer cells or it has selective antiviral activity.

As testing of this promising drug continues, people want to know; "Can I take the plant itself;" "is a hot-water infusion of the root safe and effective;" "will this plant work against other viral infections;" does Chinese cucumber somehow stimulate the immune system"?

First, it is important to emphasize here that Compound Q, which is presently only available from China, is very dangerous! It must *not be* utilized without strict and expert medical supervision owing to potential side-effects and toxicity.

Trichosanthin is chemically similar to ricin toxin, from castor beans *(Ricinus communis).* Ricin, you may recall, is one of the most potent naturally-occurring toxins. Both trichosanthin and ricin belong to a family of proteins known as single-chain ribosome-inactivating agents. In simpler terms, these highly active compounds stop all division. They therefore have the capacity of stopping the division of *healthy* cells—and they can bring about death.

It is important to recall that it is easy to kill infected monocytes with many different compounds. Chloroquine, an antimalarial, for example, is an effective agent. St John's Wort *(Hypericum perforatum)* has also been shown to be active against the AIDS virus in *test-tube experiments.* To be effective against the virus, in *a human,* relatively high concentrations of hypericin, the active ingredient, would be required—perhaps at a toxic level. At this time, we do not know if GLQ223 is any more effective that choloroquine or hypericin. Further, "Compound Q" may prove to be too large to reach the infected cells, its potency has not been established and it may also kill healthy cells.

To develop an immunotoxin for an HIV infected cell, highly specialized procedures are required. The envelope glycoproteins, GP160, for example, are found on the surface of HIV-infected cells and are the target receptors for immunotoxins. We do not know, however, if GLQ223 reaches these receptors.

Moreover, it has not yet been determined if trichosanthin is even extracted when Chinese cucumber roots are boiled. So we do not yet know if a "tea"

237

of this interesting species would have any medicinal properties, let alone be capable of killing viruses or stimulating immunity.

Further, assuming that small quantities of trichosanthin were found to occur in a hot-water extract, as an herbal tea, we do not know if this agent would be *absorbed* from the gastrointestinal tract. (It may prove to work only via the injectable route.)

For these reasons, we *cannot* recommend the self-administration of extracts of this species. Only careful human trials of the drug will answer the many questions which remain outstanding.

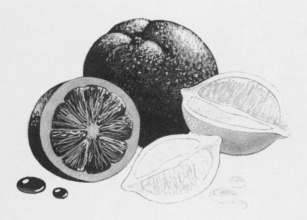

CITRUS (various species)

Here is a well-known class of essential oils with many newly discovered properties. Limonene is the major component of the essential oil of orange and other citrus fruits. It also occurs widely in the plant kingdom, particularly in those species producing essential oils, flavors and spices.

This compound belongs to a class of natural compounds known as terpenes, soon to equal the bioflavonoids and carotenoids in their applications.

About ten animal studies have been published which show that dietary limonene (the d-isomer, or d-limonene) is able to lower the incidence of chemically-induced cancers as well as delay their appearance. Elson and colleagues at the University of Wisconsin are currently the leaders in this field. In one study, they demonstrated that dietary d-limonene

markedly reduced dimethylbenzanthracene-induced mammary cancers. The dosage used in this study was 1000 parts per million, or 1 gram per kg of diet. [NOTE: humans eat about 1/2 kg per day, which translates to about 500 mg of d-limonene per day.] Using this same model system, they subsequently showed that the essential oil of orange (85% d-limonene) was more effective than pure d-limonene in preventing tumor formation. Thus, naturally-occurring terpenes in orange oil other than d-limonenes also possess anticancer activity. Further investigations by this group revealed that dietary d-limonene is effective in reversing preformed tumors, as evidenced by an increase in the tumor regression rate. Finally, Elson and associates recently observed that dietary d-limonene was effective in reducing the number of chemically-induced mammary tumors in rats when provided either during the initiation phase or during the promotion/progression phase.

The mechanism(s) of action of d-limonene against cancer are not well understood, but may involve the enhancement of drug-metabolizing systems such as *glutathione-S-transferases*. The ability of d-limonene to reverse preformed tumors and to inhibit tumor growth during the promotion/progression phase of cancer suggests an immunostimulating action, and some recent evidence does support this concept.

As an added benefit limonene is a potent, natural cholesterol-lowering compound. It acts by inhibiting the same enzyme (HMG-coenzyme A reductase) which is the target of many prescribed cholesterol-reducing drugs such as lovostatin. If these actions were not sufficient, limonene is also a powerful agent for dissolving gallstones.

COFFEE
(coffee arabica)

Sitting and drinking a home brewed cup of Kona coffee, a perfect cup at that, I wonder at the long, eventful history of this and other economic plants. Some texts says that from a region called Kaffa in Upper Ethiopia and Egypt, ancient Arabs first prepared this herbal beverage as a sharp stimulant and energizer. As Islam spread so did the use of these beans. It is said that coffee was popular because it enabled worshippers to remain awake during long and frequent prayer sessions. Known as "the wine of Islam," *Coffea arabica,* was eventually disseminated through Europe, giving rise to coffee houses in the 1500s. A Frenchman, in the 1700s, brought a cutting of the coffee plant to Martinique, a French-controlled Caribbean Island, soon spawning the great coffee industry of Brazil and Columbia.

According to some accounts, coffee was originally introduced to England as a medicine to counter the effects of drunkenness. At the time, in the early 1600s, beer was the king of drinks and taverns were popular in every town and village. Soon the sobering effects of a cup of coffee became well known. By the later part of the century coffee houses had also become very popular, not only for sobering up but also for sitting and talking.

As with tea, this new beverage was denounced by many. The early enemies of coffee were brewers of beer, who stood to lose much business if the drink became too popular, but many other citizens joined them in the assault on coffee. Idleness was said to result from too much coffee drinking, and the coffee houses, which increasingly drew male patrons, were blamed for "businesses disrupted" and "marriages weakened."

Nevertheless, coffee drinking gained in popularity. By 1700 some of the most prominent English writers became the loudest advocates of the beverage. One historian believes that coffee even affected English literature. He argues that before coffee was introduced, in Shakespeare's time, literature was "a flux of tedious words," while after coffee became popular among the writers, "keen . . . finished elegance (was) dominant."

The stimulant in coffee is caffeine. Although coffee and tea are both stimulants, some believe tea is less harmful because it promotes wakefulness without the agitation that accompanies excessive ingestion of coffee.

Coffee originated in the mountains of Ethiopia and was popular among the Arabs for centuries before it was introduced to Europe. From Mocha, an early center of the coffee trade, the plant was exported to India, Ceylon and the East Indies and later to Holland. From there seedlings were eventually brought to South America. Today Brazil grows one-half of the entire world supply. Much coffee is also grown and exported from other countries in South America, Central America, the Caribbean countries, Indonesia and Africa.

The coffee tree if left to itself grows to a height of twenty feet or more, but when cultivated it is kept to a height of eight or ten feet. It has glossy green leaves and white flowers. Its two-seeded fruits are dark purple when ripe. After roasting they become dark brown and develop the characteristic coffee aroma. Each tree bears up to six pounds of coffee "beans" each year, which after roasting and grinding is reduced to only one pound of coffee ready for the pot. Surprisingly, green coffee contains 14 percent protein, as well as 7 percent sugar, 10 to 13 percent oil, 12 percent water and 34 percent cellulose. In Turkey coffee grounds are not discarded but are mixed with sugar and eaten as a nutritious food.

Grown in the tropics, the best-quality coffee is produced by rich, well-drained soils in moist, mountainous climates. Blue Mountain coffee, grown on the island of Jamaica, is considered by many connoisseurs to be the finest variety. Espresso, popular in cafés throughout Europe and now in the United States, refers to the way in which the coffee beans are roasted, not to any particular coffee type. Espresso is dark roasted and when brewed produces a heavy, bitter beverage.

CAFFEINE AND WEIGHT LOSS

It will not surprise inveterate coffee drinkers to learn that caffeine promotes the burning of fat. A series of recent studies, most notably that of Astrup and colleagues, confirms what coffee and tea "addicts" have long known, that these beverages promote slimming in humans. It has been discovered that caffeine stimulates the expenditure of energy and the burning of fats.

Astrup's was a placebo-controlled, double-blind, dose- response study. (In other words, it met all the requirements of mainstream science.) Caffeine was tested in dosages of 100, 200, and 400 mg and compared against three different doses of ephedrine, and two placebos. Six healthy subjects were recruited from the University of Copenhagen Medical School. Excluded were people habituated to caffeine from other sources—coffee, tea, colas, chocolate, and cocoa. The test subjects were put on a weight-controlling diet, consisting of about 250 grams of carbohydrate and a fixed amount of sodium. Their body fat content was measured before and after taking the placebo (lactose) or caffeine (100, 200, or 400 mg.) in gelatin capsules. Through a series of wonderful experimental analyses, the authors discovered that caffeine has a *thermogenic* effect (i.e, raises body heat) when taken in *moderate* doses on a daily basis. "A significant thermogenic effect was found even after the *lowest* dose of caffeine (100 mg.) . . . " Interestingly, even this relatively small intake of caffeine was found to produce a lasting effect on energy expenditure. When caffeine was taken together with physical activity the thermogenic effect was enhanced.

The *mechanism* by which caffeine exerts this fat-burning effect is thought to be associated with the thermogenic cori cycle. This is where glycogen and glucose are converted to *lactate* in fat and muscle tissue. Lactate then triggers thermogenic processes in the liver.

HERBS CONTAINING CAFFEINE

Plant Name		Percent Caffeine
Common	Latin	
Arabian coffee	*Coffea arabica*	1-2%
Tea	*Camellia sinensis*	1-4%
Cacao (chocolate)	*Theobroma cacao*	less than 1%
Maté	*Ilex paraguensis*	1-2%
Cola	*Cola acuminata*	about 2.5%
Guaraná	*Paullinia cupana*	2.5-5%

COLA
(Cola acuminata)

The flavoring of many soft drinks is derived from seeds contained within the pods of the tropical African cola tree. These seeds contain more caffeine than coffee as well as some theobromine and are sometimes chewed by West African people to allay hunger and fatigue. A native cola drink is made by boiling the pulverized seeds in water for several minutes. Fresh kernels are also chewed as stimulants.

240

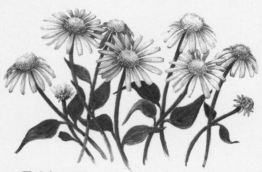

Echinacea
(Echinacea angustifolia)
(E. purpurea, E. pallida)

ECHINACEA, Coneflower
(Echinacea angustifolia)
(E. purpurea, E. pallida)

Long considered a panacea by numerous Amerind tribes, this plant of the western plains will serve mankind well into the future, based on recent scientific documentation of its immune-enhancing effects.

In 1906 a report was published by Hewett describing several case reports on the treatment of various severe conditions such as abscesses, boils, gangrenous wounds, septicemia, scarlet fever, ivy poisoning, spider bites, and ulcers. Soon thereafter, the dried roots and rhizome of the coneflower were official in the National Formulary (NF), from 1916-1950.

Then, in the 1960's reports from Eastern Europe were published on the plant's immunostimulant activity. A polysaccharide fraction increased the rate of phagocytosis and that an aqueous extract used internally was found to activate reticulo endothelium to increase alpha, beta and gamma globulin, and promote the formation of antibodies.

In 1972 an extract of the root was shown to possess significant antitumor activity in experiments with rats. Antiviral activity was reported in 1978, showing that a root extract was effective in destroying herpes influenza viruses. Work in the previous decade (1956) demonstrated the powerful antibacterial properties of coneflower. By adding an aqueous extract of the root to suspensions of penicillin activity levels of the drugs were increased.

In the 1980's interest in this Native America plant was pursued by Eastern European scientists. Wagner and co-workers reported in Germany on immunologically active polysaccharides derived from tissue cultures of this beautiful plant. Other European laboratories reported the activation of human lymphocytes, increased rate of phagocytosis and macrophage activation.

Recent work has reconfirmed that this species inhibits hyaluronidase and explains why it also possesses potent wound- healing properties.

Here we have a biologically active plant, known to the Native American to possess almost magical healing properties and now proving itself worthy of acceptance as a world-class medicine.

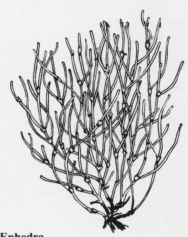

Ephedra

EPHEDRA
(Ephedra, various species)

The Ephedras have been used for relieving coughs, asthma, and allergies. Many compounds are found in this genus, most notably ephedrine and pseudo-ephedrine. Ephedrine and pseudo-ephedrine, as we will see below, are potent sympathomimetics. They excite the sympathetic nervous system causing the vaso-constriction of the nasal mucosa, dilation of the bronchioles as well as cardiac stimulation.

These natural substances produce effects similar to epinephrine (adrenaline), but are, of course, *less* stimulating to the central nervous system than amphetamine. This is why *Ephedra* is such a useful plant. It is extremely effective without being too strong in its actions, when properly utilized.

Ephedrine, the alkaloid derived from the branches of the plant, is employed as a *vasoconstrictor* and cardiac stimulant and as a *bronchodilator* in the treatment of hay fever, asthma, and emphysema. Topically, Ephedra has been used as an eyewash.

Most Ephedra species contain the alkaloid *ephedrine* in all parts of the plant. Ephedrine produces many effects when taken orally by humans, the most important being dilation of the bronchioles of the lungs and increase in blood pressure. The major use of Ephedra, therefore, is to relieve the symptoms of bronchial asthma and as a nasal decongestant.

We have all heard of *pseudoephedrine* because it often appears in over-the-counter (OTC) products.

Some confusion surrounds this alkaloid, people are not sure if it is made in the laboratory or extracted from *Ephedra*. Both may be so!

The *Ephedras* contain 0.5-20% alkaloids. Ephedrine may account for 30-90% of this alkaloid content (Marderosian and Liberti, 1988). Some plants also contain pseudoephedrine, which is an *isomer* of ephedrine.

Pseudoephedrine and ephedrine may be naturally derived or produced synthetically. Pseudoephedrine may have certain advantages. It causes fewer heart symptoms such as palpitation compared to ephedrine, but is equally effective as a bronchodilator (Roth, *et al.*, 1977).

It should be noted that the effects of either alkaloid last a few hours and that side effects may appear, including nervousness, insomnia, and vertigo (Marderosian, 1988).

EPHEDRA or ("Ma-Huang")
(Ephedra, various species)

In 1982 I pioneered the use of pseudo-ephedrine, one of the alkaloids present in the herb *Ephedra*, in the treatment of cocaine and amphetamine addiction. I also recommended the use of the "excitatory" amino acids, phenylalanine and tyrosine, because they mimic the adrenaline-like rush of the illicit drugs (see Figure 1).

FIGURE 1

COCAINE

EPHEDRINE
("SUDAFED" is psuedo–ephedrine)

AMPHETAMINE

While the chemical structures of cocaine and amphetamine are quite different they have very similiar pharmological properties.

Getting Off Cocaine: 30 Days To Freedom, M.A. Weiner, published by Avon Books, 1983, available only through Quantum Books, P.O. Box 2056, San Rafael, California 94912-2056.

Other Compounds with Biological Activity Found in Ephedra

Other compounds found in Ephedra include phenylaline, ascorbic acid, catechin, cinnamic acid, quercetrin, leucodelphinidin, quercitin, rutin, tannic acid, tannin, and terpinen-4-oL. All of these compounds exhibit anti-inflammatory or antiallergic activity (Napralert, 1990).

Thermogenesis and Weight Loss

This herb promotes weight loss (Pasquali, et al., 1987; Dulloo, 1989). Ephedra accomplishes this because it has a *thermogenic* and fat-metabolizing effect. Ephedrine also exhibits *anorectic* properties (reducing the *desire* for food).

The alkaloid is thought to activate both alpha and beta adrenoceptors, which elevates metabolic rate, increases calorie expenditure and results in weight loss. When combined with caffeine, a synergism results, yielding a *greater increase* in metabolic rate than ephedrine or caffeine alone (Dulloo, 1989).

242

For those interested in increased energy, endurance, alertness, *and* weight loss, this ancient remedy from China may hold a key.

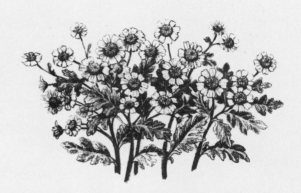

Feverfew
(Tanacetum parthenium)

FEVERFEW
(Tanacetum parthenium)

Effects of an extract of feverfew on endothelial cell integrity and on cAMP in rabbit perfused aorta. T. A. Voyno-Yasenetskaya, et al. J. Pharm. Pharmacol. 40:501-501, 1988.:

At my herbal seminars people often ask if feverfew (Tanacetum parthenium) is as effective for treating regular headaches as it is for its accepted use in the treatment of migraine headaches. For the reasons elucidated in this study, we may now understand why feverfew "works" only for migraine headaches. These researches report that crude extracts of the plant both inhibit platelet aggregation and also inhibit secretory activity in platelets, most cells, and PMN's (polymorphonuclear leucocytes). They speculate that "such activities are relevant to the medicinal properties of the plant."

We learn that feverfew contains the sesquiterpene lactones (parthenolide and parthenolide-like compounds) and that these compounds bring about the anti-clotting effects of extracts. Blood platelets are so affected because the cellular sulphydryl groups they contain are "neutralized" by this herb. Feverfew extracts also slow the spread of platelets and the formation of clot-like substances on collagen. In a series of novel experiments the authors demonstrated that extracts of this plant protected the endothelial layer of rabbit aorta from laboratory induced injury (i.e., perfusion with a salt solution).

As for headaches, it is interesting to note that by inhibiting the secretion of histamines from most cells, migraine type pain is controlled or eliminated.

In concluding their comments these authors reconfirm "feverfew being of value as an antithrombotic agent as well as being of value in migraine and arthritis."

GARLIC (and onion)
(Allium spp)

Garlic and onions have been used for thousands of years to treat cancers. Hippocrates wrote about a steam fumigation of garlic to treat cancer of the uterus. Similar usage against cancers are recorded in ancient Egypt, Greece, Rome, India, Russia, Europe and China.

Recent research in China demonstrated a significant inverse relationship between the incidence of stomach cancer and the intake of garlic and related *allium* vegetables. By interviewing 1131 controls and 564 patients with stomach cancer it was found that people with no stomach cancer ate significantly higher amounts of these vegetables (a mean intake of 19.0 kg/year) than did the cancer patients (a mean intake of 15.5 kg/year). Those people who ate less than 11.5 kg/year were found to be more than twice as likely to develop cancer of the stomach than were people who ate more than 24 kg/year. Interestingly, people in Georgia where vitalia onions are grown enjoy a stomach cancer mortality rate among whites that is one-third the average U.S. level and one-half of the average level of stomach cancer in Georgia.

Both garlic and onion oils inhibit the enzymes lipoxygenase and cyclooxygenase. Each of these enzymes is known to act on one of two parallel biochemical pathways (within the arachidonic acid cascade) and only by inhibiting these enzymes can this pathway be arrested. When arrested, the production of prostaglandin is slowed. Since many cancers are prostaglandin dependent, this may explain why the *allium* oils have anti-tumor properties.

Dr. Sydney Belman of New York University has

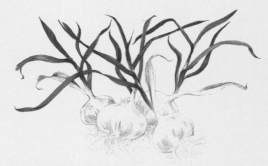

Garlic (onion)
(Allium spp)

conducted much of the cancer research on *allium* oils. He showed that onion oil inhibits PMA-induced cancer. PMA stimulates prostaglandins and platelet aggregation, the oil of onion which contains dipropenyl sulphide, inhibits both.

Garlic and onion contain over 75 different sulfur-containing compounds. While most of the medical benefits derived from supplementation with extracts of these plants are a result of these sulfurous compounds, recent studies show the additional presence of the bioflavonoids quercetin and cyanidin. Onions contain very high amounts of quercetin which has been used to treat allergies, inflammatory diseases, and diabetic cataracts.

Selenium, the cellular antioxidant, is another constituent found in the *allium* vegetables and their extracts. The antitumor effects claimed for selenium may be based on its ability to replace the sulphur in the amino acid l-cystine. Leukemic white blood cells have a rapid turnover of l-cystine, a similar amino acid, and by substituting selenium for sulphur, leukemia can be suppressed, in animals.

The amazing alliums are also effective antibacterials, killing *clostridium, pseudomonas, salmonella* and other problematic species. The fungus *candida albicans* which is frequently seen in a number of immunologic conditions (AIDS and cancer) is also destroyed by allicin and other components of garlic.

Perhaps most significant is the effect of garlic and onion and their extracts on the lipid profile of blood and tissues. They lower cholesterol, triglycerides and LDL cholesterol levels while also increasing the beneficial cholesterol, HDL.

GINGER
(Zingiber officinale)

This widely used condiment has also had important medicinal applications. It is mainly employed in gastrointestinal upsets; as a stimulant and carminative (removing gas from the gastrointestinal tract) it is used to treat indigestion and flatulence. Because of these properties, as well as its aromatic qualities, it is often combined with bitters to make them more palatable; Ginger adds an agreeable, warming feeling.

Ginger tea has become a popular remedy for colds, producing perspiration and also helping to bring on menstruation if suppressed by a cold. Externally, Ginger is a rubefacient, and has been credited in this connection with relieving headache and toothache.

The flavor is due to the presence of borneol, while gingerol imparts its pungency.

Ginger has a recorded history of medicinal usage in China dating from the 4th century B.C. Today, the condiment is commonly found in many Chinese food preparations, indicating well established culinary as well as medicinal uses.

Currently, ginger has received new attention as an aid to *prevent* motion sickness, specifically the characteristic nausea which accompanies this problem. Ginger tea has long been an American country herbal remedy for coughs and asthma, related to allergy or inflammation; the creation of the soft drink ginger ale sprang from the common folkloric usage of this herb, and still today remains a popular beverage for the relief of stomach upset.

The mechanism by which ginger produces anti-inflammatory activity is that of the typical NSAID (non-steroidal anti-inflammatory drug). This common spice is a more biologically active prostaglandin inhbitor (via cyclooxygenase inhibiton) than onion and garlic.

By slowing associated biochemical pathways an inflammatory reaction is curtailed. Ginger is used in Ayurveda, the traditional Indian System to treat arthritis, pain, fever, and blood clumping—all related to the metabolism of arachidonic acid (AA) as it affects *various eicosanoids*. In a study, Danish women between the ages of 25 to 65 years consumed either 70 grams raw onion or 5 grams raw ginger daily for a period of one week. By measuring thromboxane production during the course of this study the author

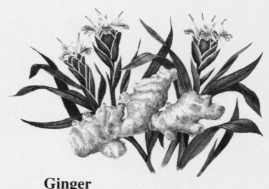

Ginger
(Zingiter officinale)

learned *that ginger, more clearly than onion, reduced thromboxane production by almost 60%*. This confirms the Ayurvedic "prescription" for this common spice and its anti-aggregatory effects. By reducing blood platelet "clumping," ginger, onion and garlic may reduce our risk of heart attack or stroke (Srivastiva, 1989). In a series of experiments with rats, scientists from Japan discovered that extracts of ginger inhibited gastric lesions by up to 97%. The authors conclude that the folkloric usage of ginger in stomachic preparations were effective owing to the constituents zingiberene, the main terpenoid and 6-gingerol, the pungent principle (Yamahara, 1988).

In an earlier look at how some of the active components of ginger (and onion) act inside our cells, it was found that the oils of these herbs inhibit the fatty acid oxygenases from platelets, thus decreasing the clumping of these blood cell components (Vanderhoek, 1980). Remember arachidonic acid (AA)? It is metabolized inside blood platelets by two fatty acid oxygenases (enzymes); a cycloxygenase and a lipoxygenase. By interfering with the cycloxygenase enzyme, ginger helps slow the production of thromboxane A_2, a key player in the platelet clumping process.

In summary ginger interferes with the manufacture of prostaglandin and so blocks inflammation.

Recent experiments (1990) have shown that gingerol completely abolished the infectivity of *schistosoma mansoni*, a major parasite in tropical and subtropical areas of the world.

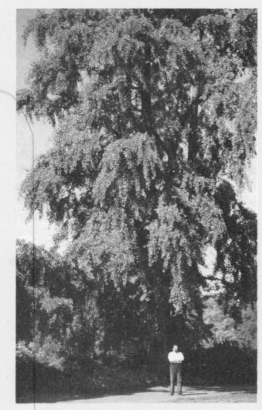

Large specimen of Ginkgo *tree. Kew Gardens, England.*

GINKGO
Ginkgo biloba)

Perhaps the most exciting new research on ginkgo was recently published in *The Journal of Urology* (Sikora *et al.*, 1989), detailing a study of sixty patients suffering from arterial erectile dysfunction. After 6 months of daily treatment with 60 mg. of an extract of ginkgo biloba, 50% of the subjects were once again able to achieve penile erections. Upwards of 45% of the remaining subjects showed some improvement.

Ginkgo, also known as maidenhair, is the oldest living tree, dating to the age of the dinosaurs. A common tree, it is very hardy and can live a thousand years! It has been recognized in Chinese medical practice for nearly 3,000 years.

Ginkgo research has proceeded in many different areas. The most interesting and important relate to:

1) Vascular diseases
2) Brain function
3) Impotency
4) Dopamine synthesis
5) Retinal lesions
6) Migraine
7) Hearing loss
8) Hemorrhoids
9) Inflammation
10) Asthma

Flavonoids extracted from the leaves of *Ginkgo biloba*, such as quercetin, kampferol and isorhamnetin, have been shown to inhibit histamine and barium chloride contractions in isolated guinea-pig intestine (Peter, 1968), and to possess antibradykininic activity on guinea-pig ileum (last portion of small intestine connecting to large intestine) (Natarajan *et al.*, 1970).

Ginkgo's effect as an anti-allergic, anti-asthmatic agent has been demonstrated by Chung, *et al.'s (1987)* paper in *The Lancet*, "Effect of a ginkgolide mixture in antagonising skin and platelet responses to platelet activating factor in man." The authors concluded that "Platelet activating factor (PAF) has been implicated in pathophysiological states including allergic inflammation, anaphylactic shock, and asthma. Ginkgolide B is the most active PAF antagonist found in this class (of ginkgolides)." It would appear that ginkgo relieves the broncho- constriction due to its PAF antagonist activity.

Of importance to allergy sufferers, a randomized,

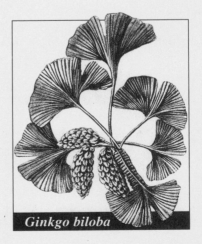

Ginkgo biloba

double-blind, placebo-controlled crossover study in 8 atopic asthmatic patients showed that a bronchial provocation test of house dust mite or pollen, preceded by 2 days of 40 mg. per day of ginkgo, *demonstrated significant inhibition* of the bronchial allergen challenge compared to placebo.

As the Asians, Germans and French all show, Ginkgo is the herb to know.

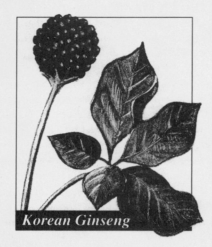
Korean Ginseng

GINGSENG
(Var. sp.)

As suggested in Section I, ginseng in used for its reputed antifatigue effects, improved performance and stamina, as well as to improve concentration and reaction times in the elderly (Takagi, 1974; Hallstrom, 1982; Schmidt, 1978; and others).

The *ginsenosides* are the main active principles of ginseng. These are classified as triterpene saponins (Carr, 1986) and consist of about 20 identified structures. Ginsenosides of the R_b grouping are *"slightly sedative"* while those of the R_g grouping are more *stimulating* (Shibata, 1977). Both types of ginsenosides show some *anti-fatigue* activity (Kaku, *et al.*, 1975).

Ginseng extracts "have a low acute or chronic toxicity" (Carr, 1986), one researcher "unable to determine a LD_{50} because the largest . . . doses orally failed to produce toxic effects in mice, rats or the mini

pig" (Berté, 1973 & 1982).

According to one supplier, "it is desirable that the ratios between R_g and R_b are monitored in ginseng roots and products along with the total concentration of ginsenoside."

The same supplier describes "quality problems in the Ginseng Market Place" and suggests that a standardized ginseng extract has clear advantages. According to a test of ginseng products selected at random, the West German Government's State Product Test Institution reported that "1/4 of all ginseng products contained little or no active ingredients" ("Shiftung Warentest," 1985).

Buying a *concentrated extract* of ginseng offers the consumer a far more reliable assurance that the active constituents are present at precise levels as stated on labels. In this case, knowing that what nature provides *is there*, is an improvement over nature herself.

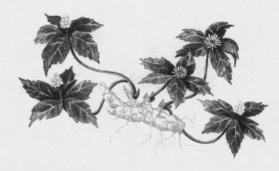

Goldenseal
(Hydrastis canadensis)

GOLDENSEAL
(Hydrastis canadensis)

Here is another Native American plant with wide usage by Indian healers. An infusion of the roots was made into an eye wash for sore eyes. It was also utilized by Indians and white settlers for skin diseases, gonorrhea, and indolent ulcers.

Three components of the plant were at one time official drugs; Hydrastine was entered in the *United States Pharmacopoeia* (USP) from 1905-1926, *Hydrastinine hydrochloride* in the USP from 1916-26 and the *National Formulary* (NF) from 1926-1950.

246

All were classified as internal hemostatics.

Recent research has corroborated these and other biological activities. The dried rhizome possesses cytotoxic activity, which indicates it is useful against viruses. Its antibacterial properties have been well-established since 1950, especially against *E. Coli* and *Staphylococcus aureus*. Not to be overlooked is goldenseal's potent hypotensive activity. In one experiment in rabbits, an extract of the root brought about a severe drop in blood pressure.

This is a potent plant which must be utilized with care. One of its constituent alkaloids, L-Canadine, reportedly paralyzes the central nervous system and causes severe peristalsis.

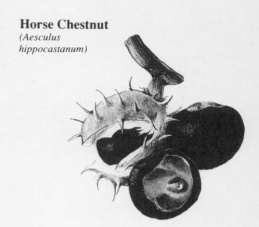

Horse Chestnut
(Aesculus hippocastanum)

GUARANÁ
(Paullinia Cupana)

Guaraná is another caffeine-rich beverage of South America. It is made from the pulverized fruits of a vinelike plant that grows wild in the Amazon Valley or is cultivated on small plantations. Sometimes called the "cola of Brazil," guaraná contains two to three times as much caffeine as coffee or tea. This makes it one of the most powerful of all caffeine drinks.

HORSECHESTNUT
(Aesculus hippocastanum)

This easily recognized, stately tree was originally found in northern Greece but is now distributed widely throughout temperate parts of the world. It is especially magnificent during May when its white or reddish flowers are in profuse bloom.

The powdered kernel of the nut causes sneezing. The oil extracted with ether from the kernels has been used in France as a topical remedy for rheumatism. A decoction of the leaves was formerly employed in the United States as a treatment for whooping cough, while the seed oil has been considered useful against sunburn. The nuts contain narcotic properties, and a tincture is very useful against hemorrhoids.

The active principle of Horsechestnut seeds is known to be the complex triterpene glycoside escin. Escin is widely used in Europe as an anti-inflammatory agent for a number of venous problems, including varicose veins and edema of the legs.

Many, many animal experiments have repeatedly confirmed the anti-inflammatory and anti-edema actions of escin. Magliulo, *et al.* (1968) studied the process of inflammation in detail and learned that *escin* inhibits the movement of inflammatory cells, especially macrophages, *without* lessening their activity or phagocytic properties.

This remarkable glycoside also has potent powers to reduce edema. It achieves this by normalizing the permeability of blood vessel walls (Siering, 1962). In human therapy, Italian researchers found this compound to be "well tolerated throughout treatments lasting 50 consecutive days" (Manca and Passarelli, 1965).

It so appears that there is ample evidence supporting the folkloric usage of horsechestnut to treat varicose veins and inflammatory disorders of the legs.

When next you gaze at these thickly armored fruits consider the sweet healing balm contained therein.

KHAT
(Catha edulis)

(Reflections on a rainbow)

When I was working towards my first graduate degree, in ethnobotany, I had the good fortune to live in a rainforest on Hawaii. In a tiny gardener's cottage on the 120 or so acres of the Lyon Arboretum in the back of Manoa Valley on Oahu, I lived, studied and raised my first child. Being a living repository of some of the world's most beautiful and interesting plants, I often strolled in nature's magical embrace. Being the late '60's, a time when experimentation took many forms, I sampled plants unusual for a "just-arrived" New Yorker. Among these was the then unheard of *Catha edulis*, growing a few hundred yards from our front porch. I remembered reading about "Abyssinian Tea" in an issue of my then bible, the *Journal of Economic Botany.* Learning of its CNS effects in the library, I drove back into the valley reflecting on a rainbow and seeking the smooth dark-green, glossy leaves reputed for their stimulant and euphoria-inducing effects.

Now, I happen to be opposed to using hallucinogenic substances and was so even then, in the heyday of "psychedelic" activities. The reason I became more interested in Khat was in part due to the literature which reported that in *moderate* doses the plant produced a stimulation similar to strong coffee, with the added benefits of euphoria and "loquacity." In *large* doses a "manic-like psychosis" could result. Being a naturalist dictated that I personally attempt to establish the dose-response curve for myself, hoping to discover a new and safe cerebral stimulant which might be introduced to the Western World. (I certainly did *not* seek added loquaciousness, the opposite necessary in my new environment.)

As I chewed my first Khat leaf beneath the jagged peaks of Manoa Valley, I wondered on the dispersal of this remarkable shrub. First mentioned in the 1300s in an Arabian medical test, the use of Khat is thought to have originated in tropical East Africa. It grows wild along riverbanks above 4,500 feet in Ethiopia and was slowly introduced into mountainous regions of South Yemen and later other African countries. Cultivated today interspersed with coffee trees at high altitudes, Khat is quite hardy and can be grown in the Mediterranean region and in the southern United States (Paris, 1958). Used as a stimulant *before* the advent of daily coffee consumption, several *million* people in South-Western Arabia and East Africa habitually chew Khat today. The habit has not spread because the desired, stimulating effect is thought to be best obtained from *fresh* leaves (Khan and Kalix, 1984). Yet we learn from an earlier source "the drug is sold in bundles of stalks in full leaf weighing about 500 g and measuring 40 cm long by

8-10 cm in diameter . . . the yellow leaves being the most sought after" (Paris, 1958). The dry plant has less potency than fresh leaves.

Long used to overcome fatigue and the need for sleep, Khat chewers "are able to dance and talk all night without feeling sleepy." As a general stimulant and "mental excitant" Khat remains the drug of choice in the African region. The active principle has been known for its "amphetamine-like properties" for many years. Many books still report that (+) norpseudoephedrine or *cathine* is the main active principle of these leaves. But pharmacological work in the 1960's and 1970's elucidated *three* major compounds isolated from the phenylalkylamine fraction. These are *cathine, cathinone* and (−)- *norephedrine* (Giannini, 1982). As you will note in the following set of structures cathine and cathinone closely resemble amphetamine.

Figure 1

It is now believed that *cathinone* is the main active principle of Khat. Both compounds produce anorexia, and behavior characteristic of amphetamine usage, including a "manic-like psychosis" when taken in *excess* (Giannini, 1982; Kalix, 1984). Another writer somewhat modifies this position giving the *whole* plant a "clean bill of health" when compared with amphetamines taken as an isolated drug. He further reports "there is evidence that amphetamines produce their pharmacological action by modulating adrenergic/dopaminergic systems at subcortical sites; it has been suggested that cathinone does *not* act upon dopaminergic systems as d-amphetamine does and is therefore less disruptive to behavior" (*Bulletin on Narcotics*, 1980).

In reviewing the literature on Khat I am impressed with the similarity of the controversy surrounding the coca leaf. In the native cultures that gave rise to these plants and continue to utilize them for their positive effects there is little trouble surrounding their *moderate*** use. When *isolated* alkaloids are *extracted* from these plants the results are often horrific, for the habitual users and the society in which they live. Nature seems to be meant to be taken whole (at least chewed!). When we try to improve on her, by refining wheat, extracting sugar cane, distilling alcohol or removing cocaine from coca leaves, we often end up expressing our own condemnation.

Of course, I did not know any of this when I chewed my first leaf of Khat. Feeling the astringent juices running back in my throat and glancing at the romantically sharp mountain range in that Hawaiian rainforest I was sure I had "discovered" Western man's next useful stimulant, from Africa. Unfortunately, a South American shrub beat Khat to our shores.

***Excessive* Khat chewing is, however, harmful. It produces constipation, weight-loss, gastritis, impotence, insomnia, and reactive depression.

LICORICE
(Glycyrrhiza glabra)

Among the ancient Greeks Licorice root had a reputation for quenching thirst. It is soothing to the mucus membrane and has been given to treat irritated urinary, bowel, and respiratory passages. It was often given in combination with Senega and Mezereon, when these drugs were used on persons with irritated or inflamed eliminatory organs. The root also reportedly had expectorant and laxative properties. Children suck on Licorice sticks both as candies and as a

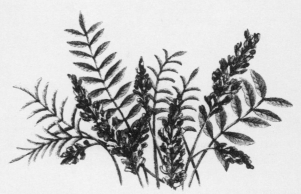

Licorice
(Glycyrrhiza glabra)

remedy for coughs. Licorice is a valuable flavoring adjunct to medicines with unpleasant tastes; and the powered root was used in the preparation of pills, both to give them more substance and to coat the surfaces to prevent their sticking together.

The multitude of pharmacological effects of Licorice rhizomes and roots are practically all attributed to the presence of a triterpene saponin called *glycyrrhizin*.

Glycyrrhizin is about fifty times sweeter than sugar, and has a powerful *cortisone-like effect*. In fact, several cases have been reported in the medical literature in which humans ingesting 6-8 ounces (a very large amount) of licorice candy daily for a period of several weeks are "poisoned" due to the cortisone-like effects of licorice extract in the candy. Proper treatment restores patients to normal. The above amount of this compound is very large compared with the relatively *small* amount found in supplements.

In addition, Licorice rhizomes and roots have a high mucilage content. When mixed with water, the resulting preparation has a very pleasant odor and taste, and acts as an effective demulcent on irritated mucous membranes, such as accompany a sore throat.

It is not surprising then, that licorice and its glycoside constituent glycyrrhizin have such wide applications. It should be noted that this chemical constitutes only 7 to 10% of the total root (on a dry weight basis) (Tyler, 1988).

Glycyrrhetic acid (G.A.) is obtained when acid hydrolysis is applied to the main component of licorice. This compound is extensively used in Europe for its anti-inflammatory properties, especially in Addison's disease and peptic ulcer (Finney, 1958; Fujita, 1980; Sugishita, 1984; Baltina, 1989).

Some European researchers concluded that this natural product (G.A.) may be preferred to cortisone because it is safer, especially when prolonged treatment is required (Gijon, 1960).

A note of caution. Side effects from the ingestion of large amounts of licorice have been reported. Glycyrrhizin in very large amounts can promote hypokalemia and hypertension. For these reasons people with heart problems and high blood pressure are advised to avoid consuming large quantities of licorice or its components.

MATÉ
(Ilex paraguensis)

Just as millions of people drink coffee and tea in other parts of the world, millions in South America enjoy maté. The characteristic aromatic flavor and the stimulant caffeine are extracted by pouring water, either hot or cold, over dried leaves. As with tea, the most expensive grade of maté is composed of the youngest leaves, while cheaper grades contain twigs, stems and older leaves. Botanically, maté is a species of holly. It is cultivated and is also found growing wild.

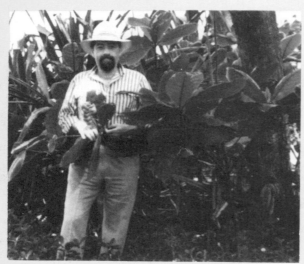

The author with young mathaké plants.

MATHAKÉ (Tropical almond)
(Terminalia catappa)

This species, widely distributed in the tropics, is one of the most effective anti-fungal plants yet is not widely known. In 1984, I introduced the tropical almond to several physicians who report strong activity against *Candida albicans* in trials with patients. My decision to bring this plant into western medicine was based on first-hand observations of its powerful anti-fungal activity when used in Fijian folk-medicine.

Subsequent literature analysis indicated that a decoction of the leaves (mixed with other plants) is used to induce abortion in New Guinea. However, *mathaké* by itself is perfectly safe, being used as a tonic in Mexico, and the nuts have been eaten by children since antiquity. The compounds found within the leaves kill *staphylococci*, which may explain its folkloric use as a tonic.

Robert F. Cathcart, III, M.D., of Los Altos, California, reports that *mathaké* should be used as an alternative to Pau D'Arco.

At this time we do not know if mathaké acts directly to kill yeast or if any of its compounds enhances the immune system. Owing to its clinical effectiveness in initial trials and its long history of usage, this plant is worth utilizing as part of an overall immune-enhancing program.

MILK THISTLE
(Silymarin marianum)

Selectivity of Silymarin on the Increase of Glutathione Content in Different Tissues of the Rat. Alfonso Valenzuela, Monica Aspillaga, Soledad Vial, and Ricardo Guerra. Planta Medica, 55:420-422, 1989.:

These Chilean scientists add another page to our understanding of how milk thistle acts to protect the liver from cellular damage. Silymarin is one active component extracted from milk thistle seeds (Silybum marianum). It is a flavonoid long recognized for its ability to benefit people with liver disorders and as a protective compound against liver-damaging agents as diverse as mushroom toxins, carbon tetrachloride, and other chemicals. This flavonoid demonstrates "good antioxidant properties, both in vivo and in

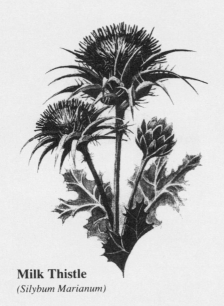

Milk Thistle
(Silybum Marianum)

hepatotoxicity may result, characterized by glutathione (GSH) depletion, suppression of GSH biosynthesis, and liver damage. "GSH," we learn, "is considered to be the most important biomolecule against chemically-induced cytotoxicity." This flavonoid is thought to exert a membrane-stabilizing action which inhibits or prevents lipid peroxidation. In reviewing this study I conclude that silybin and silymarin may be useful in protecting the liver in many cases *besides* acetaminophen overdosage. Alcohol also depletes GSH and these flavonoids will offer good protection for those who continue to drink. Interestingly, silybin dihemisuccinate remains medicine's most important antidote to poisoning by the mushroom toxins a-amantin and phalloidin.

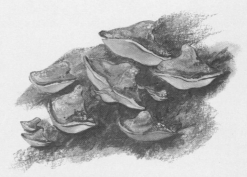

Mushrooms
Reishi
(Ganoderma lucidum)

vitro." We now learn that silymarin also *increases the content of liver glutathione (GSH), an effect not* known with other closely related flavonoids such as (+)— cyanidanol-3 (cathequin). These experiments, with rats, also showed an increase of glutathione content and the redox state (a measurement of antioxidant activity) in the intestine and stomach. The effects selectively occur, only in the digestive tract, and *not* in the kidney, lung, and spleen. For centuries folklore has told us that milk thistle acts most directly to protect the liver. We now have further scientific validation for this "old wives tale."

Silybin Dihemisuccinate Protects Against Glutathione Depletion and Lipid Peroxidation Induced by Acetaminophen on Rat Liver. Rolando Campos, Argelia Garrido, Ricardo Guerra, and Alfonso Valenzuela. Planta Medica, 55:417-419, *1989.*

In this study we learn how a herb (milk thistle) may offer us some protection against the toxic side-effects of a common pain-reliving drug (acetaminophen). Here, again, milk thistle is the subject of an intensive study by Chilean researchers. In this case, we see how *silybin*, a soluble form of silymarin, protects rats against liver glutathione depletion and lipid peroxidation. Acetaminophen is a widely used analgesic and fever medication. In *overdosage* severe

MUSHROOMS
A. Reishi
(Ganoderma lucidum)

Long regarded with suspicion by Americans, the mushrooms are now receiving renewed attention owing to the health promoting compounds found in several species. While most of the results reported thus far are based on animal studies, the historical reverence assigned reishi mushrooms by the Japanese tends to support the contention that human studies will produce equally exciting results.

The Japanese names for this member of the basidiomycetes are mannentake, meaning "tens of thousand year fungus," saiwaitake "happy fungus," or *kisshotake*, "lucky fungus." Originally utilized in

251

China as a food "to lengthen life," the reishi mushrooms have been eaten in Japan for at least 3,000 years.

Reishi mushrooms are commercially available in several varieties. *G. lucidum*, the red variety, is the type preferred in Japan. *G. japonicum*, which is darker and softer as well as cultured varieties are also sold. Chinese herb doctors tend not to distinguish these species, using them all, however, only G. lucidum has been the subject of intensive research.

A recent study from Korea showed that *Ganoderma* elicited immunopotentiation in mice. Antitumor activity in mice of polysaccharide fractions of these mushrooms was reported from Japan, while Chinese scientists described adaptogenic activity, again in mice. According to this Chinese study a hot water extract was found to enhance a self-protecting mechanism of the central nervous system, improve heart function and correct parasympathetic nerve function. Perhaps most interestingly this study also demonstrated an anti-radiation effect from a polysaccharide fraction. The immune-enhancing effects ascribed to reishi mushrooms by the Korean scientists noted above were described as enhancing macrophages and polymorphonuclear leucocytes (two types of fighting cells). Many studies have reported potent antiallergic activity, including antihistamine actions. And, it is now well-established that mushrooms such as reishi can significantly reduce serum cholesterol and "thin" the blood in a manner similar to aspirin by reducing agglutination of platelets.

From the above documentation it appears that the claims of healing properties in these (and other) mushrooms are based on fact not myth. Fears of toxicity should be allayed by the finding that reishi has an LD of greater than 5,000 mg/K, with no toxic effect at this high level of consumption even after 30 days of consumption. No toxic effects in humans are to be expected even if a person were to eat 350 grams a day, between 40-300 times the therapeutic dose.

B. Shiitake
(Lentinus edodes)

When I first studied medical mycology, over 20 years ago, Wilson and Plunkett's classic text provoked

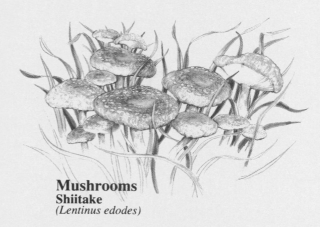

Mushrooms
Shiitake
(Lentinus edodes)

such fear and revulsion through the color photos of rare fungous diseases of man that I vowed to never eat another mushroom! All fungi became a source of dread for me.

Within the past few years I have since changed my view of these "lower" plants. The mushrooms are not only acceptable to me but have become highly coveted, owing to their documented immunostimulant, cholesterol-lowering, and antitumor activities.

Extracts of shiitake have been shown to inhibit a number of different cancerous tumors in animal experiments. A principle antitumor compound isolated from this species lentinan does not appear to kill tumor cells directly but inhibits tumor growth by stimulating immune-function.

Lentinan appears to function by activating macrophages which then engulf cancerous cells. This activation is again via an *indirect* route—T-helper cells are stimulated which increase the effectiveness of macrophages.

The AIDS epidemic has fostered interest in any helpful compounds and lentinan is now a high priority item. A highly publicized letter to the prestigious medical journal *The Lancet* (October 20, 1984) was signed by Robert Gallo, one of the co-discoverers of the HIV VIRUS, and two French researchers from the Pasteur Institute. In it the authors concluded that lentinan "may prove to be effective in AIDS or pre-AIDS or for HIV carriers." They tell of the disappearance of HTLV-I and HTLV-III antibodies after intravenous administration of lentinan in two Japanese patients.

Unfortunately, despite repeated requests to subject this drug to human trials, based on its long history of usage for cancer treatment in Japan, nothing much has been done by governmental authorities in the U.S.

This is odd considering the long list of studies showing lentinan's antiviral properties; interferon inducing, natural killer cell enhancing, phagocytosis rate enhancing, as well as numerous antitumor studies. The *in vitro* inhibition of HIV by an extract of this mushroom is not, of itself, highly significant owing to the many substances known to kill this virus. However, taken together with all of the above evidence, it is safe to assume that Shiitake is all that it is claimed to be.

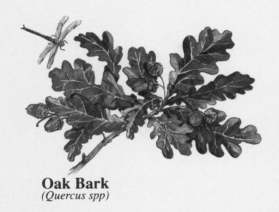

Oak Bark
(Quercus spp)

OAK BARK
(Quercus spp)

In my antique copy of The Dispensatory of the United States (1834) white oak bark is accorded all the respect that a major pharmaceutical would receive in a current textbook of pharmacology. Powdered oak bark was then taken in the form of a powder, extract or decoction, primarily for its high tannin content.

It was not used internally to a great extent, but a decoction of the bark has been found useful in treating chronic diarrhea, advanced dysentery, and other conditions. The principal use of the bark has been for external application, as an astringent wash, especially for flabby ulcers, as a gargle, and internally via injection for leucorrhea and hemorrhoids.

The inner bark of white oak is known to contain about 10 percent of a tannin complex, often referred to as quercitannic acid. As with all tannins, it predictably exerts an astringent and mild antiseptic action, the latter effect being due primarily to the phenolic nature of the tannin complex. Thus, as reported in folklore accounts, decoctions or infusions of *Quercus alba* bark, when applied locally, would have an astringent effect, which would tend to shrink hemorrhoids and accelerate the healing of skin ulcers.

Tannins, the active principle of white oak bark, are going through a revival owing to their medicinal properties. With the proliferation of intestinal parasites this class of plant-derived substances is receiving the respect once seen in older books on pharmacognosy and botanical medicine. Tannins precipitate proteins from solution, and act to protect injured tissues by precipitating their proteins to form an "antiseptic, protective coat under which the regeneration of new tissues may take place. "They are utilized in medicine as astringents in the G.I. tract, on burns, on skin abrasions, for bleeding or infected mouth sores, as a local application for hemorrhoids, and as a douche for vaginal and cervical discharges. It is not known whether tannins kill parasites directly or if they act to protect an invaded intestinal wall by the above-described mechanism. That they do work is attested to by the renewed popularity of this class of compounds.

It should be noted, however, that tannins should not be taken for prolonged periods. An increased incidence of cancer of the esophagus and buccal cavity has been noted among habitual betel-nut chewers *(Areca catechu)* in India and South Africa. This is linked to the high content of condensed catechin tannin found in the nuts of this graceful palm which are chewed for their stimulant drug content.

PAU D'ARCO
(Tabebuia impetiginosa and other species)

The inner bark of these stately, full leaved trees of Central and South America have received so much attention for their medicinal properties that sales of nearly $200 million have been reported. This is no doubt in part due to the keen marketing program undertaken by Brazilian and Argentinean suppliers of "taheebo." However, this marketing was based on solid reports of the bark's anticancer properties, first

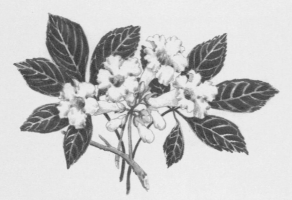

Pau D'Arco
(Tabebuia impetiginosa and other species)

simpler terms this type of naturally occurring flavo-noid acts as an *anti-histamine.* Quercetin works best when combined with vitamin C. Like quercetin, sub-stantial evidence supports the use of vitamin C in allergic diseases.

In addition, quercetin inhibits lipoxygenase, an enzyme involved in the metabolism of arachidonic acid (AA) in cells. Recall, AA is required for the inflammatory response to occur, via the production of prostaglandins and leukotrienes. Bioflavonoids such as quercetin can *block* the production of leu-kotrienes and other *pro-inflammatory* AA metabo-lites. They also act as anti-oxidants, scavenging dangerous free-radicals and protecting cells (Metz, 1981; Warso, 1983).

published in the 1960's.

The bark is rich (2-7%) in lapachol, a naphthoq-uinone, and also contains lapachone and xyloidone, both quinoids. Studies in the 1970's showed evidence that lapachol was active against mouse lymphocytic leukemia.

Currently, Pau D'Arco is widely utilized for its reputed anti-candida properties. While no direct evi-dence exists to confirm or deny this activity, the anec-dotal evidence is quite overwhelming. Moreover, a carefully controlled animal study published by a researcher at the prestigious Naval Medical Research Institute in Bethesda, Maryland demonstrated that dietary intake of lapachol is protective against penetration and infection by another deadly parasite, *Schistosoma Mansoni.*

From the available evidence it appears that this "miracle" bark from South America, which has gained wide acceptance for its anti-fungal properties will continue to gain in its applications, most notably against intestinal parasites.

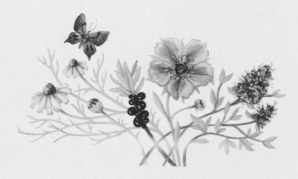

Suppressing inflammation and allergies are only some of the effects of quercetin. This potent phytopharmaceutical, made by nature and found in many plants has also been found to stimulate the immune system and kill viruses (Middleton, 1989).

QUERCETIN (a bioflavonoid)

Here we briefly look at a bioflavonoid found in *many, many* plants. It has the ability to block inflam-matory and allergic reactions which is why we are dis-cussing this compound.

Quercetin achieves these "blocking" actions by inhibiting IgE mediated allergic mediator release from mast cells (Welton, *et al.*, in Cody, 1988). In

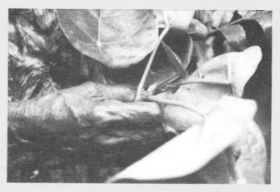

"Healing Hands." Many traditional remedies owe their activity to bioflavonoids.

254

Where can we find this remarkable herbal compound? As we stated, it is widely distributed in the vegetable kingdom. Quercetin (and other flavonoids) is found in fruits, vegetables, seeds, nuts, leaves, flowers, roots and bark.

In my many years of searching the tropical jungles for new plant remedies I've often watched local healers as they prepared and administered various folk-cures. Seeing cases of badly inflamed skin treated with plant medicine made me wonder if the almost instantaneous anti-inflammatory effects were due to the flavonoids found in the various salves and infusions.

RUE
(Ruta Chalepensis)

Al-Said MS, Tariq M, Yahya AL, Rafatullah S, Ginnawi OT & Ageel AM. Studies on **Ruta chalepensis,** *an ancient medicinal herb still used in traditional medicine. Journal of Ethnopharmacology 28: 305-312, 1990.:*

Ruta chalepensis, otherwise known as rue, is a traditional plant medicine used in many countries. The authors cite its clinical application in the management of pain, fevers, rheumatism, bleeding disorders (including menstrual dysfunction), and neurological disorders. The authors undertook the current investigations to assess the anti-inflammatory, analgesic (pain-reducing), central nervous system (CNS) depressant, and fever-reducing activity of this ancient medicinal.

Prior to testing the pharmacologic activity of an ethanol rue extract, the authors performed a phytochemical screening battery. They reported the occurrence of alkaloids, tannins, flavonoids, saponins, coumarins, volatile oil, sterols and/or triterpenes.

The anti-inflammatory activity of an ethanolic rue extract was tested against a powerful non-steroidal anti-inflammatory drug (oxyphenbutazone). An oral dose of 500 mg/kg of bodyweight of the animals was used. The rue extract inhibited inflammatory swelling by 40% in one model (61% inhibition with oxyphenbutazone), and by 24% in a second model (54% with oxyphenbutazone). Although the authors were unable to attribute the significant anti-inflammatory activity of the rue extract to a specific constituent, they speculate that this may be mediated by flavonoids present in the extract.

The ability of rue extract to depress CNS function was evidenced by a sharp fall in spontaneous movement in the rue-treated animals. Of the four dosages administered, the three highest dosages had sedative effects; the lowest dose actually *increased* spontaneous movement 90 minutes following administration. A fall in body temperature was also noted in the animals injected with the two highest dosages. No analgesic activity was seen in any of the rue-treated animals, independent of the dosage. These tests differed from the anti-inflammatory model in that mice (versus rats) were used, and the extract was injected (versus oral administration) into the abdominal cavity.

The authors parallel these findings to those seen with major tranquilizers, with rue displaying a selective sedative action in the absence of any pain-reducing properties. By contrast, tranquilizers such as Valium display both sedative and analgesic activity. Animals injected with a brewer's yeast extract (to induce a fever), and then treated with the two highest doses of rue extract displayed a normalization of body temperature, reinforcing the fever reducing potential of rue. In light of rue's effects upon the CNS, it is plausible to suggest that rue extract exerts its influence upon the temperature regulating centers within the hypothalamus of the brain, thereby resetting the "thermostat" in fever states.

The authors also evaluated the effects of the extract upon certain blood parameters. No change in blood clotting time, nor in fibrinogen levels, was noted. Fibrinogen is a blood protein with powerful platelet activating action, critical to the blood clotting cascade. Although the authors stated that blood hemoglobin levels were evaluated, no values were reported, suggesting that no change was observed.

The rich traditional medicine legacy behind rue affords a wealth of clinical support of this plant's efficacy. The current study reinforces its application in inflammatory conditions, and in states of hyper-anxiety/hyperarousal. However, the authors recommend further acute and chronic toxicology studies in order to assess its safety in humans.

SCHISANDRA

(Schisandra chinesis)

Traditional Chinese Medicine continues to offer new candidates to the annals of World Medicine. As we in the West are slowly learning, "traditional" or "folk" medicine really is the medicine of the people.

Schisandra is the source of several Oriental medicines, including "gomishi" in Japan, where it is utilized for tonic and antitussive purposes (Hikino, 1984). This interesting plant has many biological activities including:

antibacterial (equivocal results)	(Chen, 1987)
sympathomimetic (stimulant)	(Volicer, 1966)
resistance stimulation	(Shipoch Liev, 1967)
liver—protective	(Hikino, 1984; Pau, 1984)
antitoxic	(Shin, 1980)
antiallergenic	(Nishiyori, 1981; Koda, 1982)
antidepressant glycogenesis	Hancke, 1986)
stimulant	(Liu, 1979)

In addition, and perhaps most interesting from the point of view of it being a folkloric "tonic," this herb protected against the narcotic and sedative effects of alcohol (ETOH) and pentobarbital (PB) and exposure to the highly toxic ether, in mice (Hancke, 1986). As a result of these data, the authors concluded that Schisandra "may be useful clinical agents for reversal of CNS depression."

They base this "antidepressant activity" on the reasoning that depression may be due, in part, to adrenergic exhaustion following "severe psychogenic stress." It is known that MAO (monoamine oxidase) inhibitors and other selected compounds which increase noradrenergic neurotransmission within the CNS (such as imipramine) have proven benefit in depression.

The principle active compounds found in Schisandra, lignans known as *schizandrin, gamma-schisandrin,* and *deoxy-schisandrin,* are proposed as new agents in the war on depression.

This herb is also being promoted for its "stimulating effect on the nervous system without being excitatory like amphetamine or caffeine." There are some proponents who claim "the higher the degree of exhaustion, the greater is the stimulating effect."

Classed as an adaptogen (like ginseng), Schisandra has a long history of folkloric use in China and Tibet and more recent folk applications in Russia.

"Throughout the ages various groups of people have enjoyed the benefits of Schisandra. For example, in Northern China there lives a hunting tribe known as the Nanajas. Their hunting lifestyle means that they often set out on long and exhausting hunting trips under harsh conditions. But they always take along dried Schisandra fruit. A handful of the small red berries gives them the strength to hunt all day without eating.

To this day hunters in the wilds of Eastern Siberia use the berries, stalks and roots of this plants in the form of tea to provide them with extra energy when hunting.

This amazing fruit helped Russian pilots to withstand lack of oxygen in their flights during the forties. In more recent years Schisandra has contributed to the successes of the Swedish skiing team. In Russia Schisandra is a registered medicine for vision difficulties, i.e. short-sightedness and astigmatism, etc." (Wahlstrom, 1987).

A very interesting study on performance in race horses tends to confirm the folkloric claims. Polo horses given the berry extract of this species showed the following:

- a lower increase in heart rate (during exercise)
- a quicker recovery of respiratory function
- a reduction of plasma lactate
- improved performance
  (Ahumada, 1989)

It appears that this creeping herb from the Far East has valid claims to the title of a "new" anti-fatigue agent which possibly helps to accelerate "restorative processes" within the human body.

Caution

While Schisandra is a very safe herb with much historical usage one supplier of a standardized extract recommends that this herb be avoided by: epileptics, those with high intracranial pressure or severe hypertension, and those with "high acidity."

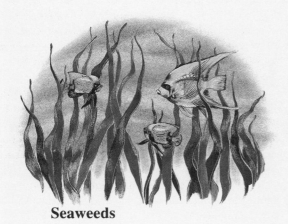

Seaweeds

SEAWEEDS
Blue-green algae
(Lyngbya lagerheimii and Phormidium tenue)

Just recently, Dr. K. R. Gustafson and other scientists at the National Cancer Institute (U.S.) reported that cellular extracts from cultured blue-green algae protected human T cells from infection with the AIDS virus. In test-tube experiments pure compounds extracted from these algae also proved to be "strikingly active against HIV-1." These algae were originally collected in Hawaii and the Palau Islands (Micronesia) and then cultured. The original technique for culturing such marine organisms and producing an extract (which later proved to be cytotoxic) was pioneered by my first professor of pharmacology, Dr. T. R. Norton. It was in Dr. Norton's basement laboratory at Leahi Hospital of the University of Hawaii School of Medicine where I was first introduced to the search for medicines from plants, back in 1968.

The AIDS virus killing compounds just discovered in the blue-green algae are classified as sulfolipids. These lipids are found within the structures of chloroplast membranes and occur widely in other algae, higher plants and microorganisms which conduct photosynthesis. Dextran sulfate, which also inhibits HIV-1 in vitro, is a sulfate ester not a sulfonic acid, as is this new AIDS antiviral compound.

Here, again, is another exciting new potential antiviral drug compound from the world of plants.

Chlorella
(Chlorella spp.)

All that has been said about the other species of seaweed is also applicable to the various unicellular marine algae, especially species of Chlorella.

Numerous animal studies have demonstrated antitumor activity, antiviral activity, and interferon inducing effects. A glycolipid fraction was tested which showed immune-enhancing effects in mice, most likely it was *chlorellin*.

These microscopic species of algae possess distinct biological activities and are certain to take their place among the better-known marine organisms.

A. Laminaria spp. (brown algae, kelp)
I first learned of the anti-cancer and antithrombotic effects of the brown algae from a Japanese colleague. True, I had long believed that mankind would once again "return to the sea," by adding the aquatic plants to his armamentarium of terrestrial medicinals. But my attention was not galvanized until I learned about fucoidan.

Recent research has shown that the main active component with antitumor activity in edible seaweeds is likely a type of sulphated polysaccharide, fucoidan. The same compound has been shown to be responsible for anticoagulant and fibrinolytic activities in animal studies. Another researcher, utilizing epidemiological and biological data, speculates that *Laminaria*, the brown kelp seaweed being discussed, is "an important factor contributing to the relatively low breast cancer rates reported in Japan."

An entire book has been written that is devoted to "marine algae in pharmaceutical science." Marine flora are shown to possess numerous medicinal properties, including antibiotic, antiviral, antimicrobial in general, and antifungal.

Not all of these activities are owing to fucoidan. Dextran sulfate, used in Japan for 30 years to treat heart disease, is shown to also inactivate the herpes simplex virus, for example. The antifungal activity found against *Candida albicans* is owing to a cycloendesmol compound.

Japanese food is in vogue in Western nations, primarily because of the low fat, low calorie, high-fiber aspects. Wakame (a brown kelp, *Undaria*), *Kombu* (Laminaria), and *Nori* (Porphyra) which is used to wrap around rice for sushi, all contain active anti-tumor compounds. These sea vegetables protect us against cancers of the digestive tract due to at least four known factors. The alginic acid content swells in the intestine thus diluting potential carcinogens; some contain beta-sitosterol, a potent anti-cancer compound; they may contain antibiotic compounds which inhibit the growth of several different gram-positive and gram-negative bacteria known to potentiate carcinogens in the colon; and they may possess anti-oxidant activity.

TEA
(Camellia sinensis)

At least half the people in the world drink "the cup that cheers but not inebriates." The beneficial qualities of tea leaves were discovered in the Orient thousands of years ago quite by accident. It is said some Buddhist priests, unable to drink the foul water near their temple, steeped in it the leaves of an aromatic shrub that grew in the vicinity, simply to mask the water's unpleasant taste. They so enjoyed the mild stimulating effects that word spread of this experiment, and the shrub was soon cultivated throughout the region.

Of course, there are other stories about the origin of this delightful beverage. None argue that it was in China that tea was first discovered. The Chinese emperor Kien Lung most aptly extolled the virtues of these leaves when on his deathbed he wrote:

Set a tea-pot over a slow fire; fill it with cold water; boil it long enough to turn a lobster red; pour it on the quantity of tea in a porcelain vessel; allow it to remain on the leaves until the vapor evaporates, then sip it slowly, and all your sorrows will follow the vapor.

Arthur Gray, *The Little Tea Book*

Dutch spice traders first introduced tea to Europe in 1610. Slowly tea became a fashionable but expensive drink. Some of the best kinds then cost as much as fifty dollars a pound. One prominent Dutch physician advised his patients to drink at least eight to ten cups of tea daily, and he even went so far as to claim that he drank fifty, one hundred and sometimes two hundred cups a day.

Not everyone was in favor of this new beverage. As with all new and popular things, there was serious opposition. Some labeled it unfit for civilized people, and others claimed that it was harmful and the source of idleness. In spite of all opposition, however, tea grew in popularity. It became the national drink in England and Russia. The Russian samovar (meaning "to boil itself," from the Greek) is a large brass urn that was devised to keep water boiling throughout the day and night so tea could be prepared at any time. Tea reached New England in 1714. Not only was tea drunk, but the boiled leaves were eaten as a vegetable with salt and butter added.

The quality of tea depends upon how carefully the plants have been grown and at what altitude. Processing also affects the quality. New tea plants are started from seeds planted in containers. They are transplanted when about a foot high, and the picking of leaves begins when the bush is four or five years old. Only the two leaves at the tip of each branch are plucked for the best tea, and this must be done by hand. Although poor- quality teas may contain other leaves and twigs as well, the highest-quality teas contain just the outermost leaves. Tea bushes are pruned back after ten years, and a plant may produce usable leaves for up to forty years.

Processing begins when the harvested leaves are dried and crushed and then spread in cool fermentation sheds. They are later dried with bursts of hot air. After this treatment the leaves develop their aroma and black color. This type of tea is known commercially as black tea, and it is the most popular in the United States because of its strong flavor. The best-known type of black tea is orange pekoe.

Green tea, an unfermented type, is produced by drying the picked leaves, rolling them to break down the tannin-containing cells and redrying them prior to grading, packing and shipping. This is the preferred type of tea in Asia, being somewhat less strongly flavored than black tea. Some important grades of green tea include gunpowder, hyson, and imperial.

Jasmine, a scented tea, is produced by drying the tea leaves together with jasmine flowers. The flowers are later removed, but the tea retains their scent. Jasmine is known as a semi-fermented tea, and it has the flavor of green tea and the color of black tea.

Tannin forms about 10 percent of dry tea leaves. It is similar to the substances used to tan leather and to make black ink. When taken in quantity, tannin interferes with the digestive processes. Steeping tea leaves for a prolonged period of time causes too much tannin to dissolve in the water and makes the tea injurious. This is the reason tea is steeped for only a short time; little of the tannin is extracted into the beverage, while nearly all the aromatic and stimulating properties are.

The stimulant in tea is known as theine. It is almost identical to caffeine, which is present in coffee and cola beverages. These stimulants act by affecting the cerebrum and give the drinker a fresh sense of alertness.

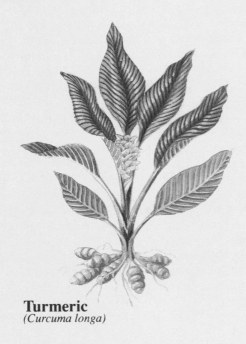

Turmeric
(Curcuma longa)

TURMERIC
(Curcuma longa)

The wisdom of ethnic diets continues to amaze me. Time tested, *authentic* ethnic foods and food combinations evolved slowly and would not have survived as part of a culture were it not for the health-benefits experienced through trial and error.

In the case of East Indian cuisine it has long been the unique use and preparation of freshly ground seasonings that set these ethnic dishes apart. To the Indian it is the *vasana*, or aroma, of food that is key.

Turmeric, ginger, pepper and chili are the major spices found in Indian food. But the list of all the spices used is quite large: cardamon, cloves, cinnamon, mace, nutmeg, saffron, various peppers, dill, cumin, fennel, bay leaf, mustard, coriander and, of course, garlic.

Regional cuisines feature different spices. East, West, South and Northern India, Pakistan and Sri Lanka all have distinctive spiced dishes; collectively they are generally called "East Indian" cuisine.

In one study turmeric extract was tested for its anti-carcinogenic and anti-mutagenic properties. In laboratory (non-human) experiments it was found that this ancient spice reduced both the number of tumors in mice and the mutagenicity of benzo(a)pyrene (BP) and two other potent mutagens, NPD and DMBA (Nagabhushan and Bhide, 1987).

Preventing cancer is now receiving the attention it has long deserved. Biochemical and epidemiological studies have demonstrated the role diet can play in modulating the development of cancer. Earlier studies by these same scientists showed that the active principle of turmeric (curcumin) is a potent anti-mutagenic agent.

For those interested in *how* curcumin may act to prevent cancer we turn again to the by-now all pervasive theory of free-radical inactivation.

The test carcinogens BP and DMBA are "metabolically activated to proximate mutagenic/carcinogenic epoxides" which then bind to macromolecules. The authors conclude that curcumin, which is a "potent anti-oxidant may scavenge these epoxides and prevent binding to macromolecules . . . " (see above reference).

Here then is an example of a spice with similar cell-protective properties as possessed by the nutrient anti-oxidants, vitamin C and vitamin E, which inhibit free radical reactions.

Which brings us to the issue of curcumin as a non-steroidal anti-inflammatory agent. The mechanism of action is unclear but the plant has long been used in folk-medicine to treat conditions such as arthritis, especially in India (Chandra and Gupta, 1972; Rao, *et al.*, 1982).

As we have seen, several other plants with anti-inflammatory activity share certain properties with turmeric. This type of herb is known as a non-steroidal anti-inflammatory (NSAID). Curcumin

259

inhibits cyclooxygenase and lipoxygenase enzymes. Curcumin has three main mechanisms of action; 1) antioxidant activity; 2) lipoxygenase inhibitor; and 3) cycloxygenase inhibition (Tønnesen, 1989). Here then is another set of benefits for a spice long considered an essential flavoring component of an ethnic cuisine.

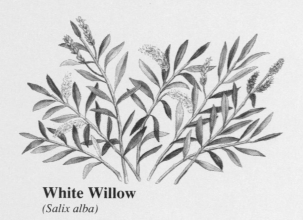

White Willow
(Salix alba)

WHITE WILLOW
(Salix alba)

Aspirin-like compounds, the nonsteroidal, anti-inflammatories, have been found to inhibit the manufacture of certain prostaglandins (PG's) from their precursor, the fatty acid arachidonic acid (AA). Prostaglandins play a key role in the regulation of immune function and compounds capable of blocking the synthesis of certain PG's probably enhance immunity, notably by stimulating the production of macrophages and lymphocytes.

It should be noted, though, that the immune system is not a one way path. Both enhancement and suppression of immunological functions have been reported for PG's! For the sake of this small discussion of aspirin-like compounds, especially willow bark's salicin, it is sufficient to note that PG's and the metabolites of AA are involved in immune reactions. They may also act as co-carcinogens, or as tumor promoters directly.

While we do not know precisely how aspirin and like compounds work, we do know they are among mankind's most useful medicines. Willow bark contains salicin which probably decomposes into salicylic

acid in the human system. The structural formulas for each are shown below.

The glucoside salicin, as obtained from various species of willow, was official in the U.S. Pharmacopoeia from 1882 to 1926.

Looking again at the immune effects of aspirin we should recall that it is a prostaglandin (PGE2) inhibitor. Since PGE2 is an immunosuppressant, when we take aspirin, or like compounds, we may stimulate our immune system by blocking PGE2 production.

By inhibiting the enzyme cyclooxygenase the known activities of aspirin-like compounds take place; namely, blocking of platelet aggregation, antipyretic, anti-inflammatory, analgesic, and immune-enhancing actions. While the PG's play paradoxical roles in each of the above actions, it can be assumed the PG cyclooxygenase inhibitors stimulate the immune response. This includes increased natural killer (NK) cell activity, increased lysing ability of cytotoxic T cells, increased "arming" of macrophages for tumor killing, and direct killing of tumors.

Finally, aspirin is now receiving wide usage to prevent heart attacks in men over 50. This may be due to the fact that cyclooxygenase inhibitors prevent platelet aggregation or blood clots. The spread of tumor cells is also thought to be associated with the clumping of platelets. Several tumor cell types can aggregate platelets and in so doing a metastasis is formed! So, in addition to preventing heart attacks, the aspirin-like compounds, including salicin may also help prevent the spread of cancer.

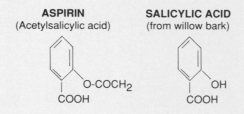

This is a long way from the simple infusions made from the willows by Native Americans. Dioscorides, the ancient Greek physician (circa A.D. 60), who described a species of willow and recommended its use for lowering fevers surely was unaware of the AA

260

pathway and the role of 20-carbon metabolites in stimulating immunity by blocking the synthesis of PG's.

Nevertheless, nature's wisdom is total and current investigations seem to elucidate rather than improve on her formulations. The next time you notice a pussy willow rustling in the breeze focus on the catkins, envision the salicin beneath their surface, and ponder this.

Table 1 Herbs Affecting Immunity

Plant	Compound	Type of Compound	Immune Effects
1. **Astragalus** (*Astragalus membranaceus*)	Not specified (From dried root)		Interferon induction natural killer cell enhancement; antiviral
2. **Citrus oils**	d-limonene	Terpene	Destroys tumors enhances drug metabolism
3. **Echinacea** (*Echinacea angustifolia*)	Echinacoside Unnamed or (Echinacin) Pentadecadiene Caffeic Acid	Glycoside Polysaccharide Hydrocarbon Phenolic	Antibacterial; Nonspecific immune stimulation antitumor effects
4. **Garlic** (*Allium sativa*)	Allicin Methyl allyl Trisulphide	Allyl sulfide	Antitumor effects; kills (candida) Cyclooxygenase & lipoxygenase inhibitor (slows tumor growth)
5. **Golden Seal** (*Hydrastis canadensis*)	Berberine; Hydrastine L-canadine	Alkaloids	Antibiotic Antiviral
6. **Mathaké** (*Terminalia species*)	Linoleic acid Palmitic acid & others	Fatty acids	Antibacterial (kills (Staphylococcus aureus); Anti yeast (kills Candida albicans)
7. **Mushrooms** A. Reishi (*Ganoderma lucidum*)	Arabinoxylo-glucan	Triterpenes Polysaccharides	Adaptogenic; Antitumor; Immuno stimulant
B. Shiitake (*Lentinus edodes*)	Lentinan; Virus-like double pachymaran	Polysaccharide; Stranded DNA	Stimulates T-helper cells; stimulates interferons, NK cells, & macrophages
8. **Oak Bark** (*Quercus* spp.)	Quercitannic acid	Tannins	Anti-parasite
9. **Pau D'Arco** (*Tabebuia impetiginosa*)	Lapachol Lapachone; Alpha & beta xyloidone	Naphthoquinone Quinone Quinone	Mild antitumor action
10. **Seaweeds** A. *Laminaria* spp.(brown algae) B. *Chlorella* spp. (micro algae) C. *Lyngbya lagerheimii* & *Phormidium tenus* (blue green algae)	Fucoidan Chlorellin containing sulfonic acid	Sulfated polysaccharide fatty acid; Glycolipid	Antitumor, antifungal Antiviral; immunostimulant kills AIDS virus
11. **White Willow** (*Salix alba*)	Salicin	Glycoside	Inhibits PG production Inhances immune response Kills cancer cells

Table 2		Herbs for Allergy and Inflammation	
Plant	**Compound**	**Type of Compound**	**Effects**
1. **Butcher's Broom** (*Ruscus aculeatus*)	ruscogenin; neo-ruscogenin and flavonoids	steroidal glycosides	anti-inflammatory; for varicose veins and edema of the legs
2. **Cayenne** (*Capsicum frutescens*)	capsaicin	phenol	topical anti-inflammatory agent
3. **Ephedra or ("Ma-Huang")** (*Ephedra*, various species)	Ephedrine; pseudo-ephedrine	Alkaloids	bronchodilation; central nervous system stimulant
4. **Garlic (and onion)** (*Allium spp*)	aliin; allicin thiosulfinate, quercetin	sulfur containing compounds; bioflavonoid	anti-inflammatory; PAF (platelet activating factor) inhibitor; see item 9
5. **Ginger** (*Zingiber officinale*)	gingerol gingerdione	sesquiterpenes	anti-inflammatory analgesic (relieves pain); antipyritic (lowers fever)
6. **Ginkgo** (*Ginkgo biloba*)	ginkgolides; quercetin	diterpene-lactones bioflavonoid	anti-allergic; treatment of asthma (PAF inhibitor)
7. **Horse Chestnut** (*Aesculus hippocastanum*)	escin	triterpene glycoside	for treatment of varicose veins and edema of the legs
8. **Licorice** (*Glycyrrhiza glabra*)	glycyrrizin	triterpene saponin	like hydrocortisone, inhibits inflammation; soothes mucus membrane; expectorant
9. **Quercetin** (*a compound*)	quercetin	bioflavonoid	anti-inflammatory (clycloxygenase and lipoxygenase inhibitor); anti-allergic (blocks histamine release); anti-oxidant
10. **Turmeric** (*Curcuma longa*)	curcumin	phenol	anti-inflammatory (cycloxygenase and lipoxygenase inhibitor); anti-oxidant
11. **White Willow** (*Salix alba*)	Salicin	phenolic glycoside	anti-inflammatory; analgesic (relieves pain); antipyritic (lowers fever)

PLANT INDEX (To Expanded Section)

English/Latin

Aloe Vera   *Aloe vera*
Angelica   *Angelica sinensis; A. acutiloba*
Astragalus   *Astragalus membranaceous*
Bilberry   *Vaccinium myrtillus*
Bupleurum
  (Shosaikoto)   *Bupleurum falcatum*
Butcher's Broom   *Ruscus aculeatus*
Cacao   *Theobroma cacao*
Cayenne   *Capsicum frutescens*
Chamomile   *Anthemis nobilis*
Chinese Cucumber (Compound Q Source)
  Trichosanthes kirilowii
Chlorella   *Chlorella, Var. spp.*
Citrus   *Var. spp.*
Coffee   *Coffee arabica*
Cola   *Cola acuminata*
Echinacea   *Echinacea angustifolia, E. purpurea,*
  E. pallida
Ephedra (Ma-Huang)   *Ephedra, Var. spp.*
Feverfew   *Tanacetum parthenium*
Garlic   *Allium spp.*
Ginger   *Zingiber officinale*
Ginkgo   *Ginkgo biloba*
Ginseng   *Var. spp.*
Goldenseal   *Hydrastis canadensis*
Guarana   *Paullinia cupana; P. sorbilis*
Horsechestnut   *Aesculus hippocastanum*
Khat   *Catha edulis*
Licorice   *Glycrrhiza glabra*
Mate   *Ilex paraguensis*
Mathake
  (Tropical Almond)   *Terminalia catappa*
Milk Thistle   *Silymarin marianum*
Mushrooms
  Reishi   *Ganoderma lucidum*
  Shiitake   *Lentinus edodes*
Oak   *Quercus spp.*
Pau d'Arco   *Tabebuia impetiginosa and other*
  species
Quercetin   *(A Bioflavanoid found in many plants)*
Rue   *Ruta chalepensis*
Schisandra   *Schisandra chinensis*

Seaweeds
  Blue-Green Algae   *Lyngbya lagerheimii &*
    Phormidium tenue
  Chlorella   *Chlorella spp.*
  Laminaria (Brown Algae, or Kelp)
    Laminaria spp.
Tea   *Camellia sinensis*
Turmeric   *Curcuma longa*
Willow, White   *Salix alba*

264

PLANT INDEX (To Expanded Section)

Latin/English

Aesculus hippocastanum   Horsechestnut
Aloe vera   Aloe Vera
Allium spp.   Garlic (& Onion)
Angelica sinensis; A. Acutiloba   Angelica
Anthemis nobilis   Chamomile
Astragalus membranaceous   Astragalus
Bioflavonoids   Quercetin
Bupleurum falcatum   Bupleurum (Shosaikoto)
Camellis sinensis   Tea
Capsicum frutescens   Cayenne
Catha edulis   Khat
Chlorella spp.   Chlorella
Coffee arabica   Coffee
Cola acuminata   Cola
Curcuma longa   Turmeric
Echinacea angustifolia   Echinacea
E. purpurea   Echinacea
E. pallida   Echinacea
Ephedra, var. spp.   Ephedra (Ma-Huang)
Ganoderma lucidum   Reishi Mushrooms
Ginkgo biloba   Ginkgo
Glycrrhiza glabra   Licorice
Hydrastis canadensis   Goldenseal
Ilex paraguenis   Mate
Laminaria spp.   Laminaria (Brown algae, kelp)
Lentinus edodes   Shiitake Mushrooms
Lyngbya lagerheimii   Blue-Green algae
Paullinia cupana, P. sorbilis   Guarana
Phormidium tenue   Blue-Green algae
Quercus spp.   Oak
Ruscus aculeatus   Butcher's Broom
Ruta chalepensis   Rue
Salix alba   Willow, White
Schisandra chinensis   Schisandra
Silymarin marianum   Milk Thistle
Tabebuia impetiginosa   Pau d'Arco
Tanacetum parthenium   Feverfew
Terminalia catappa   Mathake (Tropical almond)
Theobroma cacao   Cacao
Trichosanthes kirilowii   Chinese Cucumber (Source
   of Compound Q)
Vaccinium myrtillus   Bilberry
Zingiber officinale   Ginger

REFERENCES

Acheson, K. J., Zahorska-Markiewicz, B., Pittet, P., Anantharaman, K., and Jéquier, E. Caffeine and coffee: Their influence on metabolic rate and substrate utilization in normal weight and obese individuals. *Am. J. Clin. Nutr.*, *33*:989-997, 1980.

Ahumada, F., Hermosilla, J., Hola, Pena, R., Wittwer, F., and Wegmann, E.; Hancke, J. and Wikman, G. Studies on the effect of *Schizandra chinensis* extract on horses submitted to exercise and maximum effort. *Phytotherapy Research*, *3*(5):175-179, 1989.

Amla, V., Verma, S. L., Sharma, T. R., Guptu, O. P., and Atal, C. K. Clinical study of *Allium cepa* Linn in patients of brochial asthma. *Ind. J. Pharmacol.*, *13*:63, 1980.

Anderson, R. Ascorbate-mediated stimulation of neutrophil motility and lymphocyte transformation by inhibition of the peroxidase/H2O2/halide system in vitro and in vivo. *Am. J. Clin. Nutr.*, *34*:1906-1911, 1981.

Anonymous. Acid polysaccharide Ch-1 with physiological activity. Patent-Belg-894, 925: 16pp-, 1983.

Anonymous. *Journal of the National Cancer Institute*, *81*(2): 162- 164, 1989.

Anonymous. Stable anticiotic preparations. Patent-Ger-942,534 :.-., 1956.

Arch, J. R. S., Ainsworth, A. T., and Cawthorne, M. A. Thermogenic and anorectic effects of ephedrine and congener in mice and rats. *Life Sci.*, *30*:1817, 1982.

Astrup, A., Lundegaard, C., Madsen, J., *et al.* Enhanced thermogenic responsiveness during chronic ephedrine treatment in man. *Am. J. Clin. Nutr.*, *42*:83, 1985.

Astrup, A., Toubro, S., Cannon, S., Hein, P., Breum, L., and Madsen, J. Caffeine: A double-blind, placebo-controlled study of its thermogenic, metabolic, and cardiovascular effects in healthy volunteers. *Am. J. Clin. Nutr.*, *51*:759-767, 1990.

Austin, F. G. Schistosoma mansoni chemoprophylaxis with dietary lapachol. *The American Journal of Tropical Medicine and Hygiene*, *23*(3): 412-415, 1974.

Bak, A. A. and Brobbee, D. E. "The effect on serum cholesterol levels of coffee brewed by filtering or boiling." *New Eng. J. Med.*, *321*:1432, 1989.

Baltina, L. A., Davydova, V. A., Chikaeva, I. G., Shayakhmetova, R. M., Kapina, A. P., Lazareva, D. N., and Tolstikov, G. A. Synthesis and antiphlogistic activity of protected glycopeptides of glycyrrhizic acid. *Pharm. Chem. J.*, *226*:460-462, 1989.

Barchi, J. J., Norton, T. R., Furusawa, E. et al. Identification of a cytoxin from *Tolypothrix byssoidea* as Tubercidin. *Phytochemistry*, *22*: 2851-2852, 1983.

Barone, F., and Tansey, M. Isolation, purification, identification, synthesis, and kinetics of activity of the anticandidal component of *Allium sativum*, and a hypothesis for its mode of action. *Mycologia*, *69*: 793-825, 1977.

Bauer, R., Jurcic, K., Puhlmann, J., and Wagner, H. Immunological in vivo examinations of echinacea extracts. *Arzneim-Forsch*, 38(2): 276-281, 1988.

Belman, S. Inhibition of soybean lipoxygenase by onion and garlic oil constituents. *Proc. Am. Assoc. Cancer Res.*, *26:* 131, 1985.

Belman, S. Onion and garlic oils and tumour promotion. *Carcinogenesis*, *4:* 1063-1065, 1983.

Bernstein, I., Johnson, C., and Tse, C. Therapy with cromolyn sodium. *Annals of Internal Medicine*, *89*:223-228, 1978.

Bilyk, A., Cooper, P., and Sapers, G. Verietal differences in distribution of quercetin and kaempferol in onion (*Allium cepa*) tissue. *Journal of Agricultural Food Chemistry, 32:* 274-285, 1984.

Bønaa, K., Arnesen, E., Thelle, D. S., and Førde, O. H. Coffee and cholesterol: Is it all in the brewing? The Tromsø study. Br. Med. J., 297:1103-1104, 1988.

Bordia, A., and Verma, S. Effect of garlic feeding on regression of experimental atherosclerosis in rabbits. *Artery, 7:* 428-436, 1980.

Bordia, A., Verma, S., Khabia, B., Vyas, A., Rathore, A., Bhu, N., and Bedi, H. The effect of active principle of garlic and onion on blood lipids and experimental atherosclerosis in rabbits and their comparison with clofibrate. *Journal of the Association of Physicians of India, 25:* 509-521, 1977.

Boyd, L. J. The pharmacology of the homeopathic drugs. *J. Amer Inst Homeopathy, 21:* 312-323, 1920.

Braquet, P. (ed.). The role of platelet-activating factor in Immune Disorders. Proceedings of the Meeting of the Foundation IPSEN pour la Recherche Thrapeutique Paris, June 25-26, 1987 (Part II).

Bukowiecki, L. J., Lupien, J., Folléa, N., and Jahjah, L. Effects of sucrose, caffeine, and cola beverages on obesity, cold resistance, and adipose tissue cellularity. *Am. J. Physiol.*, *244*:R500-507, 1983.

Cahn, J., Herold, M., and Sanault, B. Antiphlogistic and anti-4 inflammatory activity of F 191. Int. Symp. Non Steroidal Anti-o inflammatory Drugs, Milano, 1964.

Capra, C. Studio farmacologico e tossicologico di componenti del Ruscus aculeatus L. *Fitoterapia, 43:*99, 1972.

Catha Edulis (Khat): Special Issue, *Bulletin on Narcotics*, *32*(3):1-95, 1980.

Caujolle, F., Meriel, P., and Stanilas, E. Sur les propriétés pharmacologiques de Ruscus aculeatus L. *Ann. Pharm. Franc.*, *11*:109, 1953.

Chabanon, R. Expérimentation du Proctolog dans les hémorroides et les fissures anales. *Gaz. Méd de France*, *83*:3013, 1976.

Chandra, Dinesh and Gupta, S. S. Anti-inflammatory and anti-arthritic activity of volatile oil of curcuma longa (haldi). *Indian J. Med. Res., 60,* 1972.

Chang, C. Y., Hou, Y. D., and Xu, F. M. Effect of astragalus membranaceus on enhancement of mouse natural killer cell activity. *Chung-kuo I Hsueh K'o Hsueh Yuan Hsueh Pao, 4*(4): 231-234, 1983.

Chang, I. H., Kim. J. H., and Han, D. S. Toxicological evaluation of medicinal plants used for herbal drugs (4). Acute toxicity and antitumor activities. *Korean J. Pharmacog, 13*(2):62-69, 1983.

Chang, J., and Lewis, A. J. Prostaglandins and cyclooxygenase inhibitors, in Immune-modulation agents and their mechanisms, E.L. Fenischel and M.A. Chirigos (Eds.) Marcel Dekker, New York, 1984.

Chen, Y. Y., Shu, Z., and Li, L. N. Studies of fructus shizanorae. IV. Isolation and determination of the active compounds (in lowering high SGPT levels) of *Schizandra chinensis. Chung-Kuo K. O. Hsueh, 19:*276-, 1976.

Cheng, H. H., et al. The anti-tumor effect of cultivated ganoderma lucidum extract. *Journal of the Chinese Oncology Society, 1*(3): 12-16, 1982.

Cheraskin, E., Ringsdorf, W. M., Setyaadmadja, A. T. S. H., and Barrett, R. A. Effect of caffeine versus placebo supplementation on blood-glucose concentration. Lancet, 2:1299-1300, 1967.

Chi, M. Effects of garlic products in lipid metabolism in cholesterol-fed rats. *Proceedings of the Society for Experimental Biology and Medicine, 171:* 174-178, 1982.

Chida, K., and Yamamoto, I. Antitumor activity of a crude fucoidan fraction prepared from the roots of kelp (*laminaria* species). *Kitasato Arch. of Exp. Med., 60*(1-2): 33-39, 1987.

Chu, D. T., Wong, W. L. and Mavligit, G. M. Immunotherapy with Chinese medicinal herbs I. immune restoration of local xenogeneic graft-versus-host react cancer patients by fractionated astragalus membranaceous in vitro. *J Clin Lab Immunol, 25*(3): 119-123, 1988.

Chung, K. F., McCusker, M., Page, C. P., Dent, G., Guinot, Ph., and Barnes, P. J. Effect of a ginkgolide mixture (BN 52063) in antagonizing skin and platelet responses to platelet activating factor in man. *The Lancet,* January 31, 1987.

Clegg, R. J., Middleton, B., Bell, G. D., and White, D. A. Inhibition of hepatic cholesterol synthesis by monoterpenes administered in vivo. *Biochem Pharmacol, 29:* 2125-2127, 1980.

Cody, V., *et al.* (eds.) *Plant Flavonoids in Biology and Medicine II,* New York, Alan R. Liss, 1988.

Coeugniet, E. G., and Elek, E. Immunomodulation with viscum album and echinacea purpurea extracts. *Onkologie, 10*(3): 27-33, 1987.

Collier, W. A., and Van De Piji, L. The antibiotic action plants, especially the higher plants, with results from Indonesian plants. *Chron Nat, 105*: 8-, 1949.

Costill, D. L., Dalsky, G. P., and Fink, W. J. "Effects of caffeine ingestion on metabolism and exercise performance." *Med. Sci. Sports, 10:*155, 1978.

Curatolo, P. W. and Robertson, D. "The health consequences of caffeine." *Ann. Intern. Med., 98:*642, 1983.

D'Amico, M. L. Investigation of the presence of substances having antibiotic action in higher plants. *Fitoterapia, 21:* 77-, 1950.

Da Consolacao, F., Linardi, M., De Oliveira, M.M. and Sampaio, M.R.P. A lapachol derivative active against mouse lymphocytic leukemia P-388. *J Med Chem, 18:* 1159-, 1975 (Sect Pharmacol Inst Biol Sau Paulo Brazil)

Dabas, Y., Rao, V., Saxena, O., and Sharma, V. Efficacy of therapy against infectious genital tract disorders in bovine. *Indian Journal of Animal Science, 53:* 81-89, 1983.

De, A. K. and Ghosh, J. J. Short and long-term effects of capsaicin on the pulmonary anti-oxidant enzyme system in rats. *Phytotherapy Research, 3*(5), 1989.

De Swarte, R. D. Drug allergy. In R. Patterson (ed.), *Allergic Diseases,* Philadelphia, J. B. Lippincott Co., 1980.

Dörling, E. Do ginsenosides influence performance? *Notabene Medici, 10*(5):241-246, 1980.

Dorsch, W., et al. Anti-asthmatic effects of onions. *Biochemial Pharmacology, 37*(23):4479-4486, 1988.

Dulloo, A. G. and Miller, A. S. "Ephedrine, caffeine and aspirin: 'Over the counter' drugs that interact to stimulate thermogenesis in the obese." *Nutrition, 5:*7, 1989.

Dulloo, A. G. and Miller, D. S. Reversal in obesity in the genetically obese fa/fa Zucker rat with an ephedrine/Methylxanthine (caffeine) thermogenic mixture. *J. Nutrition, 117:*383-389, 1987.

Dulloo, A. G. and Miller, D. S. Obesity—a disorder of the sympathetic nervous system. *World Rev. Nutr. Diet, 50:*1, 1987.

Dulloo, A. G., Geissler, G. A., Horton, T., Collins, A., and Miller, D. S. Normal caffeine consumption: Influence on thermogenic and daily energy expenditure in lean and postobese human volunteers. *Am. J. Clin. Nutr., 49:*44-50, 1989.

Eagle, R. *Eating and Allergy,* New York, Doubleday & Co. Inc., 1981.

Elden, H. R. Ginsenosides—new uses for an old root. *Drug and Cosmetic Industry,* pp. 36-40, April 1990.

Elegbede, J., Elson, C. Tanner, M., Qureshi, A., and Gould, M. Regression of rat primary mammary tumors following dietary d-i limonene. *Journal of the National Cancer Institute, 76:* 323-325, 1986.

267

Elson, C., Maltzman, T., Boston, J., Tanner, M., and Gould, M. Anti-carcinogenic activity of d-limonene during the initiation and promotion/progression stages of DMBA-induced rat mammary carcinogenesis. *Carcinogenesis, 9:* 331-332, 1988.

Evans, D., Miller, D., Jacobsen, K., and Bush, P. Modulation of immune responses in mice by d-limonene. Journal of Toxicological and Environmental Health, 20: 51-66, 1987.

Fenwich, G.. and Hanley, A. The genus *Allium-Part 2. CRC Critical Reviews in Food Science and Nutrition, 22:* 273-341, 1985.

Ferreira De Santana, C., Goncalves De Lima, O, D'Albuquerque, I.L., Lacerda, A.L., and Martins, D.G. The antitumor and toxic properties of substances extracted from the wood of tabebuia avellanedae. *Rev Inst Antibiont Univ Fed Pernambuco Recife, 8:* 89-, 1968. (Inst Antibiont Univ Fed Pernambuco Recife Brazil)

Finney, R. S. H., Somers, C. F., and Wilkinson, J. H. Pharmacological properties of glycyrrhetinic acid—a new anti-inflammatory drug. *J. Pharm. Pharmacol., 10:*687, 1958.

Forgo, I. On the question of influencing the performance of sportsmen. *Aerztliche Praxis, 33*(44):1784-1786, 1981.

Forgo, I. and Schimert, G. The duration of effect of the standardized Ginseng extract G115® in healthy competitive athletes. *Notabene Medici, 15*(9):636-640, 1985.

Frazier, C. A. Insect sting reactions in children. *Ann. Allergy 23*:37-46, 1965.

Fredholm, B. B. Gastrointestinal and metabolic effects of methylxanthines. In Dews, P. B., ed., The methylxanthine beverages and foods: Chemistry, consumption, and health effects. New York: A. R. Liss Press, 1984, pp. 331-354.

Frick, O. Immediate hypersensitivity. In H. Fudenberg, D. Stites, J. Caldwell, and J. Wells (eds.), *Basic and Clinical Immunology,* Los Altos, CA, Lange Medical Publications, 1976, pp. 204-224.

Fujita, H., Sakurai, T., Yoshida, M., and Toyoshima, S. Anti-inflammatory effects of glycyrrhizinic acid. *Oyo Yakuri, 19:*481-484, 1980.

Garcia-Leme, J. *Hormones and Inflammation.* Boca Raton, FL, CRC Press, 1989.

Giannini, A. James and Castellani, S. A manic-like psychosis due to Khat (Catha edulis Forsk.). *J. Toxicol. - Clin. Toxicol, 19*(5):455-459, 1982.

Gijon, J. R. and Murcia, C. R. Estudio farmacologico comparativo de la actividad anti-inflammatoria local del acido glicirretinico con la de la cortisona. *An. Real Acad. Farm., 26:*5, 1960.

Gong, Z. and Lin, Z. B. The pharmacological study of lingzhi (ganoderma lucidum) and the research of therapeutical principle of "fuzheng guben" in traditional Chinese medicine. *Pei-Ching I Hsueh Yuan Hsueh Pao, 13:* 6-10, 1981.

Gustafson, K. R., et al. AIDS-antiviral sulfolipids from cyanobacteria (blue-green algae). *Journal of the National Cancer Institute, 81*(16): August 16, 1989.

Haddon, A. C. Reports of the Cambridge anthropological expedition to Torres Straits. Cambridge at the University Press, Cambridge England, *Book 6:* 107-,1908.

Hammerschmidt, D. E. and Jacob, H. S. The stimulated granulocyte as a source of toxic oxygen compounds in tissue injury. In A. P. Autor (ed.), *Pathology of Oxygen,* New York, Academic Press, 1982, pp. 59-73.

Hancke, J. L., Wikman, G., and Hernandez, D. E. Antidepressant activity of selected natural products. *Planta Med., 1986*(6):542-. 543, 1986.

Hartwell, J. L. Plants used against cancer. A survey. *Lloydia, 32:* 247-296, 1969; *33:* 97-194; 288-392, 1970.

Hay, G. and Willuhn, G. Antiviral activity of aqueous extracts from medicinal plants in tissue cultures. *Drug Res, 28*(1): 1-7, 1978.

Hendrich, S. and Bjeldanes, L. F. Effects of dietary cabbage, brussels sprouts, illicium verum, *Schizandra chinensis* and alfalfa on the benzopyrene metabolic system in mouse liver. *Food Chem. Toxicol., 21*(4):479-486, 1983.

Hendrich, S. and Bjeldanes, L. F. Effects of dietary *Schizandra chinensis,* brussels sprouts and illicium verum extracts on carcinogen metabolism systems in mouse liver. *Food Chem. Toxicol., 24*(9):903-912, 1989.

Hernandez, O. E., Hancke, J. L., and Wikman, G. Evaluation of the anti-ulcer and antisecretory activity of extracts of aralia elata root and *Schizandra chinensis* fruit in the rat. *J. Ethnopharmacol., 23*(1):109-114, 1988.

Hikino, H., Kiso, Y., Taguchi, H., and Ikeya, Y. Antihepatotoxic actions of lignoids from *Schizandra chinensis* fruits. *Planta Med., 50*(3):213-218, 1984.

Hill, R. B. and La Via, M. F. (eds.) *Principles of Pathobiology* (Third Edition), New Jersey, Oxford University Press, 1980.

Hoppe, H. A., Levring, T., and Tanaka, Y. (eds.). Marine algae in pharmaceutical science. Walter de Gruyter, Berlin, New York, 1979.

Hou, Y., Ma, G. L., Wu, S. H., Li, Y. Y., and Li, H. T. Effect of radix astragali seu hedysari on the interferon system. *Chin Med J, 94*(1): 35-40, 1981.

Huxtable, R. J. Herbs along the western Mexican-

268

American border. *Proc West Pharmacol Soc, 26:* 185-191, 1983. English (Dept Pharmacol Health Sci Cent Univ Arizona Tucson, AZ 85724 USA)

Igimi, J., Hisatsugu, T., and Nishimura, M. The use of d-t limonene preparation as a dissolving agent of gallstones. *Amer J Dig Dis,* 21:926-, 1976.

Hewett, A. C. Echinacea purpurea, echinacea angustifolia, echafolta. *Dental Rev., 20:* 1218-1230, 1906.

Iizuka, C. Antiviral substance. Patent-Fr Demande Fr-2, 485,373: 30pp-, 1980.

Itoh, T., Zang, Y. F., Murai, S., and Saito, H. Effects of *Panax ginseng* on the vertical and horizontal motor activities and on brain monoamine-related substances in mice. *Planta Medica, 55:*429, 1989.

Jancsó, N., Jancsó-Gábor, A., and Szolcsányi, J. Direct evidence for neurogenic inflammation and its prevention by denervation and by pretreatment with capsaicin. *Br. J. Pharmacol., 31:*138, 1967.

Jecuier, E. and Schultz, Y. New evidence for a thermogenic defect in human obesity. *Int. J. Obesity, 9*(Suppl 2):1, 1985.

Jung, R. T., Shetty, P. S., James, W. P. T., Barrand, M. A., and Callingham, B. A. Caffeine: Its effect on catecholamines and metabolism in lean and obese subjects. *Clin. Sci., 60:*527-535, 1981.

Kabelik, J. The echinacea: Possibly an important medicinal plant? *Ziva, 13*(1): 4-5, 1965.

Kalix, P. Amphetamine psychosis due to Khat leaves. *The Lancet,* January 7, 1984.

Kaplan, G. Mononuclear phagocytes in inflammation. In P. Venge and A. Lindblom (eds.), *The Inflammatory Process. An Introduction to the Study of Cellular and Humoral Mechanisms,* Stockholm, Almqvist and Wiksell International, 1981, pp. 239-261.

Katzeff, H. L., O'Connell, M., Horton, E. S., *et al.* Metabolic studies in human obesity during overnutrition and undernutrition: Thermogenic and hormonal responses to norepinephrine. *Metabolism, 35:*166, 1988.

Khan, I. and Kalix, P. Khat, a plant with amphetamine-like effects. *Trends in Pharmaceutical Sciences, 5,* August 1984.

Paris, R. and Moyse, H. Abyssinian tea (*Catha edulis* Forssk, *Celastraceae). Bulletin on Narcotics, April-June, 1958,* pp. 29-34.

Kim, H., Jang, C., and Lee, M. Antinarcotic effects of the standardized ginseng extract G115 on morphine. *Planta Medica,* 56:158, 1990.

Kim, M. S., Lee, M. G., Lee, J. H., Byun, S. J., and Kim, Y. C. Immunopotentiating activity of water extracts of some crude drugs. *Korean J. Pharmacolog, 19*(3):193-200, 1988.

Koda, A., Nishiyori, T., Nagai, H., Matsuura, N., and Tsuchiya, H. Anti-allergic actions of crude drugs and blended Chinese traditional medicines. Effects on Type I and Type IV allergic reactions. *Nippon Yakurigaku Zasshi, 80:*31-41, 1982.

Kremer, J. M., Jubiz, W., Michalek, A., et al. Fish-oil fatty acid supplementation in active rheumatoid arthritis. *Annals of Internal Medicine, 106*(4):497-502, 1987.

Krupp, M., and Chatton, M. The leukotrienes in allergy and inflammation. *Science, 215:*1380-1383, 1982.

Kubo, M., Matsuda, H., Nogami, M., Arichi, S., and Takahashi, T. Studies on ganoderma lucidum. IV. Effects on the disseminated intravascular coagulation. *Yakugaku Zasshi, 103*(8): 871-877, 1983.

Lansberg, L., Saville, M. E., and Young J. B. Sympathoadrenal system and regulation of thermogenesis. *Am. J. Physio., 247:*181, 1984.

Lessof, M. H., (ed.). *Clinical Reactions to Food.* Chichester, England, John Wiley & Sons, 1983.

Levine, S. A. and Kidd, P. M. *Antioxidant Adaptation, Its Role in Free Radical Pathology,* San Leandro, CA, Biocurrents Division, 1986.

Lewis, R. and Austen, K. Mediation of local homeostasis and inflammation by leukotrienes and other mast cell-dependent compounds. *Nature, 293:*103-108, 1981.

Li, Y. Y., Liu, X. Y., Shi, L. Y., Li, Y. X., and Hou, Y. D. Induction characteristic of lymphoblastoid interferon. *Chung-kuo I Hsueh K'o Hsueh Yuan Hsueh Pao, 2:* 250-252, 1980.

Liu, G. T. and Wei, H. L. Protection by fructus schizanorae against acetaminophen hepatotoxicity in mice. *Yao Hsueh Hsueh Pao, 22*(9):650-654, 1987.

Liu, G. T., Wang, G. F., Wei, H. L., Bao, T. T., and Song, Z. Y. A comparison of the protective actions of biphenyl dimethyl-d dicarboxylate trans-stilbene, alcoholic extracts of fructus schizanorae and ganoderma against experimental liver injury in mice. *Yag Hsueh Hsueh Pao, 14:*598-604, 1979.

Lombardino, J. G. (ed.). *Nonsteroidal Anti-inflammatory Drugs.* New York, Wiley, 1985.

Lopes, M., et al. "Effects of caffeine on skeletal muscle function before and after fatigue." *J. App. Physio., 54:*1303.

Maeda, Y. Y., and Chihara, G. The effects of neonatal thymectomy on the antitumor activity of lentinan. *Int J Cancer, 11:* 153-161, 1973.

Magliulo, E., Carco, F. P., Gorini, S., and Barigazzi, G. M. Ricerche in vivo ed in vitro sull'azione antiflogistica dell'escina. *Arch. Sc. Med., 125:*207, 1968.

Malchow-Møller, A., Larsen, S., Hey H., Stokholm, K. H., Juhl, E., and Quaade, F. Ephedrine as an anorectic: The story of the "Elsinore pill." *Int. J. Obes., 5:*183-187, 1981.

269

Maltzman, T., Tanner, M., Elson, C., and Gould, M. Anticarcinogenic activity of specific orange peel oil monoterpenes. Federation Proceedings, *45:* 970, 1986.

Manca, P. and Passarelli, E. Aspetti farmacologici dell'escina principio attivo dell'aesculus hyppocastanum. *Clin. Terap.*, *32:*297, 1965.

Marcelon, G., Verbeuren, T. J., Lauressergues, H., and Vanhoutte, P. M. Effect of Ruscus aculeatus on isolated canine cutaneous veins. *Gen. Pharmac.*, *14:*103, 1983.

Marderosian, A. D. and Liberti, L. E. *Natural Product Medicine: A Scientific Guide to Foods, Drugs, Cosmetics.* Philadelphia, PA, Geroge F. Stickley Co., 1988.

Maruyama, H., Nakajima, J., and Yamamoto, I. A study on the anticoagulant and fibrinolytic activities of a crude fucoidan from the edible brown seaweed *laminaria religiosa*, with special reference to its inhibitory effect on the growth of a sarcoma-180 ascites cells subcutaneously implanted into mice. *Kitasato Arch. of Exp. Med.*, *60*(3), 105-121, 1987.

Massoni, G., Piovella, C., and Fratti, L. Effets microcirculatoires de la Ginkgo biloba chez les personnes ages. *Gioren. Geront.*, *20:*444, 1972.

McCaleb, R. Ginseng conference report. *Herbalgram*, No. 16, pp. 8-12, Spring 1988.

McGrath, M. S., *et al.* GLQ 223: An inhibitor of human immuno deficiency virus replication in acutely and chemically infected cells of lymphocyte and mononuclear phagocyte lineage. *Proc. Natl. Acad. Sci.*, *86:*2844-2848, April 1989.

Metz, S. A. Anti-inflammatory agents as inhibitors of prostaglandin synthesis in man. *Med. Clin. N. Am.* *65*(4)(Symposium Issue):713-757, 1981.

Middleton, E. The flavonoids. *Medical Nutrition*, 1989.

Miyazawa, Y., Murayama, T., Ooya, N., Wang, L. F., Tung, Y. C., and Yamaguchi, N. Immunomodulation by a unicellular green algae *(chlorella pyrenoidosa)* in tumor-bearing mice. *J. Ethnopharmacol*, *24*(2-3): 135-146, 1988.

Moncada, S. and Vane, J. R. (eds.). Prostacyclin, thromboxane and leukotrienes. *British Med. Bull.*, *39*(3), July 1983.

Morgan, J. B., York, D. A., Wasilewska, A., *et al.* A study of the thermogenic responses to a meal and to a sympathomimetic drug (ephedrine) in relation to energy balance in man. *Br. J. Nutr.*, *47:*21, 1982.

Moscarella, C. Contribution l'tude pharmacologique du Ruscus aculeatus L. (Fragon pineux). Thse de Pharmacie, Toulouse, 1953.

Nagabhushan, M. and Bhide, S. V. Antimutagenicity and anticarcinogenicity of turmeric (curcuma longa). *Journal of Nutrition, Growth and Cancer*, *4:*83-89, 1987.

Nanba, H., and Kuroda, H. Antitumor mechanisms of orally administered shiitake fruit bodies. *Chem Pharm Bull*, *35*(6): 2459-2464, 1987.

Natarajan, S., Murti, V. V. S., Seshadri, T., and Ramaswani, A. S. Pharmacological properties of flavonoids and biflavanoids. *Curr. Sci.*, *39:*533, 1970.

Nishiyori, T., Matsuura, N., Nagai, H., and Koda, A. Anti-a allergic action of Chinese drugs. *Jap. J. Pharmacol. Suppl.*, *31:*115-, 1981.

Nogami, M., Ito, M., Kubo, M., Takahashi, M., Kimura, H., and Matsuike, Y. Studies on ganoderma lucidum. VII. Anti-allergic effects. (2). *Yakugaku Zasshi*, *106*(7): 600-604, 1986.

Nogami, M., Kubo, M., Kimura, H., and Takahashi, M. Studies on ganoderma lucidum. V. Inhibitory activity on the release of histamine from the isolated mast cells. *Shoyakugaku Zasshi*, *40*(2): 241-243., 1986.

Nogami, M., Tsuji, Y., Kubo, M., Takahashi, M., Kimura, H., and Matsuike, Y. Studies on ganoderma lucidum. Vi. Anti-allergic effect.(i). *Yakugaku Zasshi*, *106*(7): 594-599, 1986.

Pao, T. T., Liu, K. I., Hsu, K. F., and Sung, C. Y. Studies on schizandra fruit. I. Its effect on increased SGPT levels in animals caused by hepatotoxic chemical agents. *Natl. Med. J. China*, *54:*275-, 1974.

Pasquali, R., Cesari, M. P., Melchionda, N., Stefanini, C., Raitano, A., and Labo, G. Does ephedrine promote weight loss in low-energy-adapted obese women? *International Journal of Obesity*, *11:*163-168, 1987.

Patterson, R. ed. Allergic Diseases, Philadelphia, J. B. Lippincott Co., 1980.

Peng, J., Wu, S., Zhang, L, Hou, Y., and Colby, B. Inhibitory effects of interferon and its combination with antiviral drugs on adenovirus multiplication. *Chung-kuo I Hsueh K'o Hsueh Yuan Hsueh Pao*, *6*(2): 116-119, 1984.

Peter, H. Vasoactivity of Ginkgo biloba preparation. 4th Conf. Hung. Ther. Invert. Pharmacol. Soc. Pharmacol. Hung. (Edited by Dumbovitch, B.), 177, 1968.

Powers, S. K. and Dodd, S. "Caffeine and endurance performance." *Sports Med.*, *2:*21, 1985.

Quisumbing. E. Medicinal plants of the Philippines. JMC Press, Inc. Quezon City, Philippines, 1978.

Rainsford, K. and Swann, B. The biochemistry and pharmacology of oxygen radical involvement in eicosanoid production. In J. V. Bannister and W. H. Bannister (eds.), *The Biology and Chemistry of Active Oxygen*, NY, Elsevier Publishing Co., 1984, pp. 105-127.

Ratafia, M., and Purinton, T. The untapped market in plant derived drugs. *Medical Marketing and Media*, 58-68, June 1988.

Rayner, H. C., Atkins, R. C. and Westerman, R. A. Relief of local stump pain by capsaicin cream. *The Lancet*, 1276-1277, 1989.

Robbins, S. L. and Cotran, R. S. *Pathologic Basis of Disease*. Philadelphia, W. B. Saunders Co (2nd Edition), 1979.

Roth, R. P., *et al*. Nasal decongestant activity of pseudoephedrine. Annals of OTOL. 86, 1977.

Ryan, G. B., Majno, G. *Inflammation*. Kalamazoo, MI, The Upjohn Co., 1977.

Samson, R. R. Atherosclerosis. *44*:119-120, 1092.

Samuelsson, B. Leukotrienes: mediators of immediate hypersentivity reactions and inflammation. *Science, 220*:568-575, 1983.

Schnittman, S. M., *et al*. The reservoir for HIV-1 in human peripheral blood is a T cell that maintains expression of CD4. *Science, 245*: 305-308, 1989.

Shimizu, A., Yano, T., Saito, Y., and Inada, Y. Isolation of an inhibitor of platelet aggregation from a fungus, ganoderma lucidum. *Chem Pharm Bull, 33*(7): 3012-3015, 1985.

Shin, H. W., Kim, H. W., Choi, E. C., Toh, S. H., and Kim, K. B. Studies on inorganic composition and immunopotentiating activity of ganoderma lucidum in Korea. *Korean J Pharmacog, 16*(4): 181-190, 1985.

Shin, K. H. and Woo, W. S. A survey of the response of medicinal plants on drug metabolism. *Korean J. Pharmacog, 11*:109-122, 1980.

Shipochliev, T. and Ilieva, S. Pharmacologic study of Bulgarian *Schizandra chinensis*. *Farmatseyacsofia, 17*(3):56-, 1967.

Siering, H. Die permeabilitt von Zellmembranen, fr lonen unter dem Einfluss von Aescin. *Arzneim. Forsch, 12*:376, 1962.

Sikora, R., Sohn, M., Deutz, F. J., *et al*. Ginkgo biloba extract in the therapy of erectile dysfunction. *Journal of Urology, 141*:188A, 1989.

Sone, Y., et al. Structures and antitumor activities of the polysaccharides isolated from fruiting body and the growing culture of mycelium of ganoderma lucidum. *Agricultural Biological Chemistry, 49*(9): 2641-2653, 1985.

Soothill, J. F. Food allergy in childhood. In M. H. Lessof (ed.), *Clinical Reactions to Food*, Chichester, England, John Wiley & Sons, 1983.

Spalding, B. J. Modern drugs from folk remedies. *Chemical Week*, 52-53, February 27, 1985.

Srivastiva. K. C. Effect of onion and ginger consumption on platelet thromboxane production in humans. *Prostaglandins, Leukotrienes and Essential Fatty Acids, 35*:183-185, 1989.

Stimpel, M., Proksch, A., Wagner, H., and Lohmann-Matthes, M. L. Macrophage activation and induction of macrophage cytotoxicity by purified polysaccharide fractions from the plant echinacea purpurea. *Inf Immun, 46*(3): 845-849, 1984.

Subrahmanyan, V., Sreenivasamurthy, V., and Krishnamurthy, Swamainathan, M. The effect of garlic on certain intestinal bacteria. *Food Science, 7*: 223-230, 1958.

Sugano, N., Choji, Y., Hibino, Y., Yasumura, S. and Maeda, H. Anticarcinogenic action of an alcohol-insoluble fraction (lapi) from culture medium of lentinus edodes mycelia. *Cancer Lett, 27*(1): 1-6, 1985.

Sugano, N., Hibino, Y., Choji, Y., and Maeda, H. Anticarcinogenic action of water-soluble and alcohol-insoluble fractions from culture medium of lentinus edodes mycelia. *Cancer Lett, 17*(2): 109-114, 1982.

Sugishita, E., Amagaya, S., and Ogihara, Y. Studies on the combination of glycyrrhizae radix in shakuyakukanzo-to. *J. Pharmacobio Dyn, 7*:427-435, 1984.

Suzuki, F., Koide, T., Tsunoda, A., and Ishida, N. Mushroom extract as an interferon inducer. I. Biological and physicochemical properties of spore extracts of lentinus edodes.

Svoboda, G. H. Antitumoral effects of Vinca Rosea Alkaloids, Proc., Symp. G.E.C.A., 1st Paris 1965, 9-28 (Pub. 1966).

Svoboda, G. H. *Lloydia, 24*:173-178, 1961.

Takaku, T., Kameda, K., Matsuura, Y., Sekiya, K., and Okuda, H. Studies on insulin-like substances in Korean red ginseng. *Planta Medica, 56*:27, 1990.

Takatsu, M., Tabuchi, M., Sofue, S., and Minami, J. Anticancer substances produced by basidiomycetes. *Patent-Japan Kokai-75, 12*(293): -, 1975.

Teas, J. The dietary intake of *laminaria*, a brown seaweed and breast cancer prevention. *Nutrition and Cancer, 4*: 217-22, 1983.

Terr, A. Allergic diseases. In H. Fudenberg, D. Stites, J. Caldwell, and J. Wells (eds.), *Basic and Clinical Immunology*, Los Altos, CA, Lange Medical Publications, 1976, pp. 430-448.

The drug that builds Russians. *New Scientist*, August 21, 1980.

Tochikura, T. S., Nakashima, H., Ohashi, Y., and Yamamoto, N. Inhibition (in vitro) of replication and of the cytopathic effect of the human immunodeficiency virus by an extract of culture medium of lentinus edodes mycelia. *Med Microbiol Immunol, 177*(5): 235-244, 1988.

Tønnesen, H. H. Studies on curcumin and curcuminoids. XIII. Catalytic effect of curcumin on the peroxidation of linoleic acid by 15-lipoxygenase. *International Journal of Pharmaceutics, 50*:67-69, 1989.

Tyler, V. E., *et al*. Pharmacognosy, 9th edition, Philadelphia, PA, Lea & Febiger, 1988.

Vanderhoek, J. Y. Inhibition of fatty acid oxygenases by onion and garlic oils. *Biochem. Pharmacol., 29*:3169-3173, 1980.

Vanderhoek, J. Y., Makheia, A. N., and Bailey, J. M. Inhibition of fatty acid oxygenases by onion and garlic oils: Evidence for the mechanism by which these oils inhibit platelet aggregation. *Biochemical Pharmacology*, *29*:3169-3173, 1980.

Vane, J.R. *Nature*, *231*: 232, 1971.

Voaden, D. J., and Jacobson, M. Tumor inhibitors. 3. Identification and synthesis of an oncolytic hydrocarbon from American coneflower roots. *J Med Chem*, *15*: 619-, 1972.

Vogel, V. J. American Indian Medicine. Norman, University of Oklahoma Press. 1970.

Volicer, L, Srahka, M., Jankumi, Capek, R., Smetana, R., and Ditteova, V. Some pharmacological effects of *Schizandra chinensis*. *Arch. Int. Pharmacodyn Ther.*, *163*:249-, 1966.

Wacker, A., and Hilbig, W. Virus-inhibition by echinacea purpurea. *Planta Med*, *33*: 89-, 1978.

Wadler, G. I. and Hainline, B. *Drugs and the Athlete*, F. A. Davis and Co., Philadelphia, 1989, pp. 107-113.

Wagner, H., Stuppner, H., Puhlmann, J., Jurcic, K., Zenk, M. H., and Lohmann-Matthes, M. L. Immunologically active polysaccharides from tissue cultures of echinacea purpurea. Proc 34th Annual Congress on Medicinal Plant Research-Hamburg, Sept 22-27, 1986 : -, 1986.

Wagner, H., Wierer, M., and Fessler, B. Effects of garlic constituents on arachidonate metabolism. *Planta Medica*, *53*, 1987.

Wagner, H., Zenk, M. H., and Ott, H. Polysaccharides derived from echinacea plants as immunostimulants. Patent-Ger Offen-3, 541,945 : 10pp-, 1988.

Wahlström, M. *Adaptogens*, Utgivare, Goteborg, 1987.

Watanabe, S., and Fujita, T. Immune adjuvants as antitumor agents from marine algae. Patent-Japan Kokai Tokkyo Koho-61 197,525: 3pp-, 1986.

Wattenberg, L. Inhibition of neoplasia by minor dietary components. *Cancer Research*, *43*(supplement): 2448s-2453s, 1983.

Weiner, M. A. Earth Medicine-Earth Foods: Plant Remedies, Drugs and Natural Foods of the North American Indian. New York, Macmillan 1972; 1980. New York, Random House, 1991.

Weiner, M. A. Ethnomedicine in Tonga. Economic Botany *25*(4):423-450, 1971.

Weiner, M. A. Maximum immunity. Boston, Houghton-Mifflin, 1986.

Weiner, M. A. Secrets of Fijian medicine. Government Press, Suva c/o Quantum Books USA, San Rafael, CA, 1983.

Weiner, M. A. *The Way of the Skeptical Nutritionist*. New York, Macmillan, 1981.

Whitsett, T. L., Manion, C. V., and Christensen, H. D. Cardiovascular effects of coffee and caffeine. *Am. J. Cardiol.*, *53*:918-922, 1984.

Willis, A. L., ed. *CRC Handbook of Eicosanoids: Prostaglandins and Related Lipids*, Vol. II. Boca Raton, Florida, CRC Press, 1989.

Wilson, J. W., and Plunkett, O. A. The fungus diseases of man. Berkeley, University of California, 1965.

Woo, W. S., Shin, K. H., Kih, I. C., and Lee, C. K. A survey of the response of Korean medicinal plants on drug metabolism. *Arch. Pharm. Res.*, *1*:13-19, 1978.

Yamada, Y., and Azuma, K. Evaluation of the in vitro antifungal activity of allicin. *Antimicrobial Agents and Chemotherapy*, *11*: 743-749, 1977.

Yamahara, J., *et al.*, The anti-ulcer effect in rats of ginger constituents. *Journal of Ethnopharmacology*, *23*:299-304, 1988.

Yamamoto, I. Takahashi, M., Tamura, E., Maruyama, H., and Mori, H. Antitumor activity of edible marine algae: Effect of crude fucoidan fractions prepared from edible brown seaweeds against L-. 1210 leukemia. *Hydrobiologia*, *116/117*: 145-148, 1984.

Yamamoto, I. Takahashi, M., Tamura, E., and Maruyama, H. Antitumor activity of crude extracts from edible marine algae against L-1210 leukemia. *Botanica Marina*, *XXV*: 455-457, 1982.

Yin, H. Z. A report of 200 cases of neurosis treated by "shen wei he ji" (decoction of ginseng, schisandra fruit and others). *Zhejiang-Zhongyi Zazhi*, *17*(9):411-, 1982.

Yu, J. and Chen, K. J. Clinical observations of AIDS treated with herbal formulas. *Int. J. Oriental Med.*, *14*(4):189-193, 1989.

Zhukova, G. E., Novokhatskii, A. S., and Telitchenko, M. M. Inactivation of some RNA-contained viruses with green and blue-e green algae. *Vestn Mosk Univ Biol Pochvoved*, *27*(4): 108-, 1972.

SECTION II:
GENERAL INDEX *(Includes page references to common English plant names)*

Quantum Books

Box 2056
San Rafael, CA 94912-2056

Telephone: (415) 388-1006
Fax: (415) 388-2257

ORDER FORM

SHIP TO:_____

NAME _____

STREET _____

CITY/STATE/ZIP _____

DR. WEINER'S HEALTH LINE	Retail	Order	Total
BOOKS:			
Weiner's Herbal, 276 pages • 120 Antigue Botanical Illustrations • Revised & Expanded • 8x11	17.95		
BOOKLETS:			
Herbs for Immunity, 32 pages, 4 color ilustrated throughout, 6x9	3.95		
ORDER TOTAL			
Add $3.00 per order for Shipping & Handling FREIGHT			
WE SHIP VIA US MAIL. GRAND TOTAL			

VISA or M/C accepted. Please include expiration date with
your order; or send check or money order. Taxes are included.